Comorbidities and Complications of Cerebral Palsy

Comorbidities and Complications of Cerebral Palsy

Editors

Christine Imms
Monica S Cooper

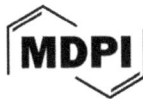

Basel • Beijing • Wuhan • Barcelona • Belgrade • Novi Sad • Cluj • Manchester

Editors
Christine Imms
The University of Melbourne
Melbourne, Australia

Monica S Cooper
The University of Melbourne
Melbourne, Australia

Editorial Office
MDPI
St. Alban-Anlage 66
4052 Basel, Switzerland

This is a reprint of articles from the Special Issue published online in the open access journal *Journal of Clinical Medicine* (ISSN 2077-0383) (available at: https://www.mdpi.com/journal/jcm/special_issues/Comorbidities_Complications_Cerebral_Palsy).

For citation purposes, cite each article independently as indicated on the article page online and as indicated below:

Lastname, A.A.; Lastname, B.B. Article Title. *Journal Name* **Year**, *Volume Number*, Page Range.

ISBN 978-3-0365-9514-6 (Hbk)
ISBN 978-3-0365-9515-3 (PDF)
doi.org/10.3390/books978-3-0365-9515-3

© 2023 by the authors. Articles in this book are Open Access and distributed under the Creative Commons Attribution (CC BY) license. The book as a whole is distributed by MDPI under the terms and conditions of the Creative Commons Attribution-NonCommercial-NoDerivs (CC BY-NC-ND) license.

Contents

About the Editors ix

Monica S Cooper and Christine Imms
Editorial Highlights from the Comorbidities and Complications of Cerebral Palsy Special Issue
Reprinted from: *J. Clin. Med.* **2023**, *12*, 5329, doi:10.3390/jcm12165329 1

Giuliana C. Antolovich, Monica S. Cooper, Michael B. Johnson, Kris Lundine, Yi Yang, Katherine Frayman, et al.
Perioperative Care of Children with Severe Neurological Impairment and Neuromuscular Scoliosis—*A Practical Pathway to Optimize Perioperative Health and Guide Decision Making*
Reprinted from: *J. Clin. Med.* **2022**, *11*, 6769, doi:10.3390/jcm11226769 5

Megan Finch-Edmondson, Madison C. B. Paton, Ingrid Honan, Petra Karlsson, Candice Stephenson, Darryl Chiu, et al.
Are We Getting It Right? A Scoping Review of Outcomes Reported in Cell Therapy Clinical Studies for Cerebral Palsy
Reprinted from: *J. Clin. Med.* **2022**, *11*, 7319, doi:10.3390/jcm11247319 15

Madison C. B. Paton, Megan Finch-Edmondson, Russell C. Dale, Michael C. Fahey, Claudia A. Nold-Petry, Marcel F. Nold, et al.
Persistent Inflammation in Cerebral Palsy: Pathogenic Mediator or Comorbidity? A Scoping Review
Reprinted from: *J. Clin. Med.* **2022**, *11*, 7368, doi:10.3390/jcm11247368 43

Jan Willem Gorter, Darcy Fehlings, Mark A. Ferro, Andrea Gonzalez, Amanda D. Green, Sarah N. Hopmans, et al.
Correlates of Mental Health in Adolescents and Young Adults with Cerebral Palsy: A Cross-Sectional Analysis of the MyStory Project
Reprinted from: *J. Clin. Med.* **2022**, *11*, 3060, doi:10.3390/jcm11113060 61

Jennifer M. Ryan, Michael Walsh, Mary Owens, Michael Byrne, Thilo Kroll, Owen Hensey, et al.
Unmet Health Needs among Young Adults with Cerebral Palsy in Ireland: A Cross-Sectional Study
Reprinted from: *J. Clin. Med.* **2022**, *11*, 4847, doi:10.3390/jcm11164847 77

Daniel G. Whitney, Tao Xu, Daniel Whibley, Dayna Ryan, Michelle S. Caird, Edward A. Hurvitz and Heidi Haapala
Post-Fracture Inpatient and Outpatient Physical/Occupational Therapy and Its Association with Survival among Adults with Cerebral Palsy
Reprinted from: *J. Clin. Med.* **2022**, *11*, 5561, doi:10.3390/jcm11195561 87

Mark D. Peterson, Allecia M. Wilson and Edward A. Hurvitz
Underlying Causes of Death among Adults with Cerebral Palsy
Reprinted from: *J. Clin. Med.* **2022**, *11*, 6333, doi:10.3390/jcm11216333 101

Alexandra Sorhage, Samantha Keenan, Jimmy Chong, Cass Byrnes, Amanda Marie Blackmore, Anna Mackey, et al.
Respiratory Health Inequities among Children and Young Adults with Cerebral Palsy in Aotearoa New Zealand: A Data Linkage Study
Reprinted from: *J. Clin. Med.* **2022**, *11*, 6968, doi:10.3390/jcm11236968 107

Roslyn Ward, Elizabeth Barty, Neville Hennessey, Catherine Elliott and Jane Valentine
Implementation of an Early Communication Intervention for Young Children with Cerebral Palsy Using Single-Subject Research Design
Reprinted from: J. Clin. Med. **2023**, 12, 232, doi:10.3390/jcm12010232 . . . . **119**

Silja Berg Kårstad, Åse Bjørseth, Johanna Lindstedt, Anne Synnøve Brenne, Helene Steihaug and Ann-Kristin Gunnes Elvrum
Parental Coping, Representations, and Interactions with Their Infants at High Risk of Cerebral Palsy
Reprinted from: J. Clin. Med. **2023**, 12, 277, doi:10.3390/jcm12010277 . . . . **145**

Ana Dos Santos Rufino, Magnus Påhlman, Ingrid Olsson and Kate Himmelmann
Characteristics and Challenges of Epilepsy in Children with Cerebral Palsy—A Population-Based Study
Reprinted from: J. Clin. Med. **2023**, 12, 346, doi:10.3390/jcm12010346 . . . . **161**

Saskia E. Kok, Joris Lemson and Frank J. A. van den Hoogen
Postoperative Airway Management after Submandibular Duct Relocation in 96 Drooling Children and Adolescents
Reprinted from: J. Clin. Med. **2023**, 12, 1473, doi:10.3390/jcm12041473 . . . . **173**

Nathalie De Beukelaer, Ines Vandekerckhove, Ester Huyghe, Geert Molenberghs, Nicky Peeters, Britta Hanssen, et al.
Morphological Medial Gastrocnemius Muscle Growth in Ambulant Children with Spastic Cerebral Palsy: A Prospective Longitudinal Study
Reprinted from: J. Clin. Med. **2023**, 12, 1564, doi:10.3390/jcm12041564 . . . . **181**

Catherine V. M. Steinbusch, Anke Defesche, Bertie van der Leij, Eugene A. A. Rameckers, Annemarie C. S. Knijnenburg, Jeroen R. J. Vermeulen and Yvonne J. M. Janssen-Potten
The Effect of Bimanual Intensive Functional Training on Somatosensory Hand Function in Children with Unilateral Spastic Cerebral Palsy: An Observational Study
Reprinted from: J. Clin. Med. **2023**, 12, 1595, doi:10.3390/jcm12041595 . . . . **199**

Aditya Narayan, Mohammad Muhit, John Whitehall, Iskander Hossain, Nadia Badawi, Gulam Khandaker and Israt Jahan
Associated Impairments among Children with Cerebral Palsy in Rural Bangladesh—Findings from the Bangladesh Cerebral Palsy Register
Reprinted from: J. Clin. Med. **2023**, 12, 1597, doi:10.3390/jcm12041597 . . . . **213**

Ingrid Honan, Emma Waight, Joan Bratel, Fiona Given, Nadia Badawi, Sarah McIntyre and Hayley Smithers-Sheedy
Emotion Regulation Is Associated with Anxiety, Depression and Stress in Adults with Cerebral Palsy
Reprinted from: J. Clin. Med. **2023**, 12, 2527, doi:10.3390/jcm12072527 . . . . **227**

Jason J. Howard, Kate Willoughby, Pam Thomason, Benjamin J. Shore, Kerr Graham and Erich Rutz
Hip Surveillance and Management of Hip Displacement in Children with Cerebral Palsy: Clinical and Ethical Dilemmas
Reprinted from: J. Clin. Med. **2023**, 12, 1651, doi:10.3390/jcm12041651 . . . . **239**

Rocío Palomo-Carrión, Caline Cristine De Araújo Ferreira Jesus, Camila Araújo Santos Santana, Raquel Lindquist, Roselene Alencar, Helena Romay-Barrero, et al.
Co-Design of an Intervention to Increase the Participation in Leisure Activities Including Adolescents with Cerebral Palsy with GMFCS Levels IV and V: A Study Protocol
Reprinted from: J. Clin. Med. **2023**, 12, 182, doi:10.3390/jcm12010182 . . . . **259**

Kayla Durkin Petkus, Garey Noritz and Laurie Glader
Examining the Role of Sublingual Atropine for the Treatment of Sialorrhea in Patients with Neurodevelopmental Disabilities: A Retrospective Review
Reprinted from: *J. Clin. Med.* **2023**, *12*, 5238, doi:10.3390/jcm12165238 . . . . **275**

About the Editors

Christine Imms

Professor Christine Imms (BAppSc(OT), MSc, PhD, Fellow OTARA) is the Apex Australia Foundation Chair of Neurodevelopment and Disability at the University of Melbourne and The Royal Children's Hospital and Honorary Researcher at the Murdoch Children's Research Institute. She is the founding Director of Healthy Trajectories, a child and youth disability research hub on the Melbourne Children's Campus. Prof. Imms is an occupational therapist, academic, and researcher who focuses on collaborative approaches that improve participation outcomes for those with child-onset neurodisability and their families. Her current role is research and knowledge translation focused. Professor Imms's research foci are (i) the effectiveness of occupational therapy and allied interventions, particularly in the field of childhood-onset disability, including cerebral palsy; (ii) the development and testing of valid, reliable outcome measures pertinent to childhood disability; (iii) the longitudinal follow-up of participation, health, and well-being outcomes for children and families; and (iv) conceptual work on 'participation' that resulted in the publication of the family of Participation Related Constructs, which underpins her related research and is used internationally to support participation research and practice in the area of childhood disability and beyond.

Monica S Cooper

Dr Monica Cooper (MBBS, BMedSc, GC-CLINTCH, PhD) is a General Paediatrician working in the Department of Neurodevelopment and Disability at The Royal Children's Hospital. Dr Cooper is affiliated with the University of Melbourne, tutors medical students, and is a Research Associate and member of the Neurodisability and Rehabilitation Group at the Murdoch Children's Research Institute. Dr Cooper was the lead author for the American Academy for Cerebral Palsy and Developmental Medicine care pathway for respiratory health in cerebral palsy. Her PhD thesis was on the epilepsies of cerebral palsy, and she is currently completing a Masters of Bioethics. Dr Cooper's scope of clinical practice is primarily focused on neurodisability. It includes optimisation of health and nutritional care, management of movement disorders, management of drooling, perioperative care, and decision making, emphasising well-being and quality of life. Dr Cooper provides care to children and adolescents with severe neurological impairment and those with medical complexity in both inpatient and outpatient settings. Her research interests include oropharyngeal dysphagia and drooling, respiratory health, epilepsy, and brain development in cerebral palsy. Dr Cooper's interest in clinical bioethics forms an important part of her work.

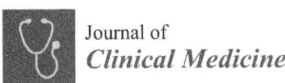

Editorial

Editorial Highlights from the Comorbidities and Complications of Cerebral Palsy Special Issue

Monica S Cooper [1,2,3] and Christine Imms [1,2,3,*]

1. Department of Neurodevelopment & Disability, Royal Children's Hospital, 50 Flemington Road, Melbourne, VIC 3052, Australia
2. Neurodisability and Rehabilitation, Clinical Sciences, Murdoch Children's Research Institute, 50 Flemington Road, Melbourne, VIC 3052, Australia
3. Department of Paediatrics, University of Melbourne, 50 Flemington Road, Melbourne, VIC 3052, Australia
* Correspondence: christine.imms@unimelb.edu.au; Tel.: +61-3-9345-5898

Cerebral palsy is a life-long condition and the most common cause of physical disability in childhood. Despite evidence of falling prevalence in some Western countries, cerebral palsy remains a global concern. Cerebral palsy is a clinical description, rather than a discrete diagnosis, and the aim of our Special Issue was to provide readers with advances in our understanding of associated comorbidities and complications. We collated research from different disciplines that addressed issues through different stages of life. In this editorial, we will draw the readers' attention to several of the papers to highlight specific life-stage issues, along with the need to address global inequities and, importantly, the long-term health consequences of growing up and living with cerebral palsy.

1. The Early Years

Starting with infants at high risk of cerebral palsy, a study of parents and their experiences with their infants found that most mothers and fathers, but not all, were able to be engaged with their infants [1]. Given the crucial nature of parent–infant interactions to child development and family wellbeing, this information highlights the need to situate our roles and interventions within a family-centred context and to provide interventions that support early and ongoing parent–child interactions. Additionally, in this early life stage, a lack of evidence-based interventions for infants with communication impairments led Ward et al. (2022) to try a multi-modal intervention with pre-linguistic infants with CP (starting at 16 months), with encouraging results in their targeted areas of language and speech production [2].

A prospective, longitudinal study on medical gastrocnemius morphology and growth showed slower rates of muscle growth, especially in the first two years of life in children with cerebral palsy functioning within the Gross Motor Function Classification System (GMFCS) level II-III, compared to those functioning within GMFCS level I. These results highlight that reduced muscle growth occurs early and that goals and treatment planning should also be considered early [3].

2. Cells, Biology and Pathophysiology

With the rising interest in stem cell infusions, a scoping review of the outcome measures used post-stem cell infusions showed that most measures did not have the requisite measurement properties to validly measure a change following the intervention. The authors' recommendations about the outcome measure selection include ensuring that the captured outcomes aligned with the priorities of the cerebral palsy community, such as quality of life [4]. Another paper focused on biomarkers and the role of inflammation in cerebral palsy, which are being increasingly studied. This paper provides supporting evidence suggestive that inflammation may persist into the adult years, likely contributing to the pathogenesis of cerebral palsy and associated complications [5].

Citation: Cooper, M.S.; Imms, C. Editorial Highlights from the Comorbidities and Complications of Cerebral Palsy Special Issue. *J. Clin. Med.* **2023**, *12*, 5329. https://doi.org/10.3390/jcm12165329

Received: 8 August 2023
Accepted: 13 August 2023
Published: 16 August 2023

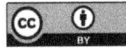

Copyright: © 2023 by the authors. Licensee MDPI, Basel, Switzerland. This article is an open access article distributed under the terms and conditions of the Creative Commons Attribution (CC BY) license (https://creativecommons.org/licenses/by/4.0/).

A review of the pathophysiology of acquired hip dysplasia in cerebral palsy provided considerations for determining the best timing and types of paediatric surgical interventions, as well as broader reflections on the hip surveillance program [6]. For the surgical correction of scoliosis, experiences of a peri-operative pathway to guide families through shared decision-making and the optimisation of post-operative care were highlighted in a publication of a multifaceted service model aimed to improve patient and caregiver experiences as well as improved outcomes [7].

3. Life Course Issues

Cerebral palsy registers continue to provide valuable information about longitudinal reporting. Data from the first population-based cerebral palsy register in Bangladesh were published. These results highlight the stark disparities in accessing education and rehabilitation services, which then impact negatively on participation and functional outcomes [8].

The unmet needs of adults with cerebral palsy were highlighted in three papers, with a reminder that we need a life-course approach to service provision [9]. Significant changes in both what health care is and how it is provided are also needed to manage the high prevalence of anxiety and depression in adults with cerebral palsy [10]. Lastly, to better delineate mortality causes in cerebral palsy, recommendations were made to detail the mechanisms of mortality in addition to the underlying associated cerebral palsy. This way, we can better understand the complications that evolve and lead to preventable early death in individuals with cerebral palsy [11].

Although we now have decades of cerebral-palsy-specific research, we still need to deepen our knowledge about the broad spectrum of impacts of the condition. We also do not yet have a suite of effective interventions that address the range of body system functions or community participation needs. There is still much work to be done.

Author Contributions: Conceptualisation, M.S.C. and C.I.; writing—original draft preparation, M.S.C.; writing—review and editing, C.I. All authors have read and agreed to the published version of the manuscript.

Acknowledgments: Thanks to the team of authors and the children and families who contributed and participated in the published studies.

Conflicts of Interest: The authors declare no conflict of interest.

References

1. Karstad, S.B.; Bjorseth, A.; Lindstedt, J.; Brenne, A.S.; Steihaug, H.; Elvrum, A.G. Parental Coping, Representations, and Interactions with Their Infants at High Risk of Cerebral Palsy. *J. Clin. Med.* **2022**, *12*, 277. [CrossRef] [PubMed]
2. Ward, R.; Barty, E.; Hennessey, N.; Elliott, C.; Valentine, J. Implementation of an Early Communication Intervention for Young Children with Cerebral Palsy Using Single-Subject Research Design. *J. Clin. Med.* **2022**, *12*, 232. [CrossRef] [PubMed]
3. De Beukelaer, N.; Vandekerckhove, I.; Huyghe, E.; Molenberghs, G.; Peeters, N.; Hanssen, B.; Ortibus, E.; Van Campenhout, A.; Desloovere, K. Morphological Medial Gastrocnemius Muscle Growth in Ambulant Children with Spastic Cerebral Palsy: A Prospective Longitudinal Study. *J. Clin. Med.* **2023**, *12*, 1564. [CrossRef] [PubMed]
4. Finch-Edmondson, M.; Paton, M.C.B.; Honan, I.; Karlsson, P.; Stephenson, C.; Chiu, D.; Reedman, S.; Griffin, A.R.; Morgan, C.; Novak, I. Are We Getting It Right? A Scoping Review of Outcomes Reported in Cell Therapy Clinical Studies for Cerebral Palsy. *J. Clin. Med.* **2022**, *11*, 7319. [CrossRef] [PubMed]
5. Paton, M.C.B.; Finch-Edmondson, M.; Dale, R.C.; Fahey, M.C.; Nold-Petry, C.A.; Nold, M.F.; Griffin, A.R.; Novak, I. Persistent Inflammation in Cerebral Palsy: Pathogenic Mediator or Comorbidity? A Scoping Review. *J. Clin. Med.* **2022**, *11*, 7368. [CrossRef] [PubMed]
6. Howard, J.J.; Willoughby, K.; Thomason, P.; Shore, B.J.; Graham, K.; Rutz, E. Hip Surveillance and Management of Hip Displacement in Children with Cerebral Palsy: Clinical and Ethical Dilemmas. *J. Clin. Med.* **2023**, *12*, 1651. [CrossRef] [PubMed]
7. Antolovich, G.C.; Cooper, M.S.; Johnson, M.B.; Lundine, K.; Yang, Y.; Frayman, K.; Vandeleur, M.; Sutherland, I.; Peachey, D.; Gadish, T.; et al. Perioperative Care of Children with Severe Neurological Impairment and Neuromuscular Scoliosis-A Practical Pathway to Optimize Peri-Operative Health and Guide Decision Making. *J. Clin. Med.* **2022**, *11*, 6769. [CrossRef] [PubMed]
8. Narayan, A.; Muhit, M.; Whitehall, J.; Hossain, I.; Badawi, N.; Khandaker, G.; Jahan, I. Associated Impairments among Children with Cerebral Palsy in Rural Bangladesh-Findings from the Bangladesh Cerebral Palsy Register. *J. Clin. Med.* **2023**, *12*, 1597. [CrossRef] [PubMed]

9. Ryan, J.M.; Walsh, M.; Owens, M.; Byrne, M.; Kroll, T.; Hensey, O.; Kerr, C.; Norris, M.; Walsh, A.; Lavelle, G.; et al. Unmet Health Needs among Young Adults with Cerebral Palsy in Ireland: A Cross-Sectional Study. *J. Clin. Med.* **2022**, *11*, 4847. [CrossRef] [PubMed]
10. Gorter, J.W.; Fehlings, D.; Ferro, M.A.; Gonzalez, A.; Green, A.D.; Hopmans, S.N.; McCauley, D.; Palisano, R.J.; Rosenbaum, P.; Speller, B.; et al. Correlates of Mental Health in Adolescents and Young Adults with Cerebral Palsy: A Cross-Sectional Analysis of the MyStory Project. *J. Clin. Med.* **2022**, *11*, 3060. [CrossRef] [PubMed]
11. Peterson, M.D.; Wilson, A.M.; Hurvitz, E.A. Underlying Causes of Death among Adults with Cerebral Palsy. *J. Clin. Med.* **2022**, *11*, 6333. [CrossRef] [PubMed]

Disclaimer/Publisher's Note: The statements, opinions and data contained in all publications are solely those of the individual author(s) and contributor(s) and not of MDPI and/or the editor(s). MDPI and/or the editor(s) disclaim responsibility for any injury to people or property resulting from any ideas, methods, instructions or products referred to in the content.

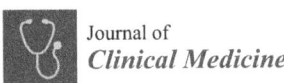

Review

Perioperative Care of Children with Severe Neurological Impairment and Neuromuscular Scoliosis—A Practical Pathway to Optimize Perioperative Health and Guide Decision Making

Giuliana C. Antolovich [1,2,3,*], Monica S. Cooper [1,2,3], Michael B. Johnson [3,4,5], Kris Lundine [3,4,5], Yi Yang [3,4,5], Katherine Frayman [3,6,7,8], Moya Vandeleur [3,6,7], Ingrid Sutherland [1,2,3], Donna Peachey [4], Tali Gadish [3,9,10], Ben Turner [3,11,12] and Adrienne Harvey [1,2,3]

1. Department of Neurodevelopment & Disability, Royal Children's Hospital, 50 Flemington Road, Melbourne, VIC 3052, Australia
2. Neurodisability and Rehabilitation, Clinical Sciences, Murdoch Children's Research Institute, 50 Flemington Road, Melbourne, VIC 3052, Australia
3. Department of Paediatrics, University of Melbourne, 50 Flemington Road, Melbourne, VIC 3052, Australia
4. Department of Orthopaedics, Royal Children's Hospital, 50 Flemington Road, Melbourne, VIC 3052, Australia
5. Gait Lab and Orthopaedics, Clinical Sciences, Murdoch Children's Research Institute, 50 Flemington Road, Melbourne, VIC 3052, Australia
6. Department of Respiratory and Sleep Medicine, Royal Children's Hospital, 50 Flemington Road, Melbourne, VIC 3052, Australia
7. Respiratory Diseases Group, Murdoch Children's Research Institute, 50 Flemington Road, Melbourne, VIC 3052, Australia
8. Centre for Health Analytics, Royal Children's Hospital, 50 Flemington Road, Melbourne, VIC 3052, Australia
9. Paediatric Intensive Care Unit, Royal Children's Hospital, 50 Flemington Road, Melbourne, VIC 3052, Australia
10. Paediatric Intensive Care, Clinical Sciences, Murdoch Children's Research Institute, 50 Flemington Road, Melbourne, VIC 3052, Australia
11. Department of Anaesthetics, Royal Children's Hospital, 50 Flemington Road, Melbourne, VIC 3052, Australia
12. Anaesthetics, Clinical Sciences, Murdoch Children's Research Institute, 50 Flemington Road, Melbourne, VIC 3052, Australia
* Correspondence: giuliana.antolovich@rch.org.au

Abstract: Neuromuscular scoliosis is a common feature in children with severe neurological impairment (SNI), including those with severe cerebral palsy. Surgical correction of scoliosis is the mainstay of treatment. This group of patients also have associated medical complexity. The complication rates post-surgery are high, although, for many, they are worth the risk. There are currently no published practice guidelines or care pathways for children with SNI who are undergoing scoliosis corrective surgery. In response to the high uptake of this surgery, coupled with the expected complication rates, our hospital established a perioperative clinic. The purpose of this paper is to describe our perioperative approach. This clinic has developed into a service beyond perioperative care and, with the collaborative meeting, enables shared decision-making to identify the right candidate for surgery. The process involves surgical expertise, understanding the family and child at the centre, and optimisation of medical care pre- and post-surgery. In this paper, we describe the process in a step-by-step manner. We provide clinical vignettes, as well as the proformas that we use, and we highlight the benefits of the team-based process.

Keywords: cerebral palsy; severe neurological impairment; scoliosis; shared decision-making

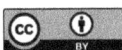

1. Introduction

Neuromuscular scoliosis is very common in children with a physical disability, particularly in those who function at the more severe end of the motor disability spectrum. The group at high risk of neuromuscular scoliosis includes children with Severe Neurological Impairment (SNI) [1], defined as children with diseases of the central nervous system, with permanent motor and cognitive impairment, with both static and progressive disorders [1], and those with cerebral palsy (CP) and who function within Gross Motor Function Classification System (GMFCS) levels IV and V [2,3]. These children also have significant medical co-morbidities [4,5]. It is likely that weaknesses in the postural muscles and diaphragm contribute to neuromuscular scoliosis, which plays a significant role in the evolution of chronic lung disease and respiratory failure in this population [6].

Advances in medical care, such as access to neonatal and paediatric intensive care, management of epilepsy and infection, and technology support (such as non-invasive ventilation and supplemental nutrition), coupled with societal changes and expectations, have substantially modified the survival of children with SNI and increased the number of children living with medical complexity [7]. For many, this increased longevity is associated with acquired morbidity and medical fragility [7]. Severe and untreated neuromuscular scoliosis is an increasingly apparent issue. Over time, the scoliosis may become stiffer, and the consequences of this include difficulties maintaining the head in the midline to continue with adequate socialisation, loss of sitting abilities, pressure sores and reduced pulmonary function [5]. Scoliosis is also a frequent cause of pain [8–11].

Whilst surgical correction is the mainstay of treatment for neuromuscular scoliosis [5,12], it is not without complications [13]. The population of children who require this surgery are medically complex, and as a consequence, decision-making to ensure optimal outcomes is important. The aim of the surgery is to align the spine and balance the head, shoulders, and trunk over a level pelvis [5]. This, in turn, improves quality of life [5,14–16]. Parents/carers have reported this surgery to be "the most beneficial intervention in their child's life" [15]. Only one study has shown improvements in lung function post-surgery [17], whilst others show pneumonia as a major complication [18]. Although the satisfaction rates postoperatively are very high, complications from surgery remain significant [19]. Overall, high-quality evidence on post-surgical outcomes is still lacking, particularly for outcomes other than curve correction [13].

Decision-making about interventions for children who are complex and medically fragile creates challenges for parents and the clinical team. Deciding when medical and surgical interventions are helping or harming a child in these circumstances is clinically and ethically complex, and there is a substantial obligation to thoughtfully approach decision-making for this group. Balancing the burdens and risks of treatments with benefits for a given child requires a collaborative multidisciplinary view, anticipatory care and active engagement with parents and carers.

This paper will describe the approach to the perioperative care of children with SNI with neuromuscular scoliosis adopted in a tertiary medical centre in Australia. The approach to care has been developed to support complex decision-making for children with SNI [1,20]. An anticipatory approach is needed to ensure that health is optimised prior to any surgical intervention. However, the goals of the surgery and broader goals of care need to be considered when deciding who will be an appropriate surgical candidate. The practical details of our approach and case vignettes are provided. The team approach to care has resulted in broader benefits, which will be described.

2. The Care Pathway

A recognition of the increasing medical complexity and frequent postoperative complications of the population requiring surgical management for spinal deformity has been a driver for the development of a clinical care pathway to address the needs of this higher-risk group [13]. A project was established to develop this pathway using the expertise of staff from the Divisions of Medicine, Surgery, Critical Care and Allied Health, and research partners from the Murdoch Children's Research Institute (MCRI). This project resulted in the establishment of two additional clinical services to support decision-making and perioperative care: the Medical Neuromuscular Scoliosis Clinic (hereafter referred to as

Clinic) and the Neuromuscular Scoliosis Multidisciplinary Meeting (hereafter referred to as Meeting).

Ambitious goals for surgical and perioperative care in surgery for children with neuromuscular scoliosis include decreasing the complication rate to <10%, reducing Intensive Care Unit admission to <24 h and reducing hospital admission lengths to <7 days [21]. Another important consideration is to address whether the institution can manage the level of medical and surgical complexity [21]. Preoperative assessment clinics have been shown to be cost-effective and paediatricians have been shown to make a number of recommendations for medical management [22,23]. The team approach, with detailed perioperative planning and postoperative management, is now considered a mainstay of the treatment for correction of neuromuscular scoliosis [21]. In a recent study, 77% of surgeons reported adhering to preoperative protocols for children with CP within their centres, although there was marked variation in the described perioperative care [24]. There are established protocols for children with neuromuscular scoliosis undergoing corrective surgery [25]. However, these are developed for children with other conditions and focus on perioperative care rather than team-based decision-making.

3. The Clinical Setting

The Orthopaedic Department provides clinical care for the assessment and management of children with scoliosis. Children are referred to this clinic from multiple sources—from within the hospital, from other major centres in the state (both metropolitan and rural), from community-based clinic services (public and private) and from interstate services. Children with a range of aetiological diagnoses are seen in this clinic. Routine care in these clinical services includes the imaging, assessment, and consideration of non-surgical (expectant care or bracing) and a range of surgical options.

4. Medical Neuromuscular Scoliosis Clinic (Clinic)

Children identified in the orthopaedic clinic as potential candidates for surgical intervention are referred to the Clinic (Figure 1). Referrals to this clinic include children with cerebral palsy, SNI, both static and progressive conditions (including Rett syndrome, cerebral palsy-like conditions, neural tube defects, genetic conditions resulting in a motor disability), and other neurodisabilities (Prader Willi Syndrome, intellectual disability syndromes). Children with neuromuscular disorders (e.g., Duchenne, Spinal Muscular Atrophy) are currently assessed in an alternative multidisciplinary setting within the hospital and are not routinely seen in the Clinic, though this process is changing. A review of referrals to the Clinic suggests that almost 40% of children referred to this clinic receive their primary care outside of our hospital.

The Clinic is led by a neurodevelopmental/complex care paediatrician and includes a respiratory physician and a neurodevelopmental clinical nurse consultant. The goals of the Clinic are to (1) identify and assess the medical comorbid conditions and risk factors for each child, (2) take the opportunity to optimise health prior to surgery and, most importantly, (3) support decision-making about proceeding with corrective surgery.

To better understand the potential benefits and risks for each child, the health, well-being and co-morbid conditions are reviewed, and the goals of the surgery as identified by the family (and the child where possible) are defined and clarified. An assessment of the potential risks and identified benefits are incorporated into both decision making and planning of perioperative care.

A detailed medical history, including respiratory history, feeding and nutrition, epilepsy control, movement disorder, sleep, and pain history, is collected. Communication, behavioural and sensory issues, schooling, and supports—both home and community based—are also elicited to better understand the issues that will face the child and family, both as inpatients and as barriers to discharge and recovery (Table S1).

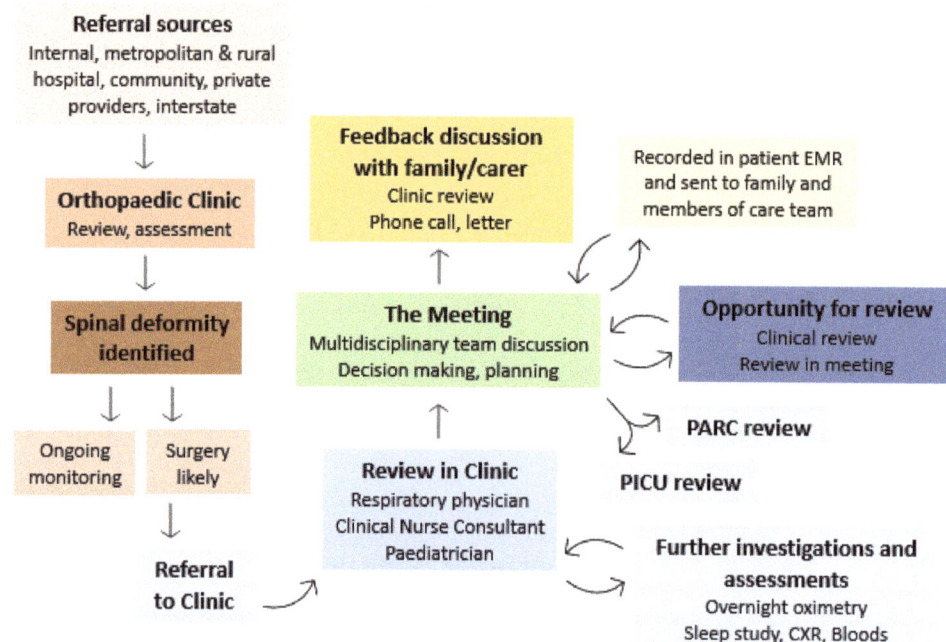

Figure 1. Description of clinical assessment and process of the Clinic and the Meeting. A summary of the outcomes of the clinical case conference, which includes further investigations and details of the perioperative plan are included in the patient Electronic Medical record (EMR), allowing for access for all members of the team as a reference point for perioperative management and admission. (PARC—pre-anaesthetic review clinic, PICU—Paediatric Intensive Care Unit, CXR—Chest X-ray).

In most cases, the child will have a baseline nutritional blood panel completed, including a capillary acid base following the appointment. Co-morbid conditions that may impact the surgery or recovery are identified and addressed to optimise the preoperative health of the child. Additional investigations—for example, chest radiograph, overnight oximetry, or polysomnography—will also be requested at this time depending on the clinical need. A perioperative care plan, which might include admission for a "tune-up", a nutritional assessment and optimisation, optimisation of respiratory health, drooling, tone and movement disorder, is prepared (File S1).

An important goal of the Clinic appointment is the exploration with the family, and child where possible, of the goals they have for the surgery, what they hope the surgery will achieve for the child, and their primary concerns or worries about the surgery. Realistic goals include reduction in pain, easier care, improved ability to perform activities of daily living, and improved social interaction [26]. This discussion also involves consideration of the overall goals of care for a child and whether there is an advanced care plan in place. If this is the case, a suspension of the advanced care plan will be required during the perioperative period, and this must be discussed not only with the family but with the broader team.

5. Neuromuscular Scoliosis Multidisciplinary Meeting (Meeting)

The Meeting follows the Clinic and brings together clinicians from different craft groups linked to the service—orthopaedic surgeons, respiratory physicians, orthopaedic clinical nurse consultant, neurodevelopmental nurse consultant, paediatricians, allied health clinicians, research allied health clinician, anaesthetist, and a paediatric intensive-care physician. In some cases, the primary or lead paediatrician of the child and other subspecialists (e.g., respiratory physician from another site, cardiologist), who are part of the child's care team, are invited to join the discussion.

The clinical history and key clinical factors, including a description of the family's and child's goals and concerns, are presented and discussed. This discussion explores and highlights the potential benefits to the child and the identified risks. If the child is a suitable candidate for surgery, a detailed perioperative plan is developed, including identification of any additional investigations or management required to optimise the health of the child (File S1).

An important goal of this discussion is to determine whether a child will benefit from an elective admission to the Paediatric Intensive Care Unit (PICU) to receive their postoperative care. There are some factors that help predict the need for postoperative PICU care: a significant respiratory history and previous admissions to PICU [27,28], an established need for non-invasive ventilation [28], and possibly a higher identified risk in certain diagnostic groups—for example, girls with Rett syndrome [29]. A history of epilepsy or a previous admission to PICU with a respiratory illness both increase the risk and length of stay in PICU post-surgery [28,30]. The surgical plan is a significant factor in this decision (minimally invasive instrumentation versus spinal fusion). Clarity regarding the need for and benefits of a PICU admission is very important. Whilst there are advantages to an elective admission to PICU for postoperative care (one-on-one nursing care, access to respiratory support allowing for the flexibility of management with sedating analgesics, and less distress to the child and family), there are also some important disadvantages. Bed availability in PICU is finite and, if no bed is available on the day of surgery, cancellation and delays can occur. Moreover, the PICU is a high-acuity and -intensity unit, and this may prove challenging to some children and families. Another consideration at our hospital is that parents cannot sleep overnight in the PICU if the patient is intubated, which may distress some families.

A plan is developed and documented in the Electronic Medical Record (EMR) as a Case Conference note and a copy sent to the family and primary care team, summarising the discussion and plan. The decision as to whether the child is safe and a suitable candidate to proceed with surgery is made at the Meeting. Sometimes there is disagreement between the clinical team and the family about whether to proceed with surgery. In these cases, the option of an additional clinical assessment, including the orthopaedic surgeon, the neurodevelopmental paediatrician and other members of the child's family and care team, is offered. If surgery is ultimately offered, the final decision to choose not to go ahead with the surgery lies with the parents. These examples highlight that the service is not just a preoperative assessment clinic. Decisions are reached from the multi-disciplinary team clinic with surgical expertise, the child and their family at the centre, and the physicians.

A letter is sent to the parents summarising the outcome of the Clinic and Meeting, and the decision. Furthermore, a pre-admission plan is prepared, covering treatment for constipation, the introduction of gabapentin if no contraindications are present, postoperative gastro-oesophageal reflux medication, and a plan as to whether a nasogastric tube will be inserted perioperatively (File S1).

Three clinical vignettes outlining typical cases and the process used to reach the decision are presented (File S2).

6. Discussion

The perioperative pathways we have developed provide a robust framework that includes parental views and hopes, recognising their role as knowledgeable caregivers, to approach this complex decision-making and ensure the best outcomes for children with SNI. The identification of medical morbidity and opportunities to optimise health and anticipatory decisions about the need for post-operative PICU care are important components of this process. The pathway brings together the skill and experience of a range of surgeons and physicians and provides an opportunity for a comprehensive assessment and planning to mitigate the risks inherent to this group. Transparency and honesty in communication is highly valued, particularly when there is uncertainty about the outcome [31–35]. This is the case when counselling for scoliosis surgery, especially when it comes to discussing evidence-based outcomes.

Deciding if an elective surgical intervention is in a child's best interests can be difficult. The "Best Interests Standard" (BIS) is an ethical, legal, and social principle that has been used to guide decision-making in children's medical care [36]. The BIS describes a broad cluster of children's interests, and includes basic needs, emotional development, play and pleasure, to live a long life and to have a relationship with a parent [37]. Multiple approaches to decision-making have been described and all focus on the key principles of the best interests of the child in the context of their family and the minimisation of harm [38].

Decision-making for children with SNI can be complex, and parents and clinicians are often faced with difficult decisions. Shared decision-making [39] in paediatrics is an ideal, in which there is collaboration and flexibility, knowledge and value-related priorities are equal [40]. Nonetheless there are ethical and practical challenges in many clinical situations. Ethical tools, such as the Zone of Parental Discretion (ZPD) [41], have been developed to help clinicians address these ethically complicated cases [38,41]. The ZPD provides a way to explore difficult decisions and uncertainty, and to balance parent authority and children's best interests. This tool is especially useful when there are disagreements. Parents may have a different view about which interests are more important, and this may create disagreement with the clinical team [42,43]. The use of ethical language to frame the clinical problems encountered has been valuable for the team.

The authority of parents as decision-makers for their child is well-described. Parents are recognised to be best placed to make decisions, as they know their child and will be bear the burden of the (medical) decisions they make, although this authority is not without limits [44]. Parents of children with SNIs have had to make many decisions throughout the lives of their children, often where there is uncertainty about the outcome [45]. Parents expect to be recognised as experts in their own child and, therefore, to warrant an important role in decision-making [42,46–49]. Parents of children with SNIs are strong advocates for their child [32,46] and emphasise the personhood of their child to the clinical team [31,47]. It is important for parents to feel heard and understood, and for their expertise as knowledgeable caregivers to be recognised. The burden and emotional impact of these complex decisions is also recognised for parents and their children [34].

The Clinic appointment allows for a more detailed discussion about the health needs of the child, and for a deeper exploration of the hopes, concerns and fears a parent has about surgery. Exploring and acknowledging hopes in decision-making is well-described and critical to the process of shared decision making [46,50]. The parental perspective and voice are important to how a decision is made. A study exploring the experience and satisfaction of parents with this process is currently being undertaken.

An additional benefit of the Clinic is that a small proportion of the children considered for orthopaedic interventions are only known to the orthopaedic team and receive their primary paediatric care outside of our hospital. This includes families who have not sought other mainstream paediatric care for their child. The Clinic assessment sometimes brings about the need for a thorough work-up, and multiple interventions prior to surgery. There are benefits for the child and family to meet the broader team and have some familiarity with the other clinical services that will be involved in the child's care in the perioperative period.

Furthermore, decisions around perioperative care are not always directly in line with previous decisions to not intervene medically. Sometimes, in order to stabilise the child for scoliosis surgery a cascade of medical investigations and interventions are undertaken; for example, a nutritional assessment in a child who is underweight and has an unsafe swallow, commencing enteral feeding or investigation of sleep-disordered breathing, which is longstanding but was previously not explored.

The planning of scoliosis surgery in a child with a clear life-limiting condition and known to the palliative care service can be seen as a confusing active intervention for families. There may also be pre-existing limitations to active interventions or resuscitation orders (although active treatments and involvement of palliative care can co-occur). Note that limitations on resuscitation orders are suspended during the perioperative period. This occurs following careful and explicit discussion with the family and team to ensure that the child can survive the surgical process.

This pathway represents a successful collaboration across multiple craft groups. Clinicians from the Divisions of Medicine, Surgery, Critical Care and Allied Health, alongside research partnerships with MCRI, are involved and meet regularly while providing clinical care. The Meeting has created a space in which the members of the clinical team have developed a greater understanding of the needs, responsibilities, and skills inherent to each other's roles. Familiarity and respect have evolved and, over time, have created an environment in which open, sometimes vigorous, and respectful discussions occur to support this complex decision-making. This relational capacity has extended beyond the meeting space and has facilitated communication between teams on the ward. The importance of establishing respectful and functional relationships in clinical care is not a new concept [51], but may be one that needs to be given a higher priority when planning complex clinical care, particularly where there is uncertainty about the outcomes. A culture of respect and open communication is recognised to improve patient safety and clinical care, and to increase the meaningfulness and joy of the work of clinicians [52,53]. The collaborative nature of this process has benefits beyond that of decision-making and planning, and has recognised benefits for clinical care, clinical relationships, and staff well-being [51,52].

7. Conclusions

The decision to go ahead with scoliosis corrective surgery in children with complex disability and medical comorbidity is a substantive one for both parents and the clinical team. Sometimes significant changes are required before the child is medically ready. The Clinic creates an opportunity to meet each child and family in a setting that is separate to the surgical clinic and allows for an additional opportunity for an exploration of parents' hopes, wishes, and fears, and to understand the values and beliefs of the family. This important information can then be shared with the broader team at the Meeting and coupled with a detailed assessment of health, potential risks and identified benefits, can be incorporated into both decision-making and planning for perioperative care. Clinical pathways of perioperative care have been developed at our hospital to provide comprehensive support for the care of children with SNI and medical complexity who need orthopaedic surgery. These pathways have created opportunities for supported, collaborative and inclusive decision-making. These pathways provide guidance for optimisation of health prior to surgery and have created improved staff relationships with positive impacts on care.

Supplementary Materials: The following supporting information can be downloaded at: https://www.mdpi.com/article/10.3390/jcm11226769/s1, Table S1—Clinic Meeting proforma. This figure shows the template used in the Medical Neuromuscular Scoliosis Clinic and the Neuromuscular Scoliosis Multidisciplinary Meeting. File S1—Letter to parents/carer proforma. This figure shows the template used in the letter for the parents. File S2—Clinical vignettes. Reference [54] are cited in the supplementary materials.

Author Contributions: Conceptualization, G.C.A., M.S.C., M.B.J., K.L., I.S., D.P. and A.H.; Writing—original draft, G.C.A. and M.S.C.; Writing—review & editing, G.C.A., M.S.C., M.B.J., K.L., Y.Y., K.F., M.V., I.S., D.P., T.G., B.T. and A.H. All authors have read and agreed to the published version of the manuscript.

Funding: This research received no external funding.

Acknowledgments: The authors would like to acknowledge the role of Louise Baker, Susan Gibb, Jenny O'Neill, Colin Robertson, and Katrina Williams in the early development of this clinical pathway.

Conflicts of Interest: The authors declare no conflict of interest.

Abbreviations

Best Interests Standard (BIS), Cerebral Palsy (CP), Electronic Medical Record (EMR), Gross Motor Function Classification Scale (GMFCS), Murdoch Children's Research Institute (MCRI), Pre-Anaesthetic Review Clinic (PARC), Paediatric Intensive Care Unit (PICU), Severe Neurological Impairment (SNI), Zone of Parental Discretion (ZPD).

References

1. Allen, J.; Brenner, M.; Hauer, J.; Molloy, E.; McDonald, D. Severe Neurological Impairment: A delphi consensus-based definition. *Eur. J. Paediatr. Neurol.* **2020**, *29*, 81–86. [CrossRef] [PubMed]
2. Saito, N.; Ebara, S.; Ohotsuka, K.; Kumeta, H.; Takaoka, K. Natural history of scoliosis in spastic cerebral palsy. *Lancet* **1998**, *351*, 1687–1692. [CrossRef]
3. Koop, S.E. Scoliosis in cerebral palsy. *Dev. Med. Child Neurol.* **2009**, *51* (Suppl. S4), 92–98. [CrossRef] [PubMed]
4. McCarthy, J.J.; D'andrea, L.P.; Betz, R.R.; Clements, D.H. Scoliosis in the Child with Cerebral Palsy. *J. Am. Acad. Orthop. Surg.* **2006**, *14*, 367–375. [CrossRef] [PubMed]
5. Howard, J.J.; Sees, J.P.; Shrader, W. Management of Spinal Deformity in Cerebral Palsy. *J. Pediatr. Orthop. Soc. N. Am.* **2019**, *1*. [CrossRef]
6. Marpole, R.; Blackmore, A.M.; Gibson, N.; Cooper, M.S.; Langdon, K.; Wilson, A.C. Evaluation and Management of Respiratory Illness in Children with Cerebral Palsy. *Front. Pediatr.* **2020**, *8*, 333. [CrossRef]
7. Berry, J.G.; Poduri, A.; Bonkowsky, J.L.; Zhou, J.; Graham, D.A.; Welch, C.; Putney, H.; Srivastava, R. Trends in Resource Utilization by Children with Neurological Impairment in the United States Inpatient Health Care System: A Repeat Cross-Sectional Study. *PLOS Med.* **2012**, *9*, e1001158. [CrossRef]
8. Wawrzuta, J.; Willoughby, K.L.; Molesworth, C.; Ang, S.G.; Shore, B.J.; Thomason, P.; Graham, H.K. Hip health at skeletal maturity: A population-based study of young adults with cerebral palsy. *Dev. Med. Child Neurol.* **2016**, *58*, 1273–1280. [CrossRef]
9. McKinnon, C.T.; Meehan, E.M.; Harvey, A.R.; Antolovich, G.C.; Morgan, P. Prevalence and characteristics of pain in children and young adults with cerebral palsy: A systematic review. *Dev. Med. Child Neurol.* **2019**, *61*, 305–314. [CrossRef]
10. McKinnon, C.T.; Morgan, P.E.; Antolovich, G.C.; Clancy, C.H.; Fahey, M.C.; Harvey, A.R. Pain in children with dyskinetic and mixed dyskinetic/spastic cerebral palsy. *Dev. Med. Child Neurol.* **2020**, *62*, 1294–1301. [CrossRef]
11. Sewell, M.D.; Malagelada, F.; Wallace, C.; Gibson, A.; Noordeen, H.; Tucker, S.; Molloy, S.; Lehovsky, J. A Preliminary Study to Assess Whether Spinal Fusion for Scoliosis Improves Carer-assessed Quality of Life for Children With GMFCS Level IV or V Cerebral Palsy. *J. Pediatr. Orthop.* **2016**, *36*, 299–304. [CrossRef] [PubMed]
12. Howard, J.J.; Farrelly, J. *Evidence-Based Treatment of Neuromuscular Scoliosis*; Springer: Cham, Switzerland, 2017.
13. Toovey, R.; Harvey, A.; Johnson, M.; Baker, L.; Williams, K. Outcomes after scoliosis surgery for children with cerebral palsy: A systematic review. *Dev. Med. Child Neurol.* **2017**, *59*, 690–698. [CrossRef] [PubMed]
14. Bohtz, C.; Meyer-Heim, A.; Min, K. Changes in Health-Related Quality of Life After Spinal Fusion and Scoliosis Correction in Patients With Cerebral Palsy. *J. Pediatr. Orthop.* **2011**, *31*, 668–673. [CrossRef] [PubMed]
15. Miyanji, F.; Nasto, L.A.; Sponseller, P.D.; Shah, S.A.; Samdani, A.F.; Lonner, B.; Yaszay, B.; Clements, D.H.; Narayanan, U.; Newton, P.O. Assessing the Risk-Benefit Ratio of Scoliosis Surgery in Cerebral Palsy: Surgery Is Worth It. *JBJS* **2018**, *100*, 556–563. [CrossRef] [PubMed]
16. Jain, A.; Sullivan, B.T.; Shah, S.A.; Samdani, A.F.; Yaszay, B.; Marks, M.C.; Sponseller, P.D. Caregiver Perceptions and Health-Related Quality-of-Life Changes in Cerebral Palsy Patients After Spinal Arthrodesis. *Spine* **2018**, *43*, 1052–1056. [CrossRef]
17. Larsson, E.-L.C.; Aaro, S.I.; Normelli, H.C.M.; Öberg, B.E. Long-Term Follow-up of Functioning After Spinal Surgery in Patients with Neuromuscular Scoliosis. *Spine (Phila Pa 1976)* **2005**, *30*, 2145–2152. [CrossRef]
18. VandenDriessche, E.; Moens, P.; Ortibus, E.; Proesmans, M. Respiratory complication rate after scoliosis surgery in children with cerebral palsy. *Eur. Respir. J.* **2020**, *56*, 1918. [CrossRef]
19. Davies, E.; Raich, A.L.; Dettori, J.R.; Sherry, N.; Legg, J. Surgical Correction of Scoliosis in Children with Spastic Quadriplegia: Benefits, Adverse Effects, and Patient Selection. *Evid.-Based Spine-Care J.* **2014**, *5*, 38–51. [CrossRef]
20. Allen, J.; Molloy, E.; McDonald, D. Severe neurological impairment: A review of the definition. *Dev. Med. Child Neurol.* **2020**, *62*, 277–282. [CrossRef]
21. Warner, W.C. Management of Spinal Deformity. *J. Pediatr. Orthop. Soc. N. Am.* **2019**, *1*. Available online: https://www.jposna.org/index.php/jposna/article/view/42 (accessed on 11 September 2022). [CrossRef]
22. Rappaport, D.I.; Adelizzi-Delany, J.; Rogers, K.J.; Jones, C.E.; Petrini, M.E.; Chaplinski, K.; Ostasewski, P.; Sharif, I.; Pressel, D.M. Outcomes and Costs Associated with Hospitalist Comanagement of Medically Complex Children Undergoing Spinal Fusion Surgery. *Hosp. Pediatr.* **2013**, *3*, 233–241. [CrossRef] [PubMed]
23. Rappaport, D.I.; Cerra, S.; Hossain, J.; Sharif, I.; Pressel, D.M. Pediatric hospitalist preoperative evaluation of children with neuromuscular scoliosis. *J. Hosp. Med.* **2013**, *8*, 684–688. [CrossRef] [PubMed]

24. Belthur, M.; Bosch, L.; Wood, W.; Boan, C.; Miller, F.; Shrader, M.W. Perioperative management of patients with cerebral palsy undergoing scoliosis surgery: Survey of surgeon practices. *J. Pediatr. Rehabil. Med.* **2019**, *12*, 205–212. [CrossRef] [PubMed]
25. Mullender, M.; Blom, N.; De Kleuver, M.; Fock, J.; Hitters, W.; Horemans, A.; Kalkman, C.; Pruijs, J.; Timmer, R.; Titarsolej, P.; et al. A Dutch guideline for the treatment of scoliosis in neuromuscular disorders. *Scoliosis* **2008**, *3*, 14. [CrossRef] [PubMed]
26. Mercado, E.; Alman, B.; Wright, J.G. Does Spinal Fusion Influence Quality of Life in Neuromuscular Scoliosis? *Spine (Phila Pa 1976)* **2007**, *32*, S120–S125. [CrossRef]
27. Sullivan, D.J.; Primhak, R.A.; Bevan, C.; Breakwell, L.M.; Humphreys, N. Complications in pediatric scoliosis surgery. *Pediatr. Anesth.* **2014**, *24*, 406–411. [CrossRef]
28. Malik, A.T.; Yu, E.; Kim, J.; Khan, S.N. Intensive Care Unit Admission Following Surgery for Pediatric Spinal Deformity: An Analysis of the ACS-NSQIP Pediatric Spinal Fusion Procedure Targeted Dataset. *Glob. Spine J.* **2020**, *10*, 177–182. [CrossRef]
29. Rumbak, D.M.; Mowrey, W.; Schwartz, S.W.; Sarwahi, V.; Djukic, A.; Killinger, J.S.; Katyal, C. Spinal Fusion for Scoliosis in Rett Syndrome with an Emphasis on Respiratory Failure and Opioid Usage. *J. Child Neurol.* **2016**, *31*, 153–158. [CrossRef]
30. Akesen, S. Predictive factors for postoperative intensive care unit admission in pediatric patients undergoing scoliosis correction surgery. *Am. J. Transl. Res.* **2021**, *13*, 5386–5394.
31. Madrigal, V.N.; Kelly, K.P. Supporting Family Decision-making for a Child Who Is Seriously Ill: Creating Synchrony and Connection. *Pediatrics* **2018**, *142*, S170–S177. [CrossRef]
32. October, T.W.; Fisher, K.R.; Feudtner, C.; Hinds, P.S. The Parent Perspective: "Being a good parent" when making critical decisions in the PICU. *Pediatr. Crit. Care Med.* **2014**, *15*, 291–298. [CrossRef] [PubMed]
33. October, T.W.; Jones, A.H.; Michals, H.G.; Hebert, L.M.; Jiang, J.; Wang, J. Parental Conflict, Regret, and Short-term Impact on Quality of Life in Tracheostomy Decision-Making. *Pediatr. Crit. Care Med.* **2020**, *21*, 136–142. [CrossRef] [PubMed]
34. Bogetz, J.; Kett, J.C.; Wightman, A. Preparing for medical decision-making in response to concerns about suffering in children with severe neurologic impairment. *Acta Paediatr.* **2021**, *110*, 755–758. [CrossRef] [PubMed]
35. Bogetz, J.F.; Hauer, J. Certainty of Decisions: A Process-Based Model for Decision Making for Children with Severe Neurological Impairment. *Clin. Pediatr.* **2018**, *57*, 1227–1231. [CrossRef] [PubMed]
36. Kopelman, L.M. The Best-Interests Standard as Threshold, Ideal, and Standard of Reasonableness. *J. Med. Philos. A Forum Bioeth. Philos. Med.* **1997**, *22*, 271–289. [CrossRef] [PubMed]
37. Bester, J.C. The Best Interest Standard Is the Best We Have: Why the Harm Principle and Constrained Parental Autonomy Cannot Replace the Best Interest Standard in Pediatric Ethics. *J. Clin. Ethics* **2019**, *30*, 223–231. [PubMed]
38. Marron, J.M. Adolescent Shared Decision-Making: Where We Have Been and Where We are Going. *J. Adolesc. Health* **2021**, *69*, 6–7. [CrossRef] [PubMed]
39. President's Commission for the Study of Ethical Problems in Medicine and Biomedical and Behavioral Research. *Making Health Care Decisions: A Report on the Ethical and Legal Implications of Informed Consent in the Patient-Practitioner Relationship*; U.S. Government Printing Office: Washington, DC, USA, 1982.
40. Adams, R.C.; Levy, S.E.; Council on Children with Disabilities. Shared Decision-Making and Children With Disabilities: Pathways to Consensus. *Pediatrics* **2017**, *139*, e20170956. [CrossRef]
41. Gillam, L. The zone of parental discretion: An ethical tool for dealing with disagreement between parents and doctors about medical treatment for a child. *Clin. Ethics* **2016**, *11*, 1–8. [CrossRef]
42. Zaal-Schuller, I.; de Vos, M.; Ewals, F.; van Goudoever, J.; Willems, D. End-of-life decision-making for children with severe developmental disabilities: The parental perspective. *Res. Dev. Disabil.* **2016**, *49–50*, 235–246. [CrossRef]
43. Zaal-Schuller, I.H.; Geurtzen, R.; Willems, D.L.; de Vos, M.A.; Hogeveen, M. What hinders and helps in the end-of-life decision-making process for children: Parents' and physicians' views. *Acta Paediatr.* **2022**, *111*, 873–887. [CrossRef] [PubMed]
44. Diekema, D. Parental refusals of medical treatment: The harm principle as threshold for state intervention. *Theor. Med. Bioeth.* **2004**, *25*, 243–264. [CrossRef] [PubMed]
45. Jonas, D.; Scanlon, C.; Bogetz, J.F. Parental Decision-Making for Children with Medical Complexity: An Integrated Literature Review. *J. Pain Symptom Manag.* **2022**, *63*, e111–e123. [CrossRef] [PubMed]
46. Feudtner, C.; Walter, J.K.; Faerber, J.A.; Hill, D.; Carroll, K.W.; Mollen, C.; Miller, V.A.; Morrison, W.E.; Munson, D.; Kang, T.I.; et al. Good-Parent Beliefs of Parents of Seriously Ill Children. *JAMA Pediatr.* **2015**, *169*, 39–47. [CrossRef] [PubMed]
47. Taylor, E.P.; Doolittle, B. Caregiver Decision-Making for Terminally Ill Children: A Qualitative Study. *J. Palliat. Care* **2020**, *35*, 161–166. [CrossRef]
48. Bogetz, J.F.; Revette, A.; DeCourcey, D.D. Clinical Care Strategies That Support Parents of Children with Complex Chronic Conditions. *Pediatr. Crit. Care Med.* **2021**, *22*, 595–602. [CrossRef]
49. Adams, S.; Beatty, M.; Moore, C.; Desai, A.; Bartlett, L.; Culbert, E.; Cohen, E.; Stinson, J.; Orkin, J. Perspectives on team communication challenges in caring for children with medical complexity. *BMC Health Serv. Res.* **2021**, *21*, 300. [CrossRef]
50. Feudtner, C. The Breadth of Hopes. *N. Engl. J. Med.* **2009**, *361*, 2306–2307. [CrossRef]
51. Leape, L.L. Hospital Readmissions Following Surgery: Turning complications into "treasures". *JAMA* **2015**, *313*, 467–468. [CrossRef]
52. Leape, L.L. Patient Safety in the Era of Healthcare Reform. *Clin. Orthop. Relat. Res.* **2015**, *473*, 1568–1573. [CrossRef]

53. Sikka, K.; Ahmed, A.A.; Diaz, D.; Goodwin, M.S.; Craig, K.D.; Bartlett, M.S.; Huang, J.S. Automated Assessment of Children's Postoperative Pain Using Computer Vision. *Pediatrics* **2015**, *136*, e124–e131. [CrossRef] [PubMed]
54. Lofti, M.; Gaume, M.; Khouri, N.; Johnson, M.; Topouchian, V.; Glorion, C. Minimally Invasive Surgery for Neuromuscular Scoliosis: Results and Complications in a Series of One Hundred Patients. *Spine* **2018**, *43*, E968–E975. [CrossRef]

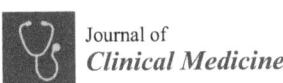

Review

Are We Getting It Right? A Scoping Review of Outcomes Reported in Cell Therapy Clinical Studies for Cerebral Palsy

Megan Finch-Edmondson [1,*], Madison C. B. Paton [1], Ingrid Honan [1], Petra Karlsson [1], Candice Stephenson [1], Darryl Chiu [1], Sarah Reedman [1], Alexandra R. Griffin [1], Catherine Morgan [1] and Iona Novak [1,2]

1 Cerebral Palsy Alliance Research Institute, Speciality of Child and Adolescent Health, Sydney Medical School, Faculty of Medicine and Health, The University of Sydney, Sydney, NSW 2050, Australia
2 Faculty of Medicine and Health, The University of Sydney, Sydney, NSW 2050, Australia
* Correspondence: mfinch-edmondson@cerebralpalsy.org.au; Tel.: +61-2-8052-2068

Abstract: Cell therapies are an emergent treatment for cerebral palsy (CP) with promising evidence demonstrating efficacy for improving gross motor function. However, families value improvements in a range of domains following intervention and the non-motor symptoms, comorbidities and complications of CP can potentially be targeted by cell therapies. We conducted a scoping review to describe all outcomes that have been reported in cell therapy studies for CP to date, and to examine what instruments were used to capture these. Through a systematic search we identified 54 studies comprising 2066 participants that were treated with a range of cell therapy interventions. We categorized the reported 53 unique outcome instruments and additional descriptive measures into 10 categories and 12 sub-categories. Movement and Posture was the most frequently reported outcome category, followed by Safety, however Quality of Life, and various prevalent comorbidities and complications of CP were infrequently reported. Notably, many outcome instruments used do not have evaluative properties and thus are not suitable for measuring change following intervention. We provide a number of recommendations to ensure that future trials generate high-quality outcome data that is aligned with the priorities of the CP community.

Keywords: cerebral palsy; cell therapies; stem cells; comorbidities; outcome measures; clinical studies

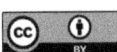

1. Introduction

Stem cell and cell therapies have been in clinical research for the treatment of cerebral palsy (CP) for more than 15 years [1]. There are a variety of cell types being investigated including umbilical cord blood, mesenchymal stem/stromal cells, and neural stem- or stem-like cells [2]. The principal target of cell therapies for the treatment of CP is remediation of the underlying brain injury thereby improving neuronal signaling, which could be achieved by either direct or indirect actions. Cell therapies are proposed to work via a variety of mechanisms for the treatment of CP. Depending on the cell type, therapeutic benefits may include reduction of inflammation, promotion of cell survival, stimulation of proliferation and migration of endogenous neural stem cells, replacement and/or regeneration of damaged brain cells, and promotion of angiogenesis [2].

Systematic reviews of randomized controlled trials have shown that improvement in gross motor skills/function, typically measured using the Gross Motor Function Measure (GMFM) [3], is the most common primary outcome assessed [4,5]. Promisingly, these studies have demonstrated that various cell therapies can produce a small but significant improvement in gross motor function [4,5], although these findings are limited by heterogeneity in various aspects (e.g., participants, interventions, outcomes). Furthermore, whilst the number of clinical studies and total number of participants with CP treated with cell therapies continues to climb (now >2427 participants across >77 published and unpublished studies) [1], there remains a high volume of lower-quality evidence employing poor study design and/or unvalidated outcome assessment tools, and thus more research is warranted.

Although CP is characterized by impairment of movement and/or posture, it is a highly heterogeneous condition, and individuals with CP often experience a range of comorbidities and/or co-occurring complications that can be just as disabling as the motor symptoms [6]. These include pain, intellectual impairment, epilepsy, behavior disorders, and vision and hearing impairments [6]. As such, there is an increasing focus within the CP field to understand these elements, and find ways to target them, with the overarching goal of improving the quality of life for people living with CP.

Individuals with CP and their families value a wide range of potential benefits following certain types of stem cell treatments [7] and other interventions [8,9]. These benefits often focus on activity and participation rather than necessarily remediating physical impairment. It is therefore important that clinical studies of cell therapies measure outcomes that are both scientifically valid and valued by individuals with CP and their families. In addition, outcomes should be measured using well-validated tools so that evidence generated from these studies can increase our confidence in study findings. To aid in this, a panel of international experts have compiled recommended CP-specific common data elements for use in clinical research studies [10]. However, these instruments may not always be consistently applied. As such, the purpose of this scoping review is to describe all outcomes that have been reported in cell therapy studies for CP to date, and to examine what instruments have been used to capture these outcomes.

2. Materials and Methods

A protocol for this review was registered on Open Science Framework (OSF) (identifier DOI 10.17605/OSF.IO/T9C8J [https://osf.io/t9c8j/?view_only=9b82c37725834a1da1a50bb199cf5091 (accessed on 14 November 2022)], registration date 8 July 2022). This scoping review was conducted according to the Preferred Reporting Items for Systematic Reviews and Meta-Analyses extension for Scoping Reviews (PRISMA-ScR) guidelines [11] (Supplementary Table S1).

2.1. Inclusion and Exclusion Criteria

We included any type of study (both controlled and non-controlled studies, including case series/reports) in which participants with CP were treated with a cell therapy intervention specifically for the treatment of CP. If studies reported participants with various diagnoses, >50% must have had CP. There was no restriction on participant age. The full text of the study must also have been published in English (due to no translation services available), in a peer-reviewed journal. Studies were excluded from this review if they reported an organ graft or transplant, or were a secondary analysis of a study that was already included in this review.

2.2. Data Sources and Search Strategy

We searched the Cochrane Central Register of Controlled Trials (CENTRAL) (The Cochrane Library, April 2022), PubMed (MEDLINE) (1946 to 6 May 2022) and EMBASE (1947 to 6 May 2022) via OVID using the search strategy described in Supplementary Table S2. The search was conducted on 10th May 2022. De-duplicated results from OVID were exported into Covidence Systematic Review Software (http://www.covidence.org (accessed on 14 November 2022)). Database searching was also supplemented by hand searching, i.e., cross checking systematic review reference lists for potentially eligible articles, and new paper alerts were monitored for potentially eligible papers published after the formal search was conducted.

2.3. Study Selection and Data Extraction

Titles and/or abstracts of studies retrieved using the search strategy were screened independently by two reviewers (split between M.F.-E., M.C.B.P., C.F.). Full texts of studies were then retrieved and independently assessed for eligibility by two reviewers (split between M.F.-E., M.C.B.P., C.F.), with any disagreements resolved by the third screener.

A data extraction form was developed specifically for this review by the research team. Data extraction was performed independently by at least two members of the research team (M.F.-E., M.C.B.P., C.F.), with any discrepancies identified and resolved through discussion with the third extractor. Extracted data included details of study design, participants, intervention/s, comparator (if relevant), and outcome instrument/s.

2.4. Assigning Level of Evidence for Included Studies

The level of evidence for each included study was assigned according to Oxford Centre for Evidence-Based Medicine: Levels of Evidence [12].

2.5. Categorization of Cell Interventions

Cell interventions were sorted into six categories: (1) Umbilical cord blood; (2) Mesenchymal stem/stromal cells; (3) Bone marrow cells, hematopoietic stem cells and peripheral blood cells (including mononuclear cell fragment, enriched/expanded cells from bone marrow or umbilical cord blood, and peripheral blood mononuclear cells); (4) Neural stem cells/neural-like cells (including neural stem cells (NSCs), neural progenitor cells, olfactory ensheathing cells and mesenchymal stem/stromal cell-derived NSC-like cells); (5) Immune cells (M2-like macrophages); and (6) Fetal cells/embryonic stem cells.

2.6. Categorization of Instruments (into Outcome Domains)

For this review, members of the research team (M.F.-E., M.C.B.P., I.H., P.K., C.S., D.C.) determined outcome domain categories and sub-categories for sorting the reported outcome instruments. This process involved consideration of all the extracted outcome instruments followed by group discussion to reach consensus on which outcome categories/sub-categories to include. All outcome instruments were then assigned to these categories/sub-categories according to the outcome domain/s they were designed to assess, again via group discussion between multiple members of the research team (M.F.-E., M.C.B.P., P.K., I.H., C.S., D.C.) to reach agreement.

Outcome instruments that spanned more than one outcome domain, i.e., encompassing multiple reported sub-domains, were assigned to various categories/sub-categories according to these sub-domains. Any instrument for which the outcome being assessed could not be determined (or agreed), the tool was a multi-domain measure but was only reported as a total score, or the instrument did not fit with any other outcome sub/category, were designated as Other. Any reported descriptive/observational outcomes were subsequently categorized into the same outcome sub/categories through discussion and agreement.

2.7. Outcome Instrument Properties

Outcome instrument properties including format (i.e., who completed the assessment and the nature of it), primary purpose (i.e., predictive, discriminative, evaluative or classification) and population designed for, were determined from various information sources including test manuals/handbooks, systematic reviews, and websites, as necessary.

The categories used for instrument format followed that of the U.S. Food and Drug Administration (FDA) types of clinical outcome assessments, namely: Patient (or self)-reported, Clinician (or therapist)-reported, Observer (e.g., parent/carer/teacher)-reported, and Performance-based measures [13]. In this review we have used the term 'Parent/other' to denote the Observer group. Additionally, the report type was specified as Questionnaire, Interview (including semi-structured interview) or Observation.

2.8. Calculating Total Number of Participants per Outcome Sub/Category

For calculating the number of participants assessed for each outcome sub/category, n's were collapsed or compounded as such: In studies that utilized multiple assessment tools within a single outcome sub-category (e.g., *Gross Motor* measured using GMFM,

Gross Motor Function Classification System Expanded and Revised (GMFCS) [14], etc.), the number of participants assessed for *Gross Motor* was collapsed, meaning that n's were not counted more than once for that sub-category. E.g., if 10 participants were evaluated using the GMFCS and GMFM, the n for *Gross Motor* would remain at 10. However, if the same 10 study participants were also assessed for *Fine Motor and Upper Limb* using the Fine Motor Function Measure (FMFM) [15], this would result in a total compounded n of 20 for the *Movement and Posture* category.

3. Results

3.1. Search Results

Following the literature search and de-duplication, 1145 records were identified. After title and abstract screening, 93 full-text reports were reviewed and 50 met eligibility [16–65]. A further four eligible reports were identified through hand searching [66–69]. In addition, during data extraction and preparation of the manuscript, two new studies were identified [70,71] that also met eligibility and were included. Moreover, a study that was initially included was retracted [30] and was therefore subsequently excluded from this review. Thus, finally, 55 reports were included. These 55 reports represented 54 studies since Amanat 2021 [17] and Zarrabi 2022 [64] are two reports of the same clinical trial (clinical trial registration identifier NCT03795974) and share the same control group. The PRISMA [72] flow chart of the search process is presented in Figure 1.

3.2. Study Characteristics

A summary of the included studies is presented in Table 1, including details of study design, participants, intervention/s and comparator/s, and outcome instrument/s.

3.3. Types of Studies

Of the 54 studies included, 17 (32%) were controlled studies: 14 were randomized controlled trials, with three of these being a cross-over design, and three were non-randomized controlled studies. A further 18 studies (33%) were single-arm and 18 (33%) were case series or case reports, including four studies [19,26,50,56] that were retrospective analyses including 'therapeutic experiments' and a 'post-registration clinical investigation'. In addition, one study (2%) [27] was a non-randomized dose comparison trial. Accordingly, the majority of included studies (n = 37, 69%) were deemed to be Level 4 evidence with n = 3 being Level 3, and n = 14 were Level 2.

3.4. Types of Participants

Collectively, data from 2066 participants was reported, and all studies exclusively included participants with CP. Most studies enrolled/treated participants of various type and topography, and all GMFCS severity levels were represented. Whilst the majority of studies recruited/treated children and youth (up to 18 years) with CP, participant ages ranged from 6 months to 35 years (Table 1).

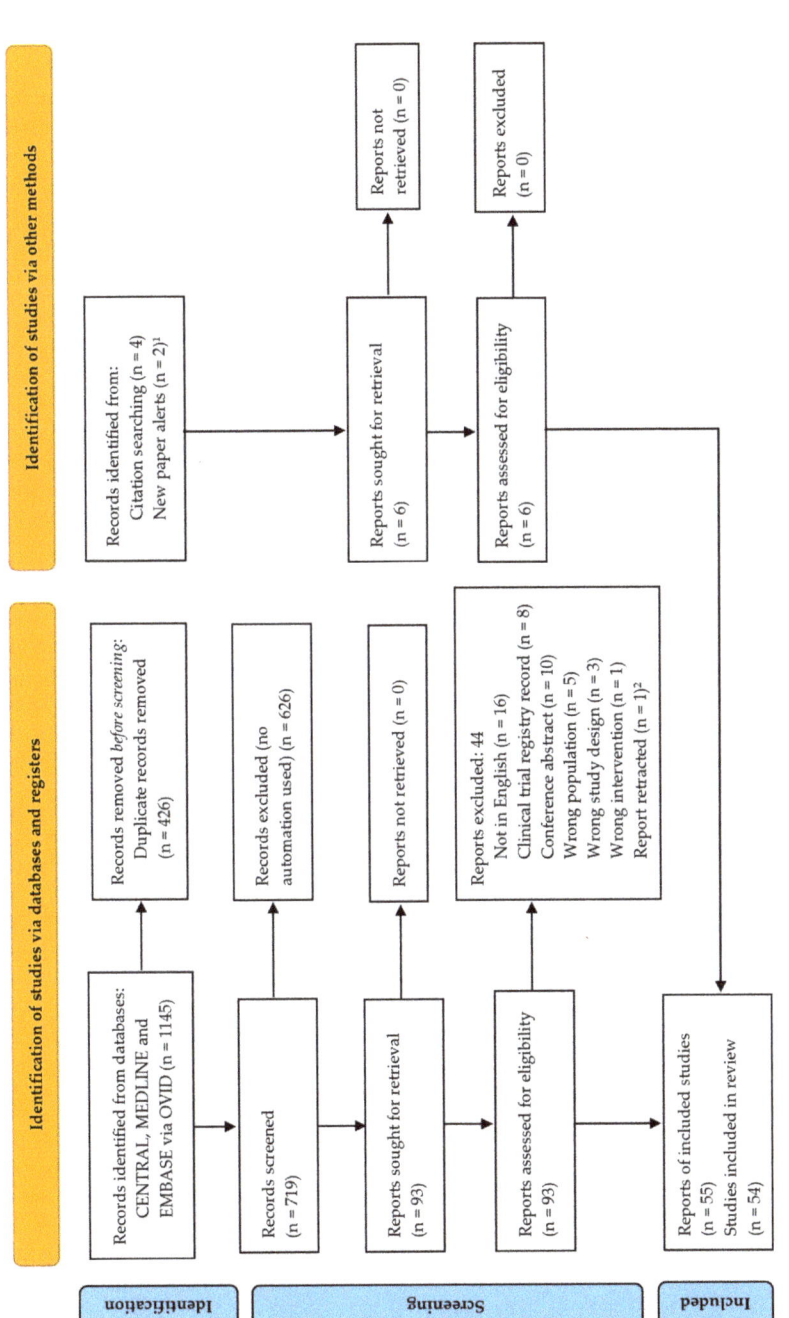

Figure 1. PRISMA flow diagram of study selection.

[1] These papers were identified after the initial searches were conducted.
[2] This paper was retracted after the initial searches were conducted.

Table 1. Details of included studies.

Study Reference	Study Design	Participant Details at Baseline	Intervention/s and Comparator/s	Cell Therapy, Donor Type and Route	Last Follow Up Post-Cell Treatment [1]	Outcome Sub-Categories: Instrument/s Reported	Level of Evidence [2]
AbiChahine 2016 [16]	Case series n = 17 n = 2 LTFU	Subtype: Various Severity: GMFCS I-II, IV-V Age: 1.5–17 years	BM-MNCs (n = 17)	Autologous, intrathecal	Not reported	Gross Motor: GMFCS Spasticity; Cognition & General Development; Activities of Daily Living; Adaptive Behavior: Descriptive Safety	4
Amanat 2021 [17] [3]	RCT n = 72 n = 5 LTFU	Subtype: Spastic quadriplegia and diplegia Severity: GMFCS II-V Age: Mean 8.5 years	Group 1: UC-MSCs + rehab (n = 36) Group 2: Sham procedure + rehab (n = 36)	Allogeneic, intrathecal	1 year	Gross Motor: GMFM-66, PEDI Spasticity: MAS Activities of Daily Living: PEDI Social-Emotional: PEDI Quality of Life: CP-QoL Neuroimaging: MRI-DTI Safety	2
Bansal 2016 [18]	Single-arm n = 10	Subtype: Not reported Severity: GMFCS II-IV Age: 2–10 years	BM-MNCs + rehab (n = 10)	Autologous, intrathecal	2 years	Gross Motor: GMFCS Fine Motor & Upper Limb: MACS Communication: CFCS Spasticity: Descriptive Neuroimaging: MRI Safety	4
Boruczkowski 2019 [19]	Case series (Retrospective) n = 107 n = 17 LTFU + n = 36–67 missing data (outcome dependent)	Subtype: Not reported Severity: Not reported Age: 1.4–17 years	UC-MSCs (n = 107)	Allogeneic, intravenous	Not reported	Gross Motor; Fine Motor & Upper Limb; Spasticity; Muscle Strength; Quality of Life; Activities of Daily Living; Cognition & General Development; Adaptive Behavior; Executive Function; Social-Emotional; Communication; Seizures/Electrical Brain Activity: Descriptive Other: Descriptive (sensory, sleep, circulation, medications) Safety	4
Chen 2010 [20]	RCT n = 33 n = 19 LTFU	Subtype: Not reported Severity: Not reported Age: 1–12 years	Group 1: Fetal OECs + rehab (n = 18) Group 2: Rehab alone (n = 15)	Allogeneic, intracerebral	6 months	Gross Motor: GMFM-66 Other: Caregiver Questionnaire Scale Safety	2
Chen 2013 [21]	Non-randomised controlled n = 60	Subtype: Not reported Severity: GMFCS III-V Age: 1–35 years	Group 1: BM-MSC-derived NSC-like cells + rehab (n = 30) Group 2: Rehab alone (n = 30)	Autologous, intrathecal	6 months	Gross Motor: GMFM-88 Language: Gesell Developmental Schedules Safety	3
Chernykh 2014 [22]	Single-arm n = 21	Subtype: Various Severity: GMFCS IV-V Age: 2–8 years	Peripheral blood expanded M2-like macrophages (n = 21)	Autologous, intrathecal	5 years	Gross Motor: GMFM-66 Fine Motor & Upper Limb: PDMS-FM Spasticity: Ashworth Scale Muscle Strength: MRC Scale Cognition & General Development; Seizures/Electrical Brain Activity: Descriptive Other: Descriptive (infections, temperatures) Biomarkers Safety	4

Table 1. Cont.

Study Reference	Study Design	Participant Details at Baseline	Intervention/s and Comparator/s	Cell Therapy, Donor Type and Route	Last Follow Up Post-Cell Treatment [1]	Outcome Sub-Categories: Instrument/s Reported	Level of Evidence [2]
Chernykh 2018 [23]	Single-arm n = 57	Subtype: Various Severity: GMFCS III-V Age: 1–10 years	Peripheral blood expanded M2-like macrophages (n = 57)	Autologous, intrathecal	5 years	Gross Motor: GMFM-66 Fine Motor & Upper Limb: PDMS-FM Spasticity: Ashworth Scale Muscle Strength: MRC Scale Cognition & General Development; Seizures/Electrical Brain Activity: Descriptive Biomarkers Safety	4
Cox 2022 [66]	RCT: Cross-over n = 20 n = 2 LITFU (longer term endpoint only)	Subtype: Various Severity: GMFCS II-V Age: 2.4–10.9 years	Group 1: UCB then placebo (n = 3) Group 2: BM-MNCs then placebo (n = 10) Group 3: Placebo then UCB (n = 2) Group 4: Placebo then BM-MNCs (n = 5)	Autologous, intravenous	2 years (1 year post cross-over)	Gross Motor: GMFM-66/-88 General Motor: VABS-2 Communication: VABS-2 Activities of Daily Living: VABS-2 Adaptive Behavior: VABS-2 Social-Emotional: VABS-2 Neuroimaging: MRI/MRI-DTI Safety	2
Crompton 2022 [24]	Single-arm n = 12 [4] n = 1 withdrew before treatment	Subtype: Various Severity: GMFCS I-V Age: 2.7–11.6 years	UCB (n = 12)	Allogeneic, intravenous	1 year	Gross Motor: GMFM-66 Fine Motor & Upper Limb: QUEST General Motor: VABS-2 Communication: VABS-2 Activities of Daily Living: VABS-2 Cognition & General Development: BSID-3, WPPSI-IV or WISC-V Adaptive Behavior: VABS-2 Executive Function: BRIEF Social-Emotional: SDQ, VABS-2 Quality of Life: CP-QoL-Child Safety	4
Dong 2018 [25]	Case report n = 1	Subtype: Not reported Severity: Not reported Age: 4 years	UC-MSCs (n = 1)	Donor type not specified, intravenous and intrathecal	Not reported	Seizures/Electrical Brain Activity: EEG Muscle Strength; General Motor; Language; Cognition & General Development: Descriptive	4
Feng 2015 [26]	Case series (Retrospective) n = 47	Subtype: Not reported Severity: "Severe" Age: 1–29 years	UCB (n = 47)	Allogeneic, intravenous then intrathecal	6 months	Safety	4
Fu 2019 [27]	Non-randomised dose comparison n = 60 n = 3 LITFU	Subtype: Spastic, topography not reported Severity: GMFCS IV-V Age: Not reported	Group 1: UC-MSCs 1 course (n = 30) Group 2: UC-MSCs 2 courses (n = 27)	Allogeneic, intrathecal	1 year	Gross Motor: GMFM-88 Fine Motor & Upper Limb: FMFM Safety	4
Gabr 2015 [67]	RCT n = 100 n = 6 withdrew before treatment	Subtype: Various Severity: GMFCS II-V Age: Mean 4.8 years	Group 1: BM-MSCs (n = 44) Group 2: Standard care (n = 50)	Autologous, intrathecal	1 year	Gross Motor: GMFCS, PEDI Quality of Life: CHQ Activities of Daily Living: PEDI Social-Emotional: PEDI Safety	2

Table 1. Cont.

Study Reference	Study Design	Participant Details at Baseline	Intervention/s and Comparator/s	Cell Therapy, Donor Type and Route	Last Follow Up Post-Cell Treatment [1]	Outcome Sub-Categories: Instrument/s Reported	Level of Evidence [2]
Gu 2020 [28]	RCT n = 40 n = 1 withdrew before treatment	Subtype: Not reported Severity: Not reported Age: Mean 4.3 years	Group 1: UC-MSCs + rehab (n = 19) Group 2: Placebo + rehab (n = 20)	Allogeneic, intravenous	1 year	Gross Motor: GMFM-88 Activities of Daily Living: ADL Neuroimaging: PET-CT Other: CFA Safety	2
Hassan 2012 [29]	Non-randomised controlled n = 52	Subtype: Athetoid and spastic, various topography Severity: GMFCS unclear [3] Age: 1–8 years	Group 1: BM-MSC (n = 26) Group 2: No treatment (n = 26)	Autologous, intrathecal	1 year	Gross Motor: GMFCS, BDPS Activities of Daily Living: BDPS Communication: BDPS Other: Descriptive ('100 points scale')	3
Hirano 2018 [68]	Case report n = 1	Subtype: Hemiplegia, type not reported Severity: GMFCS II Age: 7 years	Adipose-MSCs (n = 1)	Allogeneic, intravenous, intramuscular, subcutaneous and intra-articular	1 year	Gross Motor: GMFCS Quality of Life: SF-8 Other: Descriptive (clinical condition) Safety	4
Huang 2018 [31]	RCT n = 56 n = 2 LTFU	Subtype: Not reported Severity: Not reported Age: 3–12 years	Group 1: UCB-MSCs + rehab (n = 27) Group 2: Placebo + rehab (n = 27)	Allogeneic, intravenous	2 years	Gross Motor: GMFM-88 Neuroimaging: MRI Seizures/Electrical Brain Activity: EEG Other: CFA Safety	2
Jensen 2016 [32]	Case report n = 1	Subtype: Spastic hemiplegia Severity: GMFCS I equivalent Age: 5 years	UCB + rehab (n = 1)	Autologous, intravenous	5.5 years	Gross Motor; Fine Motor & Upper Limb; Spasticity; Muscle Strength; Cognition & General Development: Descriptive Safety	4
Kang 2015 [33]	RCT n = 36 n = 2 withdrew before treatment	Subtype: Not reported Severity: GMFCS I-V Age: 0.5–18 years	Group 1: UCB + rehab (n = 17) Group 2: Placebo + rehab (n = 17)	Allogeneic, intravenous or intra-arterial	6 months	Gross Motor: GMFM, GMPM, WeeFIM, PEDI Muscle Strength: MMT score General Motor: BSID-2 [6] Cognition & General Development: WeeFIM Activities of Daily Living: WeeFIM, PEDI Social-Emotional: PEDI Neuroimaging: PET-CT Biomarkers Safety	2
Kikuchi 2022 [70]	Single-arm n = 6	Subtype: Spastic hemiplegia, diplegia and quadriplegia Severity: GMFCS I, III-V Age: 1.7–6.7 years	UCB (n = 6)	Autologous, intravenous	3 years	Gross Motor: GMFM-66, GMFCS General Motor: KSPD Cognition & General Development: KSPD, WISC-IV Social-emotional: KSPD Neuroimaging: MRI-DTI Seizures/Electrical Brain Activity: EEG Safety	4

Table 1. Cont.

Study Reference	Study Design	Participant Details at Baseline	Intervention/s and Comparator/s	Cell Therapy, Donor Type and Route	Last Follow Up Post-Cell Treatment [1]	Outcome Sub-Categories: Instrument/s Reported	Level of Evidence [2]
Lee 2012 [34]	Single-arm n = 20	Subtype: Various topography, type not reported Severity: Not reported Age: 1.9–7.6 years	UCB (n = 20)	Autologous, intravenous	6 months	Gross Motor: GMFM-88, GMFCS, PEDI, DDST-2 Fine Motor & Upper Limb: QUEST, MACS, DDST-2 Activities of Daily Living: PEDI Social-Emotional: PEDI, DDST-2 Language: DDST-2 Neuroimaging: MRI-DTI, SPECT	4
Li 2012 [35]	Case report n = 1	Subtype: Not reported Severity: Ambulant Age: 11 years	BM-MSCs (n = 1)	Autologous, intravenous	1 year	Spasticity: Descriptive Other: Descriptive (vision) Safety	4
Liu 2017 [36]	RCT n = 105 n = 3 LTFU	Subtype: Spastic, topography not reported Severity: GMFCS II–V Age: 0.5–12.5 years	Group 1: BM-MSCs (n = 35) Group 2: BM-MNCs (n = 35) Group 3: Rehab (n = 35)	Autologous, intrathecal	1 year	Gross Motor: GMFM Fine Motor & Upper Limb: FMFM	2
Luan 2012 [37]	RCT n = 94	Subtype: Various Severity: "Severe" Age: Mean 1.3 years	Group 1: Fetal NPCs + rehab (n = 45) Group 2: Rehab alone (n = 49)	Allogeneic, intra-cerebroventricular	1 year	Gross Motor: GMFM Fine Motor & Upper Limb: PDMS-FM Cognition & General Development: Descriptive Other: Descriptive (sleep) Safety	2
Mancias-Guerra 2014 [38]	Single-arm n = 18 n = 5 LTFU	Subtype: Various Severity: Not reported Age: 2.2–5.5 years	BM-TNCs (n = 18)	Autologous, intrathecal and intravenous	6 months	General Motor: BDI Cognition & General Development: BDI Communication: BDI Adaptive Behavior: BDI Social-Emotional: BDI Neuroimaging: MRI Safety	4
Maric 2022 [39]	Single-arm n = 42	Subtype: Various types, topography not reported Severity: GMFCS I–V Age: 1–12 years	BM-MNCs (n = 42)	Autologous, intrathecal	1 year	Gross Motor: GMFCS, S-D Fine Motor & Upper Limb: LAP-D Spasticity: MAS Cognition & General Development: LAP-D Language: LAP-D Neuroimaging: MRI Seizures/Electrical Brain Activity: EEG Safety	4
Min 2013 [40]	RCT n = 105 n = 9 LTFU	Subtype: Various Severity: GMFCS I–V Age: 0.6–9.8 years	Group 1: UCB + EPO + rehab (n = 35) Group 2: Placebo UCB + EPO + rehab (n = 36) Group 3: Placebo UCB + Placebo EPO + rehab (n = 34)	Allogeneic, intravenous	6 months	Gross Motor: GMFM, GMPM, PEDI, WeeFIM Fine Motor & Upper Limb: QUEST Muscle Strength: MMST General Motor: BSID-2 Cognition & General Development: BSID-2, WeeFIM Activities of Daily Living: PEDI, WeeFIM Social-Emotional: PEDI Neuroimaging: MRI-DTI, PET-CT Safety	2

Table 1. Cont.

Study Reference	Study Design	Participant Details at Baseline	Intervention/s and Comparator/s	Cell Therapy, Donor Type and Route	Last Follow Up Post-Cell Treatment [1]	Outcome Sub-Categories: Instrument/s Reported	Level of Evidence [2]
Min 2020 [41]	RCT n = 92 n = 4 LTFU	Subtype: Various Severity: GMFCS I-V Age: 1–6.3 years	Group 1: UCB + EPO (n = 22) Group 2: UCB + Placebo EPO (n = 24) Group 3: Placebo UCB + EPO (n = 20) Group 4: Placebo UCB + Placebo EPO (n = 24)	Allogeneic, intravenous	1 year	**Gross Motor:** GMFM, GMPM, GMFCS, PEDI, SCALE **Fine Motor & Upper Limb:** QUEST **Spasticity:** MAS, Modified Tardieu Scale **Muscle Strength:** MRC Scale **General Motor:** BSID-2 **Cognition & General Development:** BSID-2, FIM **Activities of Daily Living:** FIM, PEDI **Social-Emotional:** PEDI **Neuroimaging:** MRI-DTI, PET-CT **Seizures/Electrical Brain Activity:** EEG **Other:** Descriptive (parent satisfaction), Beery VMI **Biomarkers** **Safety**	2
Nguyen 2017 [42]	Single-arm n = 40	Subtype: Spastic bilateral and unilateral Severity: GMFCS III-V Age: 1–12 years	BM-MNCs (n = 40)	Autologous, intrathecal	6 months	**Gross Motor:** GMFM-66/88 **Spasticity:** MAS **Safety**	4
Nguyen 2018 [43]	Single-arm n = 30	Subtype: Quadriplegia and hemiplegia, type not reported Severity: GMFCS II-V Age: 2–15.5 years	BM-MNCs + rehab (n = 30)	Autologous, intrathecal	6 months	**Gross Motor:** GMFM-66/88 **Spasticity:** MAS **Quality of Life:** CP-QoL-Child	4
Okur 2018 [44]	Case report n = 1	Subtype: Dystonic Severity: GMFCS V Age: 6 years	UC-MSCs + rehab (n = 1)	Allogeneic, intrathecal, intramuscular and intravenous	1.5 years	**Gross Motor:** GMFCS, TCMS **Fine Motor & Upper Limb:** MACS **Spasticity:** Modified Tardieu Scale **Communication:** CFCS **Cognition & General Development:** FIM **Activities of Daily Living:** FIM **Safety**	4
Padma Srivastava 2011 [45]	Case series n = 30	Subtype: Dystonic and spastic?, topography not reported Severity: "Moderate to severe" Age: 5–25 years	BM-MNCs (n = 30)	Autologous, intra-arterial	1 year	**Spasticity:** Ashworth Scale **Muscle Strength:** MRC Scale **Activities of Daily Living:** mBI **Other:** mRS **Safety**	4
Papadopoulos 2011 [46]	Case report n = 2	Subtype: Spastic diplegia Severity: GMFCS III Age: 1.6 and 2.7 years	Case 1: UCB + G-CSF 12 months post-infusion Case 2: UCB + G-CSF pre- and post-infusion	Autologous, intravenous	Case 1: 2.3 years Case 2: 7 months	**Gross Motor:** GMFCS **Neuroimaging:** MRI **Spasticity:** Descriptive **Safety**	4

Table 1. Cont.

Study Reference	Study Design	Participant Details at Baseline	Intervention/s and Comparator/s	Cell Therapy, Donor Type and Route	Last Follow Up Post-Cell Treatment [1]	Outcome Sub-Categories: Instrument/s Reported	Level of Evidence [2]
Purandare 2012 [47]	Case report n = 1	Subtype: Not reported Severity: GMFCS III Age: 6 years	BM-MNCs (n = 1)	Autologous, intrathecal	2 years	Gross Motor: GMFCS Neuroimaging: PET-CT Seizures/Electrical Brain Activity: EEG Fine Motor & Upper Limb; Cognition & General Development; Executive Function; Language: Descriptive Other: Descriptive (sensory)	4
Purwati 2019 [48]	Single-arm n = 14 n = 2 LTFU [8]	Subtype: Not reported Severity: GMFCS III-IV Age: 1–11 years	Adipose-derived NPCs (n = 12)	Autologous, intra-cerebroventricular	1 year	Gross Motor: GMFCS Spasticity; Cognition & General Development; Communication: Descriptive Safety	4
Rah 2017 [49]	RCT: Cross-over n = 57 n = 10 LTFU	Subtype: Various Severity: "Non-severe" Age: 2–10 years	Group 1: Peripheral blood-MNCs then placebo (n = 28) Group 2: Placebo then peripheral blood-MNCs (n = 29)	Autologous, intravenous	1 year (6 months post cross-over)	Gross Motor: GMFM-88, GMFCS, PEDI, DDST-2 [9] Fine Motor & Upper Limb: MACS, QUEST Activities of Daily Living: PEDI Social-Emotional: PEDI Neuroimaging: MRI-DTI, PET-CT General Motor; Cognition & General Development: Descriptive Safety	2
Ramirez 2006 [69]	Single-arm n = 8	Subtype: Various types, topography not reported Severity: Not reported Age: 3–12 years	Expanded UCB CD133+ cells (n = 8)	Allogeneic, subcutaneous intramuscular	6 months	Gross Motor; Fine Motor & Upper Limb; Spasticity; Cognition & General Development; Communication; Language: Descriptive Other: Descriptive (infections, vision) Safety	4
Romanov 2015 [50]	Case series (Retrospective) n = 80 n = 25 LTFU/excluded + n = 17–19 missing data (outcome dependent)	Subtype: Various Severity: GMFCS IV-V Age: 1–12 years	UCB (n = 80)	Allogeneic, intravenous	3 years post first treatment	Gross Motor: GMFCS Spasticity: MAS Muscle strength: Hand dynamometry Safety	4
Seledtsov 2005 [51]	Non-randomised controlled n = 60	Subtype: Double hemiplegia, spastic diplegia and atonic-astatia Severity: "Severe" Age: 1.5–7 years	Group 1: Fetal nervous and hematopoietic cells (n = 30) Group 2: Standard care (n = 30)	Allogeneic, intrathecal	1 year	Seizures/Electrical Brain Activity: EEG Gross Motor; Fine Motor & Upper Limb; Cognition & General Development; Communication; Language: Descriptive Other: Descriptive ('100 points scale', vision) Safety	3
Sharma 2013 [52]	Case report n = 1	Subtype: Spastic diplegia Severity: GMFCS III equivalent Age: 20 years	BM-MNC + rehab (n = 1)	Autologous, intrathecal	1 year	Cognition & General Development: FIM, IQ Score Activities of Daily Living: FIM Neuroimaging: PET-CT Other: Mental Status Examination, Descriptive (appetite) Gross Motor; Fine Motor & Upper Limb; Executive Function, Social-Emotional; Communication; Language: Descriptive	4

Table 1. Cont.

Study Reference	Study Design	Participant Details at Baseline	Intervention/s and Comparator/s	Cell Therapy, Donor Type and Route	Last Follow Up Post-Cell Treatment [1]	Outcome Sub-Categories: Instrument/s Reported	Level of Evidence [2]
Sharma 2015 [53]	Single-arm n = 40	Subtype: Various Severity: GMFCS I-V Age: 1.4–22 years	BM-MNCs + rehab (n = 40)	Autologous, intrathecal	6 months	Neuroimaging: PET-CT Gross Motor; Fine Motor & Upper Limb; Spasticity; Muscle Strength; General Motor; Activities of Daily Living; Cognition & General Development; Social-Emotional; Language: Descriptive Safety	4
Sharma 2015 [54]	Case report n = 1	Subtype: Spastic diplegia Severity: GMFCS III Age: 12 years	BM-MNCs + rehab (n = 1)	Autologous, intrathecal	1 year	Cognition & General Development: FIM Activities of Daily Living: FIM Neuroimaging: PET-CT Gross Motor; Fine Motor & Upper Limb; Muscle Strength: Descriptive Other: Descriptive (sense of smell)	4
Sharma 2020 [55]	Case report n = 1	Subtype: Spastic diplegia Severity: GMFCS III Age: 4 years	BM-MNCs + rehab (n = 1)	Autologous, intrathecal	1.3 years post first treatment	Gross Motor: GMFM, GMFCS Cognition & General Development: FIM Activities of Daily Living: FIM Neuroimaging: PET-CT Fine Motor & Upper Limb; Spasticity; Muscle Strength; General Motor; Adaptive Behavior; Executive Function: Descriptive Other: Descriptive (sensory processing) Safety	4
Shroff 2014 [56] [10]	Case series (Retrospective) n = 101 n = 10 excluded from analysis n= 25–76 LITFU between treatment phases	Subtype: Not reported Severity: GMFCS I-V Age: ≤2 to 18 years	ESCs + rehab (n = 101)	Allogeneic, multiple routes [11]	2.4 years post first treatment	Gross Motor: GMFCS Neuroimaging: SPECT Activities of Daily Living; Cognition & General Development; Executive Function; Social-Emotional; Language; Seizures/Electrical Brain Activity: Descriptive Other: Descriptive (hearing) Safety	4
Sun 2017 [57]	RCT: Cross-over n = 63	Subtype: Various Severity: GMFCS I-V Age: 1.1–7 years	Group 1: UCB then placebo (n = 32) Group 2: Placebo then UCB (n = 31)	Autologous, intravenous	2 years (1 year post cross-over)	Gross Motor: GMFM-66, PDMS Fine Motor & Upper Limb: PDMS Neuroimaging: MRI-DTI Safety	2
Sun 2021 [58]	Single-arm n = 15	Subtype: Spastic, various topography Severity: GMFCS II-IV Age: 1-6 years	UCB (n = 15)	Allogeneic; intravenous	2 years	Gross Motor: GMFM-66, PDMS Fine Motor & Upper Limb: AHA, PDMS Safety	4

Table 1. Cont.

Study	Design	Subtype/Severity/Age	Groups	Cell source, route	Follow-up	Outcomes	Level
Sun 2022 [71]	RCT n = 91 n = 1 withdrew before treatment + n = 22 LTFU incl. 18 due to COVID-19	Subtype: Hypertonic, various topography Severity: GMFCS I–IV Age: 2.1–5 years	Group 1: UCB (n = 31) Group 2: UC-MSCs (n = 28) Group 3: Control (n = 31)	Allogeneic, intravenous	1 year	Gross Motor: GMFM-66, PDMS, PEDI-CAT Fine Motor & Upper Limb: PDMS Activities of Daily Living: PEDI-CAT Adaptive Behavior: PEDI-CAT Social-Emotional: PEDI-CAT Safety	2
Thanh 2019 [59]	Single-arm n = 25	Subtype: Spastic bilateral Severity: GMFCS II–V Age: 2–15 years	BM-MNCs + rehab (n = 25)	Autologous, intrathecal	1 year	Gross Motor: GMFM-66/-88 Spasticity: MAS	4
Wang 2013 [60]	Case report n = 1	Subtype: Not reported Severity: Not reported Age: 5 years	UC-MSCs + rehab (n = 1)	Allogeneic, intravenous and intrathecal	2.3 years	Cognition & General Development: FIM Activities of Daily Living: FIM Muscle Strength; Communication: Descriptive Other: Descriptive (immunity)	4
Wang 2013 [61]	Single-arm n = 52 n = 6 withdrew before treatment + n = 6 LTFU	Subtype: Spastic and/or athetoid, topography not reported Severity: GMFCS I–V Age: 0.5–15 years	BM-MSC (n = 46)	Autologous, intrathecal +/− intra-parenchymal	1.5 years	Gross Motor: GMFM-66/-88 Safety	4
Wang 2015 [62]	Single-arm n = 16	Subtype: Spastic, topography not reported Severity: Not reported Age: 3–12 years	UC-MSC (n = 16)	Allogeneic, intrathecal	6 months	Gross Motor: GMFM-88 Fine Motor & Upper Limb: FMFM	4
Zali 2015 [63]	Single-arm n = 13 n = 1 LTFU	Subtype: Various types, topography not reported Severity: GMFCS III–V Age: 4–10 years	BM-CD133+ cells (n = 13)	Autologous, intrathecal	6 months	Gross Motor: GMFM-66, GMFCS, BBS Spasticity: MAS Activities of Daily Living: UK FIM + FAM Cognition & General Development: UK FIM + FAM Seizures/Electrical Brain Activity: EEG Safety	4
Zarrabi 2022 [64] [3]	RCT n = 72 n = 6–9 LTFU (outcome dependent)	Subtype: Spastic quadriplegia and diplegia Severity: GMFCS II–V Age: Mean 9 years	Group 1: UCB + rehab (n = 36) Group 2: Sham procedure + rehab (n = 36)	Allogeneic, intrathecal	1 year	Gross Motor: GMFM-66, PEDI Spasticity: MAS Activities of Daily Living: PEDI Social-Emotional: PEDI Quality of Life: CP-QoL Neuroimaging: MRI-DTI Safety	2

Table 1. Cont.

Zhang 2015 [65]	Case report n = 1	Subtype: Not reported Severity: Not reported Age: 0.5 years	UCB-MSCs + rehab (n = 1)	Allogeneic, intravenous	5 years	**Gross Motor:** GMFM-88 **Spasticity:** Ashworth Scale **Neuroimaging:** MRI **Seizures/Electrical Brain Activity:** EEG **Other:** CDCC Infant Mental Development Scale, CFA **Safety**	4

Bolded text denotes outcome sub-categories. Abbreviations: ADL, Activities of Daily Living assessment; AHA, Assisting Hand Assessment; BBS, Berg Balance Scale; BDI, Battelle Developmental Inventory; BDPS, Boyd's Developmental Progress Scale; Beery VMI, Beery-Buktenica Developmental Test of Visual-Motor Integration 6th edition; BM, bone marrow; BRIEF, Behavior Rating Inventory of Executive Function; BSID-2, Bayley Scales of Infant and Toddler Development 2nd edition; BSID-3, Bayley Scales of Infant and Toddler Development 3rd edition cognitive scale; CDCC, Child Development Center of China; CFA, Comprehensive Functional Assessment; CFCS, Communication Function Classification System; CHQ, Child Health Questionnaire Parent Form 50; COVID-19, coronavirus disease pandemic; CP QOL-Child, Cerebral Palsy Quality of Life Questionnaire for Children; DDST-2, Denver Development Screening Test 2nd edition; DTI, diffusion tensor imaging; EEG, electroencephalogram; ESC, embryonic stem cell; Ex-UCB, expanded umbilical cord blood cells; FIM, Functional Independence Measure; FMFM, Fine Motor Function Measure; G-CSF, granulocyte-colony stimulating factor; GMFCS, Gross Motor Function Classification System; GMFM-66/-88, Gross Motor Function Measure-66 or -88; GMPM, Gross Motor Performance Measure; KSPD, Kyoto Scale of Psychological Development; LAP-D, Learning Accomplishment System Diagnostic Score; LTFU, lost to follow-up; MACS, Manual Ability Classification Scale; MAS, Modified Ashworth Scale; mBI, Modified Barthel Index; MMST, Manual Muscle Strength Test; MMT score, Manual Muscle Testing score; MNC, mononuclear cells; MRC Scale, Medical Research Council Scale; MRI, Magnetic resonance imaging; mRS, Modified Rankin Scale; MSC, mesenchymal stem/stromal cell; n, number of participants; NPC, neural progenitor cell; NSC, neural stem cell; OEC, olfactory ensheathing cell; PB, peripheral blood; PDMS, Peabody Developmental Motor Scales (2nd edition); PDMS-FM, PDMS Fine Motor Test/Quotient; PEDI/-CAT, Pediatric Evaluation of Disability Inventory (Computer Adaptive Test); PET-CT, positron emission tomography and computed tomography scan; QUEST, Quality of Upper Extremity Skills Test; RCT, randomized controlled trial; rehab, rehabilitation; SCALE, Selective Control Assessment of Lower Extremity; SDQ, Strengths and Difficulties Questionnaire; SF-8, Short Form 8 (SF-8) Health Survey Quality of Life questionnaire; SPECT, single photon emission computed tomography scan; TCMS, Trunk Control Measurement Scale; TNC, total nucleated cell; UCB, umbilical cord blood; UK FIM + FAM, UK Functional Independence Measure and Functional Assessment Measure; VABS-2, Vineland Adaptive Behavior Scales 2nd edition; WeeFIM, Functional Independence Measure for Children; WISC-IV/V, Wechsler Intelligence Scale for Children 4th/5th edition; WPPSI-IV, Wechsler Preschool & Primary Scale of Intelligence 4th edition. [1] Most studies captured outcomes at multiple timepoints and not all outcomes were assessed at this timepoint. Some studies that administered multiple cell doses calculated follow-up from after the last cell administration. [2] Level according to The Oxford Levels of Evidence 2 [12]. [3] These are two reports of the same clinical trial (NCT03795974) and share a control group (sham procedure + rehab). [4] Participant that withdrew was replaced, so total number of recruited participants was 13. [5] GMFCS reported as mean and standard deviation. [6] BSID-2 used for motor only. [7] Ascertained from text. [8] Timing of LTFU (before/after treatment) not clear. [9] DDST-2 used for gross motor only. [10] An editorial expression of concern was raised in September 2017 regarding the ethics of this study and the potential association of the risk of teratoma formation with the transplantation of embryonic stem cells [73]. [11] Routes included intravenous, intrathecal and intramuscular in addition to eye drops, nasal spray, oral drops, ear drops, deep spinal muscle injections and retro bulbar injections, according to the participant's clinical characteristics.

3.5. Types of Interventions

The majority of studies administered one cellular intervention, however four studies in five reports [17,36,64,66,71] investigated two different cell therapies head-to-head to give a total of 58 cell regimens administered.

For these 58 cell regimens, the classification into the various cell therapy types was: 31% bone marrow cells, hematopoietic stem cells and peripheral blood cells (n = 18); 29% mesenchymal stem/stromal cells (n = 17); 26% umbilical cord blood (n = 15); 7% neural stem cells/neural-like cells (n = 4); 3% immune cells (n = 2); and 3% fetal cells/embryonic stem cells (n = 2). The source of cells was autologous in 32 studies (55%) and allogeneic in 25 studies (43%). The donor origin of the cells could not be determined in one study (2%) [25].

Cell interventions were delivered by various routes. Intrathecal (n = 25, 43%) or intravenous (n = 20, 34%) delivery was the most common. A further three studies (5%) used a combination of the two. Exclusive direct transplantation into the brain (intracerebral, intra-cerebroventricular) was used infrequently (n = 3, 5%), and all were for studies that administered neural stem cells/neural-like cells. In addition, one study (2%) [61] used intrathecal +/− intra-parenchymal brain administration for mesenchymal stem/stromal cells. The remainder of the studies (n = 6, 10%) utilized various routes (or a combination of routes) including but not limited to intra-arterial or intramuscular delivery (Table 1).

3.6. Types of Outcome Measures

Instruments measuring treatment outcomes were grouped into ten categories: (1) Movement and Posture; (2) Cognition and General Development; (3) Communication and Language; (4) Behavior; (5) Activities of Daily Living; 6) Quality of Life; (7) Brain Structure and Function; (8) Biomarkers; (9) Safety and (10) Other. Four of these categories were further split into a total of 12 sub-categories (Table 1, Figure 2). The 12 sub-categories were Gross Motor, Fine Motor and Upper Limb, Spasticity, Muscle Strength and General Motor within Movement and Posture; Communication and Language within Communication and Language; Adaptive Behavior, Executive Function and Social-Emotional within Behavior; and Neuroimaging and Seizures/Electrical Brain Activity within Brain Structure and Function.

Unsurprisingly, *Movement and Posture* was the most frequently reported outcome category (n = 4195) (Figure 2). Indeed, all included studies reported on *Movement and Posture* except Feng 2015 [26], which exclusively reported safety. Within *Movement and Posture*, measures of *Gross Motor* were the most common, followed by *Fine Motor and Upper Limb* then *Spasticity*. Safety was the next most common category (n = 1705) and was specifically reported in all but 11 studies. Reported safety data included adverse event reporting, routine laboratory and clinical assessments (e.g., bloods/biochemistry, X-ray), and neuroimaging conducted exclusively for safety. *Brain Structure and Function* (n = 1083), *Behavior* (n = 1010) and *Activities of Daily Living* (n = 865) were all also commonly reported outcome categories (Figure 2). In contrast, a relatively small proportion of participants were assessed for *Biomarkers* and *Quality of Life*. Of the four studies that conducted biomarker analysis these comprised assessment of various cytokine and growth factor levels including interferon (IFN)-γ, interleukin (IL)-17, IL-4, brain-derived neurotrophic factor (BDNF), and vascular endothelial growth factor (VEGF) [22], BDNF [23], pentraxin 3 (PTX-3), IL-8, and IL-10 [33] and PTX-3, IL-8, tumor necrosis factor (TNF)-α, and IL-1β [41].

Examining the data by either study design or cell intervention type revealed a similar pattern, with *Movement and Posture* consistently the most frequently reported outcome category, followed by *Safety*, and a relatively similar distribution of participants across outcome sub/categories (Supplementary Figures S1 and S2).

Across the included studies there were 53 unique instruments reported, although not all were true outcome measure, i.e., responsive to change (Tables 1 and 2). This number does not include measures of *Safety* or *Biomarkers* since these are commonly reported in various ways and could not be synthesized, nor descriptive/observational outcomes. The categorization of all instruments into outcome sub-/categories is shown in Table 2. Notably,

12/53 of the captured instruments had multiple sub-domains that were reported and hence were included across several outcome categories/sub-categories in Table 2.

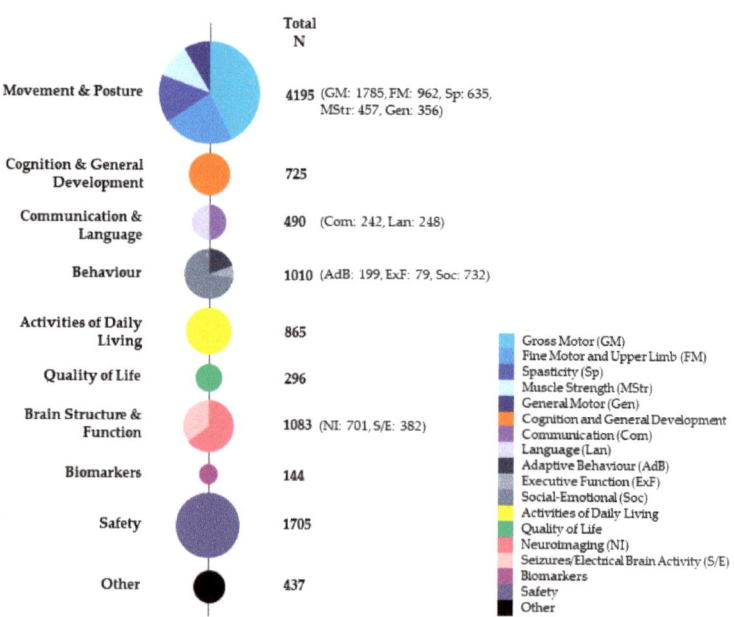

Figure 2. Number of participants assessed for each outcome category and sub-category across all included studies. N, number of participants.

Table 2. Outcome instruments used in cerebral palsy cell therapy studies with details.

Outcome Sub-Category	Instrument [Subdomain] [1]	n [2]	Format	Primary Purpose	Population Designed for
			Movement & Posture		
Gross Motor	Gross Motor Function Measure (GMFM) -66/-88	1163	Performance-based	E	CP
	Pediatric Evaluation of Disability Inventory (PEDI)/PEDI-Computer Adaptive Test (CAT) [Mobility]	573	Clinician Observation +/− Parent/other Interview	E, D	General
	Gross Motor Function Classification System (GMFCS)	533	Clinician Observation (or Parent/other/Self Interview)	C	CP
	Gross Motor Performance Measure (GMPM)	218	Performance-based	E	CP
	Peabody Developmental Motor Scales-2 (PDMS-2) [Gross Motor Quotient]	132	Performance-based	D (2nd E)	General
	The Functional Independence Measure for Children (WeeFIM) [Mobility]	130	Clinician Observation +/− Parent/other Interview	E	Pediatric Rehab
	Selective Control Assessment of Lower Extremity (SCALE)	88	Performance-based	D, E	CP
	Denver Developmental Screening Test 2 (DDST-II) [Gross Motor]	67	Performance-based +/− Parent/other Interview	D	General
	Boyd Developmental Progress Scale (BDPS) [Motor]	52	Performance-based + Clinician Observation +/− Parent/other Interview	D	General
	Learning accomplishment system diagnostic (LAP-D) Score [Sitting and Standing]	42	Performance-based/Parent/other Observation	D	General
	Berg Balance Scale (BBS)	12	Performance-based	P (2nd D, E)	Adult Rehab
	Trunk Control Measurement Scale (TCMS)	1	Performance-based	D, E	CP

Table 2. Cont.

Outcome Sub-Category	Instrument [Subdomain] [1]	n [2]	Format	Primary Purpose	Population Designed for
Fine Motor and Upper Limb	PDMS-2 [Fine Motor Quotient]	304	Performance-based	D (2nd E)	General
	Quality of Upper Extremity Skills Test (QUEST)	262	Performance-based	E	CP (Spastic)
	Fine Motor Function Measure (FMFM)	176	Performance-based	E	CP
	Manual Ability Classification Scale (MACS)	78	Clinician Observation (or Parent/other/Self Interview)	C	CP
	LAP-D [Fine Motor Skills]	42	Performance-based/Parent/other Observation	D	General
	DDST-II [Fine Motor-Adaptive]	20	Performance-based +/− Parent/other Interview	D	General
	Assisting Hand Assessment (AHA)	15	Performance-based	E	CP (Hemiplegia)
Muscle Strength	Medical Research Council (MRC) Scale for Muscle Strength; MRC Summed Scores	196	Performance-based	D, E	General
	Manual Muscle Strength Test	96	Performance-based	D, E	General
	Manual Muscle Testing (MMT) Score	34	Performance-based	D, E	General
	Hand dynamometry	15	Performance-based	D, E	General
Spasticity	Modified Ashworth Scale	381	Performance-based	D, E	CP (Spastic)
	Ashworth Scale	109	Performance-based	D, E	CP (Spastic)
	Modified Tardieu Scale	89	Performance-based	D, E	CP (Spastic)
General Motor [3]	Bayley Scales of Infant and Toddler Development 2nd Edition (BSID-II) [Motor Scale]	218	Performance-based	D (2nd E)	General
	Vineland Adaptive Behavior Scales 2nd Edition (VABS-2), parent report questionnaire [Motor Skills Domain]	30	Parent/other Questionnaire	D (2nd P, E)	General
	Battelle Developmental Inventory (BDI) [Motor]	13	Performance-based +/− Parent/other Observation/Interview	D (2nd P, E)	General
	Kyoto Scale of Psychological Development (KSPD) [Postural-Motor]	6	Performance-based	D, E	General
Activities of Daily Living					
Activities of Daily Living	PEDI/PEDI-CAT [Self-care/Daily Activities]	573	Clinician Observation +/− Parent/other Interview	E, D	General
	WeeFIM [Self Care]	130	Clinician Observation +/− Parent/other Interview	E	Pediatric Rehab
	Functional Independence Measure (FIM) [Motor Subscale]	93	Clinician Observation	E	General & Rehab
	BDPS [Independence]	52	Performance-based + Clinician Observation +/− Parent/other Interview	D	General
	Activities of Daily Living (ADL) [4]	39	Unknown	Unknown	Unknown
	Modified Barthel Index (mBI)	30	Performance-based/Self/Parent/other Observation/Interview/Questionnaire	E	Adult Rehab
	VABS-2 parent report questionnaire [Daily Living Skills Domain]	30	Parent/other Questionnaire	D (2nd P, E)	General
	UK Functional Independence Measure and Functional Assessment Measure (UK FIM + FAM) [Total Motor Subscore]	12	Clinician Observation	E	Rehab
Behavior					
Social-Emotional	PEDI/PEDI-CAT [Social Function/Social/Cognitive]	573	Clinician Observation +/− Parent/other Questionnaire	E, D	General
	VABS-2 parent report questionnaire [Socialization Domain]	30	Parent/other Questionnaire	D (2nd P, E)	General
	DDST-II [Personal-Social]	20	Performance-based +/− Parent/other Interview	D	General
	BDI [Social-Emotional]	13	Clinician Observation +/− Parent/other Observation/Interview	D (2nd P, E)	General
	Strengths and Difficulties Questionnaire (SDQ)	8	Parent/other Questionnaire +/− Interview	D, E	General
	KSPD [Language-Social]	6	Clinician Observation	D, E	General

Table 2. *Cont.*

Outcome Sub-Category	Instrument [*Subdomain*] [1]	n [2]	Format	Primary Purpose	Population Designed for
Behavior					
Adaptive Behavior	PEDI-CAT [*Responsibility*]	86	Parent/other Questionnaire	E, D	General
	VABS-2 parent report questionnaire [*Maladaptive Behavior Domain*]	30	Parent/other Questionnaire	D (2nd P, E)	General
	BDI [*Adaptive*]	13	Clinician Observation +/− Parent/other Observation/Interview	D (2nd P, E)	General
Executive Function	Behavior Rating Inventory of Executive Function (BRIEF)	7	Parent/other Questionnaire	D (2nd E)	General
Brain Structure & Function					
Neuroimaging	Magnetic resonance imaging (MRI); MRI with Diffusion tensor imaging (DTI)	525	Clinician Observation	D, P	General
	Positron emission tomography and computed tomography scan (PET-CT)	293	Clinician Observation	D, P	General
	Single photon emission computed tomography scan (SPECT)	111	Clinician Observation	D, P	General
Seizures/Electrical brain activity	Electroencephalogram (EEG)	255	Clinician Observation	D, P	General
	Seizure burden/frequency	128	Clinician Observation	D, P	General
Cognition & General Development					
Cognition and General Development	BSID-II [*Mental Scale*]	184	Performance-based	D (2nd E)	General
	WeeFIM [*Cognition*]	130	Clinician Observation +/− Parent/other Interview	E	Pediatric Rehab
	FIM [*Cognition Subscale*]	93	Clinician Observation	E	General & Rehab
	LAP-D [*Cognitive Skills*]	42	Performance-based/Parent/other Observation	D	General
	BDI [*Cognitive*]	13	Clinician Observation +/− Parent/other Observation/Interview	D (2nd P, E)	General
	UK FIM + FAM [*Total Cognitive Subscore*]	12	Clinician Observation	E	Rehab
	Wechsler Intelligence Scale for Children 4th/5th Edition (WISC-IV/-V)	7	Performance-based	D (2nd P)	General
	KSPD [*Cognitive-Adaptive*]	6	Performance-based	D, E	General
	Bayley Scales of Infant and Toddler Development 3rd Edition (BSID-III) [*Cognitive Scale*]	1	Performance-based	D (2nd P, E)	General
	Intelligence Quotient (IQ) Score	1	Performance-based	D (2nd P)	General
	Wechsler Preschool & Primary Scale of Intelligence 4th Edition (WPPSI-IV)	1	Performance-based	D (2nd P)	General
Quality of Life					
Quality of Life	Cerebral Palsy Quality of Life Questionnaire for Children (CP QOL-Child), Primary Caregiver Questionnaire	147	Parent/other Questionnaire	D, E	CP
	Child Health Questionnaire Parent Form 50 (CHQ)	94	Parent/other Questionnaire	D, E	General
	Short Form 8 (SF-8) Health Survey Quality of Life Questionnaire	1	Self/Parent/other Questionnaire	D, E	General
Language & Communication					
Language	Gesell Developmental Schedules	60	Clinician Observation	D	General
	LAP-D [*Speech skills*]	42	Performance-based/Parent/other Observation	D	General
	DDST-II [*Language Skills*]	20	Performance-based +/− Parent/other Interview	D	General
Communication	BDPS [*Communication*]	52	Performance-based + Clinician Observation +/− Parent/other Interview	D	General
	VABS-2 parent report questionnaire [*Communication Domain*]	30	Parent/other Questionnaire	D (2nd P, E)	General
	BDI [*Communication*]	13	Performance-based +/− Parent/other Observation/Interview	D (2nd P, E)	General
	Communication Function Classification System (CFCS)	11	Clinician Observation	C	CP

Table 2. Cont.

Outcome Sub-Category	Instrument [Subdomain] [1]	n [2]	Format	Primary Purpose	Population Designed for
			Other		
Other	Comprehensive Functional Assessment (CFA) Scale	94	Unknown	Unknown	Unknown
	Beery-Buktenica Developmental Test of Visual-Motor Integration 6th Edition	88	Performance-based	D	General
	Modified Rankin Scale (mRS)	30	Self (Clinician-led) Interview	E	Adult Rehab
	Caregiver Questionnaire Scale	14	Parent/other Questionnaire	Unknown	General
	CDCC Infant Mental Development Scale for general development status	1	Performance-based	D (2nd E)	General
	Mental Status Examination	1	Clinician Observation	D, E	General
			Safety		
Safety	Safety reports/AEs/Routine laboratory and clinical assessments (including neuroimaging for safety exclusively)	1705	N/A	D	General
			Biomarkers		
Biomarkers	Biomarkers (various)	144	N/A	D	General

Abbreviations: C, classification; CP, cerebral palsy; D, discriminative; E, evaluative; n, number of participants; P, predictive; Rehab, rehabilitation. [1] Does not include descriptive outcomes or investigator-developed, non-validated tools. [2] Number of participants across all studies assessed using instrument. [3] General motor could not be designated as either gross or fine. Includes oromotor function. [4] Review authors were unable to find information about this assessment.

More than one instrument was used across the studies for the majority of outcome categories/sub-categories. For example, *Gross Motor* was assessed using 12 different tools, *Cognition and General Development* by 11, and *Activities of Daily Living* by eight different instruments (Table 2). In contrast, *Executive Function* was assessed using just a single instrument, the Behavior Rating Inventory of Executive Function (BRIEF) [74], in a single study.

The most commonly reported instrument was the GMFM (n = 1163), with this measure reported for 56% of all included participants in this review. The Pediatric Evaluation of Disability Inventory (PEDI)/PEDI-Computer Adaptive Test (PEDI-CAT) [75] (n = 573), GMFCS (n = 533) and magnetic resonance imaging (MRI) with or without diffusion tensor imaging (DTI) (n = 525) were also frequently used (Table 2).

Of note, study participants were often assessed using more than one instrument within an outcome category/sub-category (Table 1). This was particularly true for *Gross Motor*. For example, Rah 2017 [49] assessed participants using the GMFM, GMFCS, PEDI and Denver Development Screening Test (DDST) [76], all measures of gross motor capacity and/or performance. Although many studies also just used single instruments to assess various outcome domains (Table 1). Furthermore, the total number of instruments used per study varied substantially. Whereas Feng 2015 [26] only assessed safety, Min 2020 [41] administered 18 instruments (including safety and biomarker assessments) (Table 1).

Descriptive Outcomes

In addition to the above reported outcome instruments, there were numerous descriptive/observational outcomes reported. For instance, 24/54 (44%) studies included purely descriptive outcome/s for at least one outcome category/sub-category (Table 1). Some studies were heavily weighted to reporting descriptive outcomes almost exclusively, particularly case series/reports or single-arm studies. Moreover, some outcome sub-categories were more often reported via descriptive means than an outcome instrument. For example, as mentioned above, although *Executive Function* was assessed using the BRIEF in only one study, it was captured descriptively in another five studies.

Of particular note are the descriptive/observational outcomes classified under the *Other* category. These covered a range of outcomes including sleep, sensory (sensory processing/smell), vision, hearing, appetite and immunity, as well as overarching/comprehensive assessments of participant condition/well-being (Table 1).

3.7. Outcome Instrument Properties

The properties of all reported instruments including format, primary purpose and population designed for are shown in Table 2. The largest proportion of instruments (55%) were either exclusively, or partially, Performance-based measures. Clinician-reported measures were the next most commonly utilized, representing 26% of instruments, and these were typically Observations. Other measures were either Parent/other-reported or could be completed interchangeably by a clinician, parent/other or the participant themselves. Only one instrument was exclusively Self-reported (Modified Rankin Scale). In general, across the various outcome sub-/categories, there was a mix between Performance-based and Clinician-reported measures, although *Brain Structure and Function* was exclusively Clinician Observation. The three Quality of Life instruments were all Parent/other or Self-reported, and most *Behavior* and *Activities of Daily Living* assessment tools included input from Parent/other (Table 2).

Of the 53 instruments, 33 (62%) were determined to be evaluative measures, 14 discriminative and/or predictive, and three were classification systems. Of particular note, all instruments within *Brain Structure and Function* were designated as discriminative/predictive, and the *Language and Communication* outcome tools were also primarily non-evaluative. Finally, 14 (26%) of the instruments were specifically designed for a CP-population, mostly within the *Movement and Posture* category. An additional six were designed for adult and/or pediatric rehabilitation and the remainder are for non-specific (general) populations.

When comparing the 53 reported outcome instruments against the highly recommended tools within the common data elements for CP [10], only six instruments overlapped: the GMFM, Tardieu Scale [77], Bayley Scales of Infant and Toddler Development (BSID) [78], Wechsler Intelligence Scale for Children (WISC) [79], BRIEF, and the Cerebral Palsy Quality of Life Questionnaire (CP QOL) [80]. Of note, the GMFCS, MACS and CFCS are also recommended in the common data elements, but as classification systems.

4. Discussion

Stem cells and cell therapies offer great potential as a treatment for CP, with efficacy demonstrated in systematic reviews [4,5]. Improvements in gross motor function have been the most commonly studied outcome in randomized controlled trials, however individuals with CP and their families cite improvements in various domains to be of value [7,9]. We conducted this scoping review to describe all outcomes reported in cell therapy studies for CP to date. From this, we wanted to understand whether clinical study outcomes align with common comorbidities and complications of CP, and hence whether they are meeting the expectations of trial participants and their families. Furthermore, we aimed to examine the instruments that are being used to assess these outcomes, to determine whether they are being captured appropriately.

We found that, across 54 included studies comprising >2000 participants, a large range of outcome domains/categories were reported. Notably, *Movement and Posture* was the most commonly assessed outcome category, captured in 98% of included studies. This is understandable given that CP is clinically characterized by motor and postural impairments. Movement and posture are routinely measured within CP clinical studies investigating a whole host of interventions, with several validated instruments with good psychometric properties available for the CP population [81]. *Safety* was the next most common outcome domain. Again, not surprising since clinical studies must necessarily focus on assessing and reporting the safety of experimental intervention/s. Specifically, Phase 1, 2 clinical trials are important for understanding how a drug interacts with the human body, and to identify adverse events. Subsequent Phase 3 clinical trials, including larger numbers of participants, are important to show long-term or rare side effects. Importantly, previous systematic reviews have reported an encouraging safety profile for cell therapy treatments in individuals with CP [4,5], giving confidence to the field in pursuing these novel interventions.

4.1. Alignment of Reported Outcomes with Symptoms, Comorbidities and Complications of CP

Some interesting observations were noted when evaluating the reported outcome categories against frequently occurring symptoms, comorbidities and complications of CP [6]. Firstly, whilst many common impairments and functional limitations were captured in the included studies (e.g., walking, talking, epilepsy (seizures), intellect and behavior), the frequency with which these were reported often differed markedly from their prevalence in the CP population. For example, as previously mentioned, gross motor was captured for 86% of participants as expected for a condition defined by limitations to movement and posture. However, other comorbidities/functional limitations with high prevalence in CP were underrepresented. These include intellectual disability (1 in 2 children with CP, but only assessed for 35% of participants), speech impairment (1 in 3 children with CP, but only assessed for 24% of participants), behavior disorders (1 in 4 children with CP, but only assessed for 49% of participants) and epilepsy (seizures) (1 in 4 children with CP, but only assessed for 18% of participants) [6]. In addition, some comorbidities and complications were reported for only a minority of participants using primarily descriptive measures, or not reported at all, despite being commonly occurring, in particular vision impairment (1 in 4 children with CP), pain (3 in 4 children with CP) and sleep disorders (1 in 5 children with CP) [6]. While questions relating to pain and sleep are included in measures of quality of life, these contribute towards the construct of quality of life rather than being assessments of pain or sleep in their own right. *Quality of Life* was captured for only 14% of participants, and of these, more than a third were assessed using health-related-specific quality of life measures. We know that quality of life is influenced by a broad array of factors (i.e., more than health), including socioeconomic status and community life, impacted by social policy such as inclusion, participation, community, and accessibility [82]. Given that quality of life was identified as the most important domain for improvement following intervention via a Delphi survey of youth with CP, parents of children with CP, and medical professionals [9], it is interesting that this was not captured more broadly. We advocate that outcome measures that assess overarching quality of life, with responsiveness to change, such as the CPCHILD [83] for children with severe physical disability [10,84], should be included in future studies.

Important to consider is why many of these prevalent comorbidities, complications and functional limitations are not typically reported in clinical studies of cell therapies to date. Whilst it may be due to a lack of availability or knowledge of suitable/appropriate measurement tools for these outcomes, it is also possible that it is not scientifically plausible for cell therapies to target all of these domains. Indeed, there is some debate in the field as to what potential benefits various cell therapies are actually capable of bestowing [85]. Whilst cell therapies have been under investigation for decades (both clinically and pre-clinically), a comprehensive understanding of the mechanism/s of action for each cell type is still being uncovered. For example, it is accepted that neural stem cells can differentiate into neurons, oligodendrocytes and astrocytes to potentially replace lost or damaged brain cells. On the other hand, cell types including mesenchymal stem/stromal cells and hematopoietic stem cells, which were frequently administered in the studies included in this review, are more ambiguous in their mechanism/s of action for CP [4]. Moreover, how various potential mechanisms of action may relate to the likelihood of improvement across different outcome domains (e.g., gross motor vs. cognition vs. pain) remains unknown. Despite these uncertainties, accumulating high-quality evidence exists to support the efficacy of various cell therapies for improving gross motor function in CP, and there is lower-quality evidence suggesting that cell therapies can have wide-ranging effects across many other domains. This includes various anecdotes and descriptive measures, and while this information can be useful in providing hints at potential areas of efficacy, these subjective reports should be verified using valid tools, in well-designed and powered clinical trials, to determine if they are indeed true effects of a cell treatment. Furthermore, a thorough review of the clinical literature across various conditions that share some of the common comorbidities and complications of CP may help identify additional beneficial effects of cell therapies on these treatment targets.

Another reason why common comorbidities, complications and functional limitations of CP are absent in clinical trials may be a 'carry-over' from preclinical (primarily rodent/small animal) research. A known limitation of many animal models is the inadequacy to faithfully replicate the complexity of human disease [86], in addition to difficulties assessing traditionally self-reported outcomes, such as pain [87]. Thus, some outcomes may get overlooked when translating promising cell therapies from the 'bench' to the clinic. This highlights the importance of consumer engagement and co-design in medical research, to ensure that research, in particular clinical trials, are informed by community priorities, whilst remaining balanced with what scientists believe, and evidence tells us, cell therapies can feasibly achieve. We therefore recommend that future trials are designed in collaboration with consumer and community representatives to ensure included outcomes are aligned with consumer priorities.

4.2. Appropriate Outcome Instrument Selection in Cell Therapy Clinical Studies for CP

Regardless of the outcome domain/s being assessed, it is vitally important that psychometrically sound and appropriate instruments are utilized. This will ensure that data generated from costly and time-consuming clinical trials is high quality and will not lead to incorrect conclusions about the efficacy (or lack thereof) of a particular intervention. This review revealed a large number (>50) of instruments used across the included studies. Encouragingly, many were 'gold standard' CP outcome measures, with responsiveness to change, such as the GMFM and the PEDI/PEDI-CAT, which were the two most frequently utilized measures. In contrast, it was concerning that the GMFCS was used to capture change following intervention for a substantial number of participants (the third most frequent outcome tool used). Whilst the GMFCS is a widely used tool for the classification of gross motor function in children with CP, it is not an evaluative measure (i.e., it was not designed, nor shown to be, responsive to change), and is thus not appropriate to be used as an instrument to detect change following an intervention. Interestingly, two other classification tools were also used: the Manual Ability Classification Scale (MACS) [88] and the Communication Function Classification System (CFCS) [89]. We recommend that these classification systems are not used as outcome assessment instruments in future studies.

Excluding the classification tools, two-thirds of all instruments reported had evaluative properties, making them suitable as outcome assessment instruments. Some outcome categories however, were primarily assessed using inappropriate instruments in terms of their evaluative properties, e.g., *Language and Communication*. There are various reasons why inappropriate instruments may be used in clinical trials, including a lack of knowledge, training, or access (e.g., funding). Alternatively, there may as yet be no widely accepted, and validated, evaluative tools for assessing that particular outcome in CP. There are excellent reviews that have identified valid and reliable measures for use in studies of children and youth with CP [81]. However, if suitable tools do not exist, we propose that these areas are not ready for measurement within clinical trials or that individualized goal setting tools might be considered.

Another consideration for selection of outcome domain/s and assessment tools relates to the heterogeneity of CP. Some may argue that the inherent variability between individuals with CP precludes the inclusion and measurement of particular outcomes because they may not be relevant for a large proportion of trial participants, e.g., hearing or vision impairment, or epilepsy. Yet, there is precedent for the use of individualized outcome measures, for example the Goal Attainment Scale (GAS) [90] or Canadian Occupational Performance Measure (COPM) [91] within clinical trials to importantly capture change that matters to the child and family. The use of such measures may enhance the relevancy of captured outcomes for a given participant, help to limit the total number of assessments, thereby reducing respondent burden, and improve sensitivity to detect meaningful change. Thus, it would be interesting to see whether such measures could be used in future trials.

4.3. Mechanisms of Cell Therapies and Ensuing Effects

CP is caused by an interference, lesion, or abnormality of the developing brain which manifests as a disorder of movement and/or posture. Repairing the underlying brain injury, via direct or indirect mechanisms, to promote increased neuronal signaling and function is the aim of cell therapies for CP. As such, it is recognized that improvements in brain structure or connectivity following cell intervention could directly improve motor function. It is important to acknowledge however that links exist between motor skills and some comorbidities of CP. Figure 3 shows a schema of the proposed effects of stem cells for CP including therapeutic targets leading to remediation of the underlying brain injury, and resultant effects on various comorbidities, leading to the ultimate goal of improving quality of life. We wish to specifically highlight that changes in brain structure and connectivity producing improvements in motor function may have secondary effects on a number of motor-associated CP comorbidities (e.g., pain, sleep, drooling and speech). This may therefore mean that, in fact, improvements in various outcomes of importance to individuals with CP and their families may be more achievable than widely believed. In addition, the non-motor-associated comorbidities of CP (e.g., cognition, behavior) may be indirectly targeted by cell treatments.

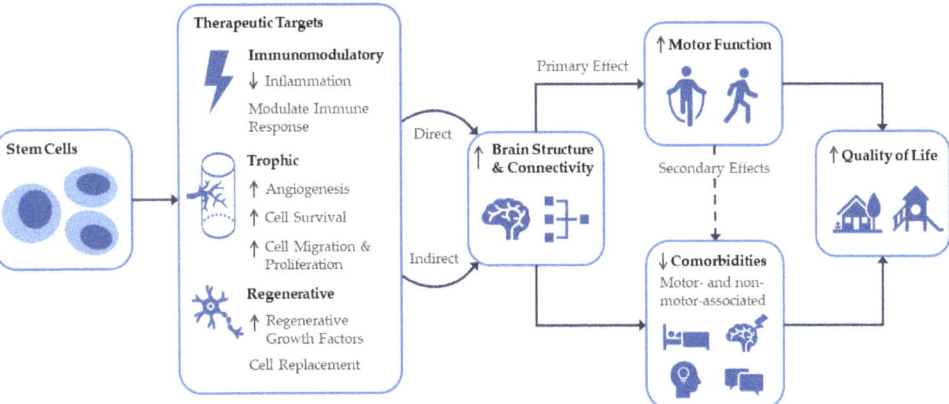

Figure 3. Schematic representation of cell intervention effects and interlinked outcomes for CP including quality of life.

4.4. Limitations

We acknowledge some limitations of this scoping review including that due to our decision to include all study designs, there is a significant amount of lower-quality evidence included. In addition, extracted outcome instruments may have been categorized in varying ways, and, for simplicity of reporting, some sub-categories of outcomes were consolidated during the sorting process, despite arguably representing distinct outcome sub-domains. Finally, we did not extract nor report on the efficacy of cell therapies for any of the outcome categories, as this was outside the scope of this review.

5. Conclusions

Stem cells are an emerging intervention for CP with potential to target a wide variety of outcome domains. We found that movement and posture and safety were the predominant outcomes assessed in cell therapy clinical studies, despite many other outcomes, including quality of life, being of high importance to individuals with CP and their families. Moreover, amongst the considerable number of outcome instruments employed in clinical studies, many are not appropriate for use as measures of change following intervention. We provide several recommendations to ensure that future trials collect scientifically valid, high-quality outcome data that also meets the expectations of the CP community.

Supplementary Materials: The following supporting information can be downloaded at: https://www.mdpi.com/article/10.3390/jcm11247319/s1, Figure S1: Number of participants assessed for each outcome category and sub-category split by study design, excluding the dose comparison study, Figure S2: Number of participants assessed for each outcome category and sub-category split by intervention type, Table S1: PRISMA-ScR Checklist, Table S2: Search strategy.

Author Contributions: Conceptualization, M.F.-E., M.C.B.P. and I.N.; methodology, M.F.-E., M.C.B.P., I.H., P.K., C.S., D.C. and S.R.; formal analysis, M.F.-E.; investigation, M.F.-E. and M.C.B.P.; data curation, M.F.-E., M.C.B.P., I.H., P.K., C.S., D.C., S.R., A.R.G., C.M. and I.N.; writing—original draft preparation, M.F.-E.; writing—review and editing, M.C.B.P., I.H., P.K., C.S., D.C., S.R., A.R.G., C.M. and I.N.; visualization, M.F.-E.; supervision, M.F.-E., P.K., S.R. and I.N.; project administration, M.F.-E. All authors have read and agreed to the published version of the manuscript.

Funding: This research received no external funding.

Institutional Review Board Statement: Not applicable.

Informed Consent Statement: Not applicable.

Data Availability Statement: The data presented in this study are openly available in Open Science Framework https://osf.io/t9c8j/?view_only=9b82c37725834a1da1a50bb199cf5091 (accessed on 14 November 2022).

Acknowledgments: The authors would like to thank Charlotte Frazer (C.F.) for assistance with study screening and data extraction.

Conflicts of Interest: The authors declare no conflict of interest.

References

1. Paton, M.C.B.; Finch-Edmondson, M.; Fahey, M.C.; London, J.; Badawi, N.; Novak, I. Fifteen years of human research using stem cells for cerebral palsy: A review of the research landscape. *J. Paediatr. Child Health* **2021**, *57*, 295–296. [CrossRef] [PubMed]
2. Sun, J.M.; Kurtzberg, J. Stem cell therapies in cerebral palsy and autism spectrum disorder. *Dev. Med. Child Neurol.* **2021**, *63*, 503–510. [CrossRef] [PubMed]
3. Russell, D.J.; Avery, L.M.; Rosenbaum, P.L.; Raina, P.S.; Walter, S.D.; Palisano, R.J. Improved Scaling of the Gross Motor Function Measure for Children with Cerebral Palsy: Evidence of Reliability and Validity. *Phys. Ther.* **2000**, *80*, 873–885. [CrossRef] [PubMed]
4. Eggenberger, S.; Boucard, C.; Schoeberlein, A.; Guzman, R.; Limacher, A.; Surbek, D.; Mueller, M. Stem cell treatment and cerebral palsy: Systemic review and meta-analysis. *World J. Stem Cells* **2019**, *11*, 891–903. [CrossRef] [PubMed]
5. Novak, I.; Walker, K.; Hunt, R.W.; Wallace, E.M.; Fahey, M.; Badawi, N. Concise Review: Stem Cell Interventions for People with Cerebral Palsy: Systematic Review with Meta-Analysis. *Stem Cells Transl. Med.* **2016**, *5*, 1014–1025. [CrossRef] [PubMed]
6. Novak, I.; Hines, M.; Goldsmith, S.; Barclay, R. Clinical Prognostic Messages from a Systematic Review on Cerebral Palsy. *Pediatrics* **2012**, *130*, e1285–e1312. [CrossRef]
7. Smith, M.J.; Finch-Edmondson, M.; Miller, S.L.; Webb, A.; Fahey, M.C.; Jenkin, G.; Paton, M.C.B.; McDonald, C.A. Acceptability of neural stem cell therapy for cerebral palsy: Survey of the Australian cerebral palsy community. *Stem Cell Res. Ther.* **2022**, *provisionally accepted*. [CrossRef]
8. Almoajil, H.; Toye, F.; Dawes, H.; Pierce, J.; Meaney, A.; Baklouti, A.; Poverini, L.; Hopewell, S.; Theologis, T. Outcomes of importance to children and young adults with cerebral palsy, their parents and health professionals following lower limb orthopaedic surgery: A qualitative study to inform a Core Outcome Set. *Health Expect.* **2022**, *25*, 925–935. [CrossRef]
9. Vargus-Adams, J.N.; Martin, L.K. Measuring what matters in cerebral palsy: A breadth of important domains and outcome measures. *Arch. Phys. Med. Rehabil.* **2009**, *90*, 2089–2095. [CrossRef]
10. Schiariti, V.; Fowler, E.; Brandenburg, J.E.; Levey, E.; McIntyre, S.; Sukal-Moulton, T.; Ramey, S.L.; Rose, J.; Sienko, S.; Stashinko, E.; et al. A common data language for clinical research studies: The National Institute of Neurological Disorders and Stroke and American Academy for Cerebral Palsy and Developmental Medicine Cerebral Palsy Common Data Elements Version 1.0 recommendations. *Dev. Med. Child Neurol.* **2018**, *60*, 976–986. [CrossRef]
11. Tricco, A.C.; Lillie, E.; Zarin, W.; O'Brien, K.K.; Colquhoun, H.; Levac, D.; Moher, D.; Peters, M.D.J.; Horsley, T.; Weeks, L.; et al. PRISMA Extension for Scoping Reviews (PRISMA-ScR): Checklist and Explanation. *Ann. Intern. Med.* **2018**, *169*, 467–473. [CrossRef] [PubMed]
12. OCEBM Levels of Evidence Working Group. The Oxford Levels of Evidence 2. Available online: https://www.cebm.ox.ac.uk/resources/levels-of-evidence/ocebm-levels-of-evidence (accessed on 24 October 2022).
13. U.S. Food and Drug Administration. Clinical Outcome Assessment. Available online: https://www.ncbi.nlm.nih.gov/books/NBK338448/def-item/glossary.clinical-outcome-assessment/ (accessed on 27 October 2022).
14. Palisano, R.J.; Rosenbaum, P.; Bartlett, D.; Livingston, M.H. Content validity of the expanded and revised Gross Motor Function Classification System. *Dev. Med. Child Neurol.* **2008**, *50*, 744–750. [CrossRef] [PubMed]

15. Shi, W.; Li, H.; Su, Y.; Yang, H.; Zhang, J. Study on reliability and unidimension of the Fine Motor Function Measure Scale for children with cerebral palsy. *Chin. J. Evid.-Based Pediatr.* **2008**, *3*, 110–118.
16. Abi Chahine, N.H.; Wehbe, T.W.; Hilal, R.A.; Zoghbi, V.V.; Melki, A.E.; Habib, E.B.B. Treatment of Cerebral Palsy with Stem Cells: A Report of 17 Cases. *Int. J. Stem Cells* **2016**, *9*, 90–95. [CrossRef] [PubMed]
17. Amanat, M.; Majmaa, A.; Zarrabi, M.; Nouri, M.; Akbari, M.G.; Moaiedi, A.R.; Ghaemi, O.; Zamani, F.; Najafi, S.; Badv, R.S.; et al. Clinical and imaging outcomes after intrathecal injection of umbilical cord tissue mesenchymal stem cells in cerebral palsy: A randomized double-blind sham-controlled clinical trial. *Stem Cell Res. Ther.* **2021**, *12*, 439. [CrossRef]
18. Bansal, H.; Singh, L.; Verma, P.; Agrawal, A.; Leon, J.; Sundell, I.B.; Koka, P.S. Administration of autologous bone marrow-derived stem cells for treatment of cerebral palsy patients: A proof of concept. *J. Stem Cells* **2016**, *11*, 37–49.
19. Boruczkowski, D.; Zdolinska-Malinowska, I. Wharton's jelly mesenchymal stem cell administration improves quality of life and self-sufficiency in children with cerebral palsy: Results from a retrospective study. *Stem Cells Int.* **2019**, *2019*, 7402151. [CrossRef]
20. Chen, L.; Huang, H.; Xi, H.; Xie, Z.; Liu, R.; Jiang, Z.; Zhang, F.; Liu, Y.; Chen, D.; Wang, Q.; et al. Intracranial transplant of olfactory ensheathing cells in children and adolescents with cerebral palsy: A randomized controlled clinical trial. *Cell Transplant.* **2010**, *19*, 185–191. [CrossRef]
21. Chen, G.; Xu, Z.; Fang, F.; Xu, R.; Wang, Y.; Hu, X.; Fan, L.; Liu, H. Neural stem cell-like cells derived from autologous bone mesenchymal stem cells for the treatment of patients with cerebral palsy. *J. Transl. Med.* **2013**, *11*, 21. [CrossRef]
22. Chernykh, E.R.; Kafanova, M.Y.; Shevela, E.Y.; Sirota, S.I.; Adonina, E.I.; Sakhno, L.V.; Ostanin, A.A.; Kozlov, V.V. Clinical experience with autologous M2 macrophages in children with severe cerebral palsy. *Cell Transplant.* **2014**, *23*, S97–S104. [CrossRef]
23. Chernykh, E.; Shevela, E.; Kafanova, M.; Sakhno, L.; Polovnikov, E.; Ostanin, A. Monocyte-derived macrophages for treatment of cerebral palsy: A study of 57 cases. *J. Neurorestoratol.* **2018**, *6*, 41–47. [CrossRef]
24. Crompton, K.; Novak, I.; Fahey, M.; Badawi, N.; Lee, K.J.; Mechinaud-Heloury, F.; Edwards, P.; Colditz, P.; Soosay Raj, T.; Hough, J.; et al. Safety of sibling cord blood cell infusion for children with cerebral palsy. *Cytotherapy* **2022**, *24*, 931–939. [CrossRef]
25. Dong, H.; Li, G.; Shang, C.; Yin, H.; Luo, Y.; Meng, H.; Li, X.; Wang, Y.; Lin, L.; Zhao, M. Umbilical cord mesenchymal stem cell (UC-MSC) transplantations for cerebral palsy. *Am. J. Transl. Res.* **2018**, *10*, 901–906.
26. Feng, M.; Lu, A.; Gao, H.; Qian, C.; Zhang, J.; Lin, T.; Zhao, Y. Safety of Allogeneic Umbilical Cord Blood Stem Cells Therapy in Patients with Severe Cerebral Palsy: A Retrospective Study. *Stem Cells Int.* **2015**, *2015*, 325652. [CrossRef]
27. Fu, X.; Hua, R.; Wang, X.; Wang, P.; Yi, L.; Yu, A.; Yang, J.; Li, Y.; An, Y. Synergistic Improvement in Children with Cerebral Palsy Who Underwent Double-Course Human Wharton's Jelly Stem Cell Transplantation. *Stem Cells Int.* **2019**, *2019*, 7481069. [CrossRef]
28. Gu, J.; Huang, L.; Zhang, C.; Wang, Y.; Zhang, R.; Tu, Z.; Wang, H.; Zhou, X.; Xiao, Z.; Liu, Z.; et al. Therapeutic evidence of umbilical cord-derived mesenchymal stem cell transplantation for cerebral palsy: A randomized, controlled trial. *Stem Cell Res. Ther.* **2020**, *11*, 43. [CrossRef]
29. Hassan, M.A.; Gabr, H.; Fathi, S.; Ramzy, G.M.; El-Hassany, A.H.; Abd El-Ghaffar, N.A. Stem cell transplantation in Egyptian patients with cerebral palsy. *Egypt. J. Neurol. Psychiatry Neurosurg.* **2012**, *49*, 117–122.
30. He, S.; Luan, Z.; Qu, S.; Qiu, X.; Xin, D.; Jia, W.; Shen, Y.; Yu, Z.; Xu, T. Ultrasound guided neural stem cell transplantation through the lateral ventricle for treatment of cerebral palsy in children. *Neural Regen. Res.* **2012**, *7*, 2529–2535. [CrossRef]
31. Huang, L.; Zhang, C.; Gu, J.; Wu, W.; Shen, Z.; Zhou, X.; Lu, H. A Randomized, Placebo-Controlled Trial of Human Umbilical Cord Blood Mesenchymal Stem Cell Infusion for Children with Cerebral Palsy. *Cell Transplant.* **2018**, *27*, 325–334. [CrossRef]
32. Jensen, A.; Hamelmann, E. First Autologous Cord Blood Therapy for Pediatric Ischemic Stroke and Cerebral Palsy Caused by Cephalic Molding during Birth: Individual Treatment with Mononuclear Cells. *Case Rep. Transplant.* **2016**, *2016*, 1717426. [CrossRef]
33. Kang, M.; Min, K.; Jang, J.; Kim, S.C.; Kang, M.S.; Jang, S.J.; Lee, J.Y.; Kim, S.H.; Kim, M.K.; An, S.A.; et al. Involvement of Immune Responses in the Efficacy of Cord Blood Cell Therapy for Cerebral Palsy. *Stem Cells Dev.* **2015**, *24*, 2259–2268. [CrossRef] [PubMed]
34. Lee, Y.H.; Choi, K.V.; Moon, J.H.; Jun, H.J.; Kang, H.R.; Oh, S.I.; Kim, H.S.; Um, J.S.; Kim, M.J.; Choi, Y.Y.; et al. Safety and feasibility of countering neurological impairment by intravenous administration of autologous cord blood in cerebral palsy. *J. Transl. Med.* **2012**, *10*, 58. [CrossRef] [PubMed]
35. Li, M.; Yu, A.; Zhang, F.; Dai, G.; Cheng, H.; Wang, X.; An, Y. Treatment of one case of cerebral palsy combined with posterior visual pathway injury using autologous bone marrow mesenchymal stem cells. *J. Transl. Med.* **2012**, *10*, 100. [CrossRef] [PubMed]
36. Liu, X.; Fu, X.; Dai, G.; Wang, X.; Zhang, Z.; Cheng, H.; Zheng, P.; An, Y. Comparative analysis of curative effect of bone marrow mesenchymal stem cell and bone marrow mononuclear cell transplantation for spastic cerebral palsy. *J. Transl. Med.* **2017**, *15*, 48. [CrossRef] [PubMed]
37. Luan, Z.; Liu, W.; Qu, S.; Du, K.; He, S.; Wang, Z.; Yang, Y.; Wang, C.; Gong, X. Effects of neural progenitor cell transplantation in children with severe cerebral palsy. *Cell Transplant.* **2012**, *21*, S91–S98. [CrossRef]
38. Mancias-Guerra, C.; Marroquin-Escamilla, A.R.; Gonzalez-Llano, O.; Villarreal-Martinez, L.; Jaime-Perez, J.C.; Garcia-Rodriguez, F.; Valdes-Burnes, S.L.; Rodriguez-Romo, L.N.; Barrera-Morales, D.C.; Sanchez-Hernandez, J.J.; et al. Safety and tolerability of intrathecal delivery of autologous bone marrow nucleated cells in children with cerebral palsy: An open-label phase I trial. *Cytotherapy* **2014**, *16*, 810–820. [CrossRef]

39. Maric, D.M.; Radomir, M.; Milankov, Z.; Stanojevic, I.; Vojvodic, D.; Velikic, G.; Susnjevic, S.; Maric, D.L.; Abazovic, D. Encouraging effect of autologous bone marrow aspirate concentrate in rehabilitation of children with cerebral palsy. *Eur. Rev. Med. Pharmacol. Sci.* **2022**, *26*, 2330–2342. [CrossRef]
40. Min, K.; Song, J.; Kang, J.Y.; Ko, J.; Ryu, J.S.; Kang, M.S.; Jang, S.J.; Kim, S.H.; Oh, D.; Kim, M.K.; et al. Umbilical cord blood therapy potentiated with erythropoietin for children with cerebral palsy: A double-blind, randomized, placebo-controlled trial. *Stem Cells* **2013**, *31*, 581–591. [CrossRef]
41. Min, K.; Suh, M.R.; Cho, K.H.; Park, W.; Kang, M.S.; Jang, S.J.; Kim, S.H.; Rhie, S.; Choi, J.I.; Kim, H.J.; et al. Potentiation of cord blood cell therapy with erythropoietin for children with CP: A 2 × 2 factorial randomized placebo-controlled trial. *Stem Cell Res. Ther.* **2020**, *11*, 509. [CrossRef]
42. Nguyen, L.T.; Nguyen, A.T.; Vu, C.D.; Ngo, D.V.; Bui, A.V. Outcomes of autologous bone marrow mononuclear cells for cerebral palsy: An open label uncontrolled clinical trial. *BMC Pediatr.* **2017**, *17*, 104. [CrossRef]
43. Nguyen, T.L.; Nguyen, H.P.; Nguyen, T.K. The effects of bone marrow mononuclear cell transplantation on the quality of life of children with cerebral palsy. *Health Qual. Life Outcomes* **2018**, *16*, 164. [CrossRef]
44. Okur, S.C.; Erdogan, S.; Demir, C.S.; Gunel, G.; Karaoz, E. The effect of Umbilical Cord-derived Mesenchymal stem cell transplantation in a patient with cerebral palsy: A case report. *Int. J. Stem Cells* **2018**, *11*, 141–147. [CrossRef]
45. Padma, M.V.; Bhasin, A.; Mohanty, S.; Sharma, S.; Kiran, U.; Bal, C.S.; Gaikwad, S.; Singh, M.B.; Bhatia, R.; Tripathi, M.; et al. Restorative therapy using autologous bone marrow derived mononuclear cells infusion intra-arterially in patients with cerebral palsy: An open label feasibility study. *Neurol. Asia* **2011**, *16*, 231–239.
46. Papadopoulos, K.I.; Low, S.S.S.; Aw, T.C.; Chantarojanasiri, T. Safety and feasibility of autologous umbilical cord blood transfusion in 2 toddlers with cerebral palsy and the role of low dose granulocyte-colony stimulating factor injections. *Restor. Neurol. Neurosci.* **2011**, *29*, 17–22. [CrossRef]
47. Purandare, C.; Shitole, D.G.; Belle, V.; Kedari, A.; Bora, N.; Joshi, M. Therapeutic potential of autologous stem cell transplantation for cerebral palsy. *Case Rep. Transplant.* **2012**, *2012*, 825289. [CrossRef]
48. Purwati; Fauzi, A.A.; Gunawan, P.I.; Susilo, I.; Rini, D.P. The role of autologous adipose derived neural progenitor cells with cognitive and motoric function in cerebral palsy. *J. Glob. Pharma Technol.* **2019**, *11*, 163–169.
49. Rah, W.J.; Lee, Y.H.; Moon, J.H.; Jun, H.J.; Kang, H.R.; Koh, H.; Eom, H.J.; Lee, J.Y.; Lee, Y.J.; Kim, J.Y.; et al. Neuroregenerative potential of intravenous G-CSF and autologous peripheral blood stem cells in children with cerebral palsy: A randomized, double-blind, cross-over study. *J. Transl. Med.* **2017**, *15*, 16. [CrossRef]
50. Romanov, Y.A.; Tarakanov, O.P.; Radaev, S.M.; Dugina, T.N.; Ryaskina, S.S.; Darevskaya, A.N.; Morozova, Y.V.; Khachatryan, W.A.; Lebedev, K.E.; Zotova, N.S.; et al. Human allogeneic AB0/Rh-identical umbilical cord blood cells in the treatment of juvenile patients with cerebral palsy. *Cytotherapy* **2015**, *17*, 969–978. [CrossRef]
51. Seledtsov, V.I.; Kafanova, M.Y.; Rabinovich, S.S.; Poveshchenko, O.V.; Kashchenko, E.A.; Fel'de, M.A.; Samarin, D.M.; Seledtsova, G.V.; Kozlov, V.A. Cell therapy of cerebral palsy. *Bull. Exp. Biol. Med.* **2005**, *139*, 499–503. [CrossRef]
52. Sharma, A.; Sane, H.; Paranjape, A.; Gokulchandran, N.; Kulkarni, P.; Nagrajan, A.; Badhe, P. Positron emission tomography-computer tomography scan used as a monitoring tool following cellular therapy in cerebral palsy and mental retardation-a case report. *Case Rep. Neurol. Med.* **2013**, *2013*, 141983. [CrossRef]
53. Sharma, A.; Sane, H.; Gokulchandran, N.; Kulkarni, P.; Gandhi, S.; Sundaram, J.; Paranjape, A.; Shetty, A.; Bhagwanani, K.; Biju, H.; et al. A clinical study of autologous bone marrow mononuclear cells for cerebral palsy patients: A new frontier. *Stem Cells Int.* **2015**, *2015*, 905874. [CrossRef] [PubMed]
54. Sharma, A.; Sane, H.; Kulkarni, P.; D'sa, M.; Gokulchandran, N.; Badhe, P. Improved quality of life in a case of cerebral palsy after bone marrow mononuclear cell transplantation. *Cell J.* **2015**, *17*, 389–394.
55. Sharma, A.; Gokulchandran, N.; Kulkarni, P.; Kiran Mullangi, S.; Bhagawanani, K.; Ganar, V.; Sane, H.; Badhe, P. Multiple cellular therapies along with neurorehabilitation in spastic diplegic cerebral palsy: A case report. *Innov. Clin. Neurosci.* **2020**, *17*, 31–34. [PubMed]
56. Shroff, G.; Gupta, A.; Barthakur, J.K. Therapeutic potential of human embryonic stem cell transplantation in patients with cerebral palsy. *J. Transl. Med.* **2014**, *12*, 318. [CrossRef] [PubMed]
57. Sun, J.M.; Song, A.W.; Case, L.E.; Mikati, M.A.; Gustafson, K.E.; Simmons, R.; Goldstein, R.; Petry, J.; McLaughlin, C.; Waters-Pick, B.; et al. Effect of Autologous Cord Blood Infusion on Motor Function and Brain Connectivity in Young Children with Cerebral Palsy: A Randomized, Placebo-Controlled Trial. *Stem Cells Transl. Med.* **2017**, *6*, 2071–2078. [CrossRef]
58. Sun, J.M.; Case, L.E.; Mikati, M.A.; Jasien, J.M.; McLaughlin, C.; Waters-Pick, B.; Worley, G.; Troy, J.; Kurtzberg, J. Sibling umbilical cord blood infusion is safe in young children with cerebral palsy. *Stem Cells Transl. Med.* **2021**, *10*, 1258–1265. [CrossRef]
59. Thanh, L.N.; Trung, K.N.; Duy, C.V.; Van, D.N.; Hoang, P.N.; Phuong, A.N.T.; Ngo, M.D.; Thi, T.N.; Viet, A.B. Improvement in gross motor function and muscle tone in children with cerebral palsy related to neonatal icterus: An open-label, uncontrolled clinical trial. *BMC Pediatr.* **2019**, *19*, 290. [CrossRef]
60. Wang, L.; Ji, H.; Zhou, J.; Xie, J.; Zhong, Z.; Li, M.; Bai, W.; Li, N.; Zhang, Z.; Wang, X.; et al. Therapeutic potential of umbilical cord mesenchymal stromal cells transplantation for cerebral palsy: A case report. *Case Rep. Transplant.* **2013**, *2013*, 146347. [CrossRef]
61. Wang, X.; Cheng, H.; Hua, R.; Yang, J.; Dai, G.; Zhang, Z.; Wang, R.; Qin, C.; An, Y. Effects of bone marrow mesenchymal stromal cells on gross motor function measure scores of children with cerebral palsy: A preliminary clinical study. *Cytotherapy* **2013**, *15*, 1549–1562. [CrossRef]

62. Wang, X.; Hu, H.; Hua, R.; Yang, J.; Zheng, P.; Niu, X.; Cheng, H.; Dai, G.; Liu, X.; Zhang, Z.; et al. Effect of umbilical cord mesenchymal stromal cells on motor functions of identical twins with cerebral palsy: Pilot study on the correlation of efficacy and hereditary factors. *Cytotherapy* **2015**, *17*, 224–231. [CrossRef]
63. Zali, A.; Arab, L.; Ashrafi, F.; Mardpour, S.; Niknejhadi, M.; Hedayati-Asl, A.A.; Halimi-Asl, A.; Ommi, D.; Hosseini, S.E.; Baharvand, H.; et al. Intrathecal injection of CD133-positive enriched bone marrow progenitor cells in children with cerebral palsy: Feasibility and safety. *Cytotherapy* **2015**, *17*, 232–241. [CrossRef]
64. Zarrabi, M.; Akbari, M.G.; Amanat, M.; Majmaa, A.; Moaiedi, A.R.; Montazerlotfelahi, H.; Nouri, M.; Hamidieh, A.A.; Badv, R.S.; Karimi, H.; et al. The safety and efficacy of umbilical cord blood mononuclear cells in individuals with spastic cerebral palsy: A randomized double-blind sham-controlled clinical trial. *BMC Neurol.* **2022**, *22*, 123. [CrossRef]
65. Zhang, C.; Huang, L.; Gu, J.; Zhou, X. Therapy for Cerebral Palsy by Human Umbilical Cord Blood Mesenchymal Stem Cells Transplantation Combined With Basic Rehabilitation Treatment: A Case Report. *Glob. Pediatr. Health* **2015**, *2*, 2333794X15574091. [CrossRef]
66. Cox, C.S., Jr.; Juranek, J.; Kosmach, S.; Pedroza, C.; Thakur, N.; Dempsey, A.; Rennie, K.; Scott, M.C.; Jackson, M.; Kumar, A.; et al. Autologous cellular therapy for cerebral palsy: A randomized, crossover trial. *Brain Commun.* **2022**, *4*, fcac131. [CrossRef]
67. Gabr, H.; El-Kheir, W.A.; Ghannam, O.; El-Fiki, M.E.; Salah, Y. Intrathecal Autologous Bone Marrow Derived MSC Therapy in Cerebral Palsy: Safety and Short Term Efficacy. *Am. J. Biosci. Bioeng.* **2015**, *3*, 24–29. [CrossRef]
68. Hirano, A.; Sano, M.; Urushihata, N.; Tanemura, H.; Oki, K.; Suzaki, E. Assessment of safety and feasibility of human allogeneic adipose-derived mesenchymal stem cells in a pediatric patient. *Pediatr. Res.* **2018**, *84*, 575–577. [CrossRef]
69. Ramirez, F.; Steenblock, D.A.; Payne, A.G.; Darnall, L. Umbilical Cord Stem Cell Therapy for Cerebral Palsy. *Med. Hypothesis Res.* **2006**, *3*, 679–686.
70. Kikuchi, H.; Saitoh, S.; Tsuno, T.; Hosoda, R.; Baba, N.; Wang, F.; Mitsuda, N.; Tsuda, M.; Maeda, N.; Sagara, Y.; et al. Safety and feasibility of autologous cord blood infusion for improving motor function in young children with cerebral palsy in Japan: A single-center study. *Brain Dev.* **2022**, *44*, 681–689. [CrossRef]
71. Sun, J.M.; Case, L.E.; McLaughlin, C.; Burgess, A.; Skergan, N.; Crane, S.; Jasien, J.M.; Mikati, M.A.; Troy, J.; Kurtzberg, J. Motor function and safety after allogeneic cord blood and cord tissue-derived mesenchymal stromal cells in cerebral palsy: An open-label, randomized trial. *Dev. Med. Child Neurol.* **2022**, *64*, 1477–1486. [CrossRef]
72. Page, M.J.; McKenzie, J.E.; Bossuyt, P.M.; Boutron, I.; Hoffmann, T.C.; Mulrow, C.D.; Shamseer, L.; Tetzlaff, J.M.; Akl, E.A.; Brennan, S.E.; et al. The PRISMA 2020 statement: An updated guideline for reporting systematic reviews. *Br. Med. J.* **2021**, *372*, n71. [CrossRef]
73. Shroff, G.; Gupta, A.; Barthakur, J.K. Expression of Concern to: Therapeutic potential of human embryonic stem cell transplantation in patients with cerebral palsy. *J. Transl. Med.* **2017**, *15*, 193. [CrossRef] [PubMed]
74. Gioia, G.A.; Isquith, P.K.; Guy, S.C.; Kenworthy, L. *Behavior Rating Inventory of Executive Function: BRIEF*; Psychological Assessment Resources: Odessa, FL, USA, 2000.
75. Haley, S.M.; Coster, W.; Dumas, H.M.; Fragala-Pinkham, M.A.; Moed, R. *PEDI-CAT: Pediatric Evaluation of Disability Inventory Computer Adaptive Test Manual 1-3-6*; Trustees of Boston University: Boston, MA, USA, 2011; under license to CREcare, LLC.
76. Frankenburg, W.K.; Dodds, J.B. *Denver Developmental Screening Test II (DDST-II)*; Denver Developmental Materials: Denver, CO, USA, 1990.
77. Gracies, J.M.; Burke, K.; Clegg, N.J.; Browne, R.; Rushing, C.; Fehlings, D.; Matthews, D.; Tilton, A.; Delgado, M.R. Reliability of the Tardieu Scale for assessing spasticity in children with cerebral palsy. *Arch. Phys. Med. Rehabil.* **2010**, *91*, 421–428. [CrossRef] [PubMed]
78. Bayley, N. *Bayley Scales of Infant and Toddler Development*, 3rd ed.; Pearson Clinical: San Antonio, TX, USA, 2005.
79. Wechsler, D. *The Wechsler Intelligence Scale for Children*, 5th ed.; Pearson: Bloomington, MN, USA, 2014.
80. Waters, E.; Davis, E.; Mackinnon, A.; Boyd, R.; Graham, H.K.; Kai Lo, S.; Wolfe, R.; Stevenson, R.; Bjornson, K.; Blair, E.; et al. Psychometric properties of the quality of life questionnaire for children with CP. *Dev. Med. Child Neurol.* **2007**, *49*, 49–55. [CrossRef] [PubMed]
81. Schiariti, V.; Tatla, S.; Sauve, K.; O'Donnell, M. Toolbox of multiple-item measures aligning with the ICF Core Sets for children and youth with cerebral palsy. *Eur. J. Paediatr. Neurol.* **2017**, *21*, 252–263. [CrossRef] [PubMed]
82. Dickinson, H.O.; Parkinson, K.N.; Ravens-Sieberer, U.; Schirripa, G.; Thyen, U.; Arnaud, C.; Beckung, E.; Fauconnier, J.; McManus, V.; Michelsen, S.I.; et al. Self-reported quality of life of 8-12-year-old children with cerebral palsy: A cross-sectional European study. *Lancet* **2007**, *369*, 2171–2178. [CrossRef]
83. Narayanan, U.G.; Fehlings, D.; Weir, S.; Knights, S.; Kiran, S.; Campbell, K. Initial development and validation of the Caregiver Priorities and Child Health Index of Life with Disabilities (CPCHILD). *Dev. Med. Child Neurol.* **2006**, *48*, 804–812. [CrossRef]
84. Difazio, R.L.; Vessey, J.A.; Zurakowski, D.; Snyder, B.D. Differences in health-related quality of life and caregiver burden after hip and spine surgery in non-ambulatory children with severe cerebral palsy. *Dev. Med. Child Neurol.* **2016**, *58*, 298–305. [CrossRef]
85. Montague, J. The 'Unwarranted Hype' of Stem Cell Therapies. Available online: https://www.bbc.com/future/article/20190819-the-unwarranted-hype-of-stem-cell-therapies-for-autism-ms (accessed on 1 November 2022).
86. Akhtar, A. The flaws and human harms of animal experimentation. *Camb. Q. Healthc. Ethics* **2015**, *24*, 407–419. [CrossRef]
87. Klinck, M.P.; Mogil, J.S.; Moreau, M.; Lascelles, B.D.X.; Flecknell, P.A.; Poitte, T.; Troncy, E. Translational pain assessment: Could natural animal models be the missing link? *Pain* **2017**, *158*, 1633–1646. [CrossRef]

88. Eliasson, A.C.; Krumlinde-Sundholm, L.; Rösblad, B.; Beckung, E.; Arner, M.; Ohrvall, A.M.; Rosenbaum, P. The Manual Ability Classification System (MACS) for children with cerebral palsy: Scale development and evidence of validity and reliability. *Dev. Med. Child Neurol.* **2006**, *48*, 549–554. [CrossRef]
89. Hidecker, M.J.; Paneth, N.; Rosenbaum, P.L.; Kent, R.D.; Lillie, J.; Eulenberg, J.B.; Chester, K., Jr.; Johnson, B.; Michalsen, L.; Evatt, M.; et al. Developing and validating the Communication Function Classification System for individuals with cerebral palsy. *Dev. Med. Child Neurol.* **2011**, *53*, 704–710. [CrossRef]
90. Kiresuk, T.J.; Sherman, R.E. Goal attainment scaling: A general method for evaluating comprehensive community mental health programs. *Community Ment. Health J.* **1968**, *4*, 443–453. [CrossRef]
91. Law, M.; Baptiste, S.; McColl, M.; Opzoomer, A.; Polatajko, H.; Pollock, N. The Canadian occupational performance measure: An outcome measure for occupational therapy. *Can. J. Occup. Ther.* **1990**, *57*, 82–87. [CrossRef]

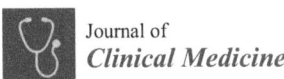

Review

Persistent Inflammation in Cerebral Palsy: Pathogenic Mediator or Comorbidity? A Scoping Review

Madison C. B. Paton [1,*], Megan Finch-Edmondson [1], Russell C. Dale [2,3], Michael C. Fahey [4], Claudia A. Nold-Petry [4,5], Marcel F. Nold [4,5,6], Alexandra R. Griffin [1] and Iona Novak [1,7]

1. Cerebral Palsy Alliance Research Institute, Speciality of Child and Adolescent Health, Sydney Medical School, Faculty of Medicine and Health, The University of Sydney, Sydney, NSW 2050, Australia
2. Children's Hospital at Westmead Clinical School, Faculty of Medicine and Health, Sydney Medical School, University of Sydney, Sydney, NSW 2145, Australia
3. Kids Neuroscience Centre and T Y Nelson Department of Neurology and Neurosurgery, Children's Hospital at Westmead, Sydney, NSW 2145, Australia
4. Department of Paediatrics, Monash University, Melbourne, VIC 3168, Australia
5. The Ritchie Centre, Hudson Institute of Medical Research, Melbourne, VIC 3168, Australia
6. Monash Newborn, Monash Children's Hospital, Melbourne, VIC 3168, Australia
7. Faculty of Medicine and Health, The University of Sydney, Sydney, NSW 2050, Australia
* Correspondence: madison.paton@cerebralpalsy.org.au

Abstract: Research has established inflammation in the pathogenesis of brain injury and the risk of developing cerebral palsy (CP). However, it is unclear if inflammation is solely pathogenic and primarily contributes to the acute phase of injury, or if inflammation persists with consequence in CP and may therefore be considered a comorbidity. We conducted a scoping review to identify studies that analyzed inflammatory biomarkers in CP and discuss the role of inflammation in the pathogenesis of CP and/or as a comorbidity. Twelve included studies reported a range of analytes, methods and biomarkers, including indicators of inflammatory status, immune function and genetic changes. The majority of controlled studies concluded that one or more systemic biomarkers of inflammation were significantly different in CP versus controls; most commonly serum or plasma cytokines such as tumor necrosis factor, Interleukin (IL)-6 and IL-10. In addition, differences in inflammation were noted in distinct subgroups of CP (e.g., those with varying severity). The available evidence supports the pathogenic role of inflammation and its ongoing role as a comorbidity of CP. This review shows that inflammation may persist for decades, driving functional impairment across development and into adulthood. However, inflammation is complex, thus further research will increase our understanding.

Keywords: inflammation; biomarker; cerebral palsy; comorbidity; scoping review

1. Introduction

Cerebral palsy (CP) describes a group of permanent motor and postural disorders, causing activity limitations, that are attributed to non-progressive disturbances in the developing brain [1]. The motor disorders of CP are commonly accompanied by sensation, perception, cognition, behavior and communication disturbances, with epilepsy and secondary musculoskeletal issues. Inflammation is detailed in the pathogenesis of most perinatal brain injury that contributes to the risk of developing CP, including neonatal stroke, preterm birth, birth asphyxia and infection [2,3]. Systematic reviews of the clinical literature now support an association between higher circulating levels of pro-inflammatory mediators and the diagnosis of CP, particularly in the setting of prematurity [4]. However, the duration and extent of this inflammation, as well as the implications in people with CP, remain unclear.

Inflammation in CP may comprise changes in cytokines [4]; altered immune response with a dysregulated response to stimuli (e.g., lipopolysaccharide (LPS)) [5]; adaptive immune changes including T- and B- cell distribution and function [6], and other genetic and non-genetic changes to signaling pathways [7]. It is commonly reported that inflammation following perinatal brain injury changes over time, between the acute to chronic phases of injury [8]. However, persistent inflammation (i.e., inflammation extending months-to-years after the primary injury phase) has been postulated to have detrimental effects on the brain and may contribute to ongoing sequelae of CP [9,10]. This is supported by the *sustained inflammation hypothesis*, also known as programming effects, whereby prenatal, antenatal or neonatal pro-inflammatory cytokines induce inflammation that contributes to long-term cytokine dysregulation [11]. Whilst it has been discussed that persistent inflammation may be present in people with CP [5,7], there is ongoing debate about the strength of this evidence and its implications. There are currently two main streams of thought:

(1) *Inflammation persists well after the original brain injury with long-term consequence in CP.* If inflammation persists, other commonly characterized symptoms of CP, including pain and cognition may be confounded or exacerbated. For example, systemic immune disturbances in innate and cellular immunity increase brain glial cell responsiveness, which may worsen neurological deficits [12]. In this context, inflammation may be viewed as a contributing factor to the symptoms experienced by people with CP, and present with the motor and movement impairments, in other terms be a "comorbidity" of CP.

(2) *Inflammation persists in CP without long-term consequence or indeed, does not persist at all.* If inflammation is not a comorbidity of CP, it may instead standalone as a pathogenic feature of CP; meaning that the original inflammatory insult that causes the motor and postural impairment exists with no other long-term implications on health or outcomes. Alternatively, that inflammation does not persist.

When considering either stream of thought, there are many unknowns around how and why inflammation may or may not persist. Crosstalk between inflammation arising from the central nervous and systemic immune system are also unclear, along with the possible contribution of epigenetic programming from the initial insult [13].

Interestingly, the role of inflammation in the pathogenesis of CP is frequently investigated; many publications report on inflammatory biomarkers either collected close to the time of birth (e.g., umbilical cord blood) or during the neonatal period up to 4 weeks of age, or study a mixed at-risk population which are then correlated with outcomes such as CP [14,15]. Early inflammatory biomarkers and associations with neurodevelopmental outcome can be seen as indirect measures that allude to the impact of inflammation, genetic and immune changes in the pathogenesis of brain injury. However, direct measures of inflammation in children and adults with CP is lacking and the extent and duration of inflammation is not understood. The need for more research in this space has been previously stated [7].

Hence, this scoping review aims to identify and synthesize results from clinical studies that analyze biomarkers of inflammation in established CP and discuss the role of inflammation in the pathogenesis of CP and as a comorbidity. In addition, as CP is highly heterogenous, we also aim to elucidate any effects within subgroups of CP, including etiology, age and type and topography of CP. Adequate identification of those with higher inflammation may open the potential for personalized medicine and targeted therapeutics, as well as identify responders/non-responders to treatments with an inflammation-modulating mechanism of action.

2. Materials and Methods

We followed the Joanna-Briggs Institute *Population, Concept, and Context* keywords search method to formulate our scoping review question [16]. The study protocol was published on the Open Science Framework, July 2022 (DOI 10.17605/OSF.IO/6ZVUN (accessed on 17 November 2022)). This scoping review is reported in accordance with the *Preferred Reporting Items for Systematic Reviews and Meta-Analyses extension for Scoping Reviews Guidelines (PRISMA-ScR*, [17]). The PRISMA-ScR Checklist can be found in Supplementary File S1.

2.1. Study Eligibility Criteria

We included all study types (controlled and non-controlled) that reported on participants with CP. Studies were required to include the analysis of biomarkers that measured changes in inflammation, or markers of immune or inflammatory pathways, including genetic. Full text records, published in English in a peer-reviewed journal were eligible for inclusion. No limits were placed on the date of publication.

We excluded studies that measured inflammation in infant populations prior to a CP diagnosis; captured biomarkers only for the purpose of analysis of risk factors susceptibility, associations and causal pathways to CP; or used neuroimaging, neuropathology or indirect functional measures as a biomarker.

2.2. Search Strategy

We ran searches on 28 June 2022 using MEDLINE (1946 to 28 June 2022), Cochrane Central (The Cochrane Library, June 2022) and Embase (1947 to 28 June 2022) via Ovid using the following strategy: (Cerebral palsy.tw) AND (Inflamm*.tw). Searches were limited to English language articles and de-duplicated.

2.3. Study Selection

De-duplicated search results were exported into Covidence Systematic Review Software (Veritas Health Innovation, Melbourne, Australia, available at: http://www.covidence.org (accessed on 17 November 2022)). Additional de-duplication was conducted before titles and abstracts were screened by two independent reviewers (MCBP and MFE). Full texts of studies were then retrieved and independently assessed for eligibility.

2.4. Data Extraction

Data was extracted by two independent review authors (MCBP and MFE) into a Microsoft Excel spreadsheet which was developed specifically for this review. Extracted information included study details, participants and groups, method of biomarker analysis, analyte details, significant study findings including subgroup analyses (comprising severity, type/topography, age and etiology).

2.5. Defining Reportable Inflammatory Biomarkers

Consistent with the inclusion criteria and scope of this review, only biomarkers related to inflammation were included. We defined biomarkers as molecules, proteins (including cytokines and chemokines, as well as their receptors) or cells and characteristics of cellular function. This also included quantitative PCR as a biomarker of the amount of cytokine expression, at the RNA level. Whilst we did not limit on the type of analytes, we do not report on growth factors, hormones or neuropeptides.

2.6. Data Synthesis

Results are reported as a summary of included studies and in relation to three biomarker result types of (1) cytokine analysis, (2) immune function and/or (3) genetic changes and gene expression. Briefly, we define immune function to mean changes in immune or blood cells upon stimulation; changes in cytokine analysis is defined by the differences in unstimulated expression of inflammatory markers including quantitative PCR at the RNA level; and, genetic changes and gene expression refer to an alteration or variation (including polymorphisms) in nucleotide sequences and DNA expression. Results of findings within CP subgroups related to inflammation and age, CP type, severity, topography and etiology are also synthesized, reported and discussed.

3. Results

3.1. Search Results

A total of 1489 records were identified following the search procedure shown in Figure 1. After 556 duplicates were removed, 933 studies were screened by title and abstract with 895 studies subsequently excluded. Following full-text screening for eligibility, 12 studies were included in this review [5,6,9,18–26].

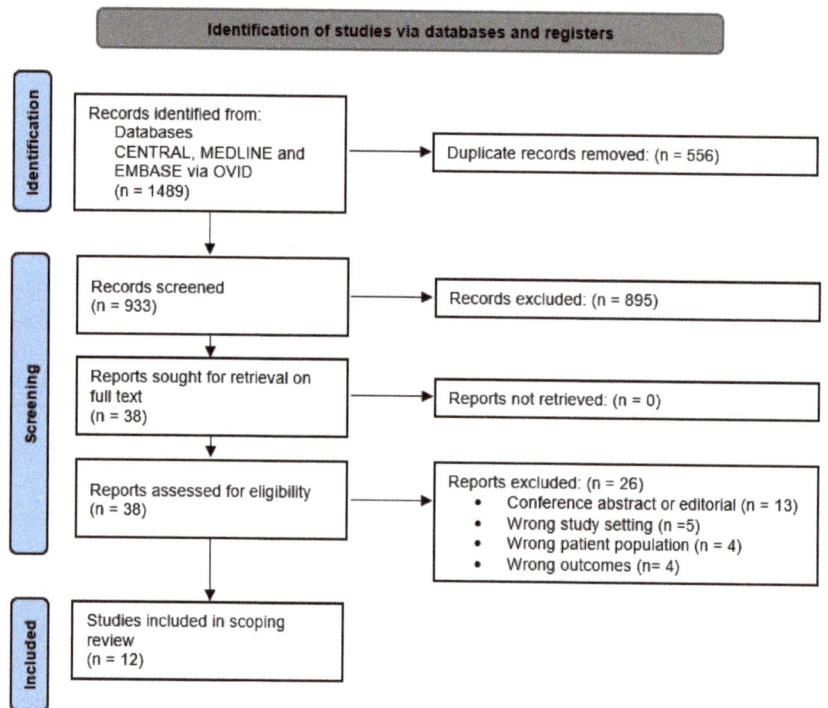

Figure 1. PRISMA Flow Diagram.

3.2. Study Characteristics

Studies that had reportable information on inflammatory biomarkers indicating directionality of inflammation and immune responses compared to a control were synthesized and presented (Table 1) [5,6,9,18,19,21,22,24–26]. The two studies without a control group could not be summarized and reported in Table 1 [20,23]. However, their study characteristics and outcome data are presented below (see Section 3.4. *Additional findings in single arm studies*) and in Table 2, which describes sub-group differences.

Table 1. Study characteristics and main findings.

Citation	CP Group/s and Comparator Details	Etiology of CP Group	Result Type / Sample Type / Method of Analysis: Inflammatory Markers	Reported Significant Findings Related to CP
Tao 2008 [19]	Children with CP: Type/topography/severity: not reported Mean age 5.2 years, range 0–10 (n = 31, 55% male) Neonatal controls with asphyxia or infection: Mean age 6.3 days, range 0–10 (n = 37, 54% male) Age-matched controls, no CP: Mean age 4.8 years, range 0–10 (n = 40, 58% male)	HIE and/or infection	*Cytokine analysis* Serum ELISA: TNF, IL-6	↑TNF in CP vs. neonatal controls ↑TNF in CP vs. age-matched controls ↑IL-6 in CP vs. age-matched controls
Lin 2010 [5]	Children and adolescents with CP: Spastic/di, tri or quad/GMFCS II–V: Mean age (SD) 7.2 (±3.6) years (n = 32, 59% male) GA-matched controls, no CP: Mean age (SD) 6.2 (±2.2) years (n = 32, 44% male)	Preterm with PVL	*Cytokine analysis* Plasma ELISA: TNF, IL-6 *Immune function* Supernatant from PBMCs, +/− LPS ELISA: TNF, IL-6 Flow cytometry: TNF *Immune function* RNA from PBMCs, +/− LPS RT-PCR: 84 TNF genes (TNF ligand/receptor signalling)	↑TNF in CP vs. GA-matched controls ↑TNF (ELISA) after LPS in CP vs. GA-matched controls ↑TNF (flow cytometry) before vs. after LPS in CP group ↑10 genes (CAD, CASP2, CRADD, EDA2R, IKBKG, TAK1/TGF1α, JNK/JNK1, 4-1BB/CD137, TL1/TL1A, TRAF3) in CP vs. GA-matched controls
Koh 2015 [21]	Children with CP: Type/topography/severity: not reported Mean age not reported (n = 14, sex not reported) Adult controls, no CP: Mean age not reported (n = 14, sex not reported) Cord blood from healthy neonates (n = 14, sex not reported)	Not reported	*Immune function* Mobilised PBMCs, +LPS/PMA and ionomycin Flow cytometry: TNF, IL-1β, IL-2, IL-3, IL-6, IL-8, IL-9, GM-CSF	↓IL-1β in CP vs. adult controls ↑GM-CSF in CP vs. adult controls ↑IL-8 in CP vs. adult controls
Wu 2015 [24]	Children with CP: Spastic/tri, quad, di, mono, hemi/GMFCS I–V Mean age (SD) 3.7 (±2.3) years (n = 54, 59% male) Age-matched controls, no CP: Mean age (SD) 4.6 (±3.1) years (n = 28, 54% male)	Not reported	*Cytokine analysis* Plasma ELISA: TNF	↑TNF in CP vs. age matched-control

Table 1. *Cont.*

Citation	CP Group/s and Comparator Details	Etiology of CP Group	Result Type / Sample Type / Method of Analysis: Inflammatory Markers	Reported Significant Findings Related to CP
Von Walden 2018 [26]	Children and adolescents with CP: Spastic/topography not reported/GMFCS I-II, IV-V Mean age 15.5 years, range 9-18 (n = 18, another n = 2 with ABI, 85% male) Children and young adult controls, no CP: Mean age 15.1 years, range 7-21 (n = 10, 80% male)	Not reported	*Cytokine analysis* Skeletal muscle biopsy RT-PCR: IL-1β, IL-1R, IL-6, IL-6R, TNF, TWEAK, IL-8, IL-10	↑ IL-1β in CP vs. controls ↑ IL-6 in CP vs. controls ↑ TNF in CP vs. controls
Xia 2018 [25]	Infants and children with CP: Spastic and non-spastic/hemi, di, quad /GMFCS not reported Mean age for genotyping/plasma collection (SD) 16.2 (±12.7) months; 20.8 (±14.4) months (n = 282, 65% male) Infant and children controls, no CP: Mean (SD) age for genotyping/plasma collection 24.0 (±16.4) months; 21.6 (±13.8) months (n = 197, 77% male)	Mixed: HIE, PVL, other/not specified	*Cytokine analysis* Plasma [1] ELISA: IL-10	↑ IL-10 in CP vs. controls
Pingel 2019 [22]	Children and adolescents with CP: Type not reported/hemi, di, quad/GMFCS I-V: Mean age (SEM) 10.31 (±1.1) years (n = 14, 50% male) Adults with CP: 38.8 (±3.6) years (n = 10, 60% male) Adult controls, no CP: Mean age (SEM) 36.53 (±3.8) years (n = 10, sex not reported)	Not reported	*Cytokine analysis* Plasma ELISA: TGFβ1, CRP, IL-6	↑ TGFβ1 and CRP in children with CP vs. adult controls [2]
Ng 2021 [18]	Adults with CP: Type/topography/severity: not reported Mean age (SD) 25 (±5.39) years (n = 64, 55% male) Older adults' with mild cognitive impairment, no CP (mean age (SD) 66.95 (±4.29) years) (n = 40, 30% males) Older adults' controls, no MCI, no CP: (mean age (SD) 71.8 (±5.66) years) (n = 56, 20% males)	Not reported	*Cytokine analysis* Plasma ELISA: CRP	None

Table 1. Cont.

Citation	CP Group/s and Comparator Details	Etiology of CP Group	Result Type Sample Type Method of Analysis: Inflammatory Markers	Reported Significant Findings Related to CP
Taher 2021 [6]	Children and adolescents with CP: Type/topography/severity: not reported Mean age: "School-aged children", age not reported (n = 10, 80% male) School aged children post NE, no CP (n = 10, 70% male) Mean age: not reported School aged children no NE, no CP (n = 23, 78% male) Mean age: not reported Neonates with NE (n = 30, 50% male) Mean age: not reported Neonates, no NE (n = 17, 53% male) Mean age: not reported	NE	*Proportions of immune cell types* Whole blood Flow cytometry: T cells (CD3+), B cells (CDCD3- CD19+), NK cells (CD3-/CD56+), MAIT cells (CD3+/Vα7.2+/CD161+), iNKT cells (CD3+/Vα24Jα18+) Vδ1 TCRs (CD3+/ Vδ1+), Vδ 2 TCRs (CD3+/ Vδ2+) *Cytokine analysis* Serum ELISA: IFN-γ, TNF, IL-2, IL-5, IL-6 IL-8, IL-9, IL-10, IL-15, IL-17A, IL-21, IL-22, IL-23	↑T-cells (absolute and % freq) in children with CP vs. school-aged children ↑Vδ2 T cells (absolute and % freq) in children with CP vs. school-aged children ↑iNKT cells (absolute and % freq) in children with CP vs. school-aged children ↑CD4− CD8− T cell frequencies in children with CP vs. school aged children ↓Vδ1 T cells (absolute and % freq) in children with CP vs. school aged children ↓MAIT cell (% freq) in children with CP vs. school aged children ↑B cell (% freq) in children with CP vs. school aged children ↓IL-8 in children with CP vs. school aged children post NE

Table 1. Cont.

Citation	CP Group/s and Comparator Details	Etiology of CP Group	Result Type / Sample Type / Method of Analysis: Inflammatory Markers	Reported Significant Findings Related to CP
Zareen 2010 [9]	Children and adolescents with CP: Type not reported/topography not reported/GMFCS II, III, V Mean age (SD) 10.08 (±1.67) years, range 1–16 (n = 12, 67% male) Age-matched controls, no CP Mean age (SD) 9.08 (±1.08) years, range 6–14 (n = 12, 67% male)	Mixed: NE, congenital infection and stroke	*Cytokine analysis* Serum ELISA: IL-1α, IL-1β, IL-6, IL-8, IL-10 IL-18, IL-1Ra, TNF INF-γ, GM-CSF *Immune function* Supernatant from whole blood + LPS ELISA IL-1α, IL-1β, IL-6, IL-8, IL-10, IL-18, IL-1Ra, TNF, IFN-γ, GM-CSF	None ↑ IL-1α, IL-1β, IL-2, IL-6 after stim in CP vs. age-matched controls

Significance is defined as reported in the included papers ($p < 0.05$). "Infants" (<1 year); "children" (1–9 years); "adolescents" (10–19 years); "adults" (20–59 years), "older adults" (60+ years). [1] Whole blood DNA Genotyping SNPs excluded from table as results were not relevant. [2] Additional significant finding detected comparing children with CP to adults with CP. Results appear as a subgroup finding in Table 2 related to age. ↑ increase; ↓ decrease; ABI, acquired brain injury; CD, cluster of differentiation; CP, cerebral palsy; CRP, C-reactive protein; CSF, cerebrospinal fluid; ELISA, enzyme-linked immunosorbent assay; di, diplegia; FACS, fluorescence activated cell sorting; freq, frequency; G-CSF, granulocyte-colony stimulating factor; GMFCS, gross motor function classification system; HIE, hypoxic ischemic encephalopathy; ID, intellectual disability; IKK-γ, inhibitor of nuclear factor kappa-B kinase subunit γ; hemi, hemiplegia; IFN, interferon; IL, interleukin; iNKT, Invariant natural killer T; IP, interferon γ-induced protein; JNK, c-Jun N-terminal kinases; LPS, lipopolysaccharide; MAIT, Mucosal-associated invariant T; MIP1β, macrophage inflammatory protein; MCP, monocyte chemotactic protein; n, sample; NE, neonatal encephalopathy; NLR, neutrophil to lymphocyte ratio; PBMCs, peripheral blood mononuclear cells; PMA, phorbol 12-myristate 13-acetate; PROM, premature rupture of membranes; RA, receptor antagonist; RANTES, regulated on activation normal T expressed and secreted; RNA, ribonucleic acid; RT-PCR, reverse transcription polymerase chain reaction; SD, standard deviation; SEM, standard error of the mean; SNP, Single nucleotide polymorphism; TNF, tumor necrosis factor; TLR, Toll-like receptor; TCR, T-cell receptor; TAK, transforming growth factor-β-activated kinase; TWEAK, tumor necrosis factor-like weak inducer of apoptosis; quad, quadriplegia; vs., versus.

Table 2. Main findings related to subgroups of cerebral palsy.

Theme	Reported Significant Findings in Subgroups of Those with CP	Citation
Age	↑ plasma TNF in CP vs. younger (1–3 years) and older (4–12 years) controls ↑ plasma TNF in younger subjects (1–3 years) with CP vs. older subjects (4–12 years) with CP ↑ TGFβ1 and CRP in children with CP vs. adults with CP	Wu 2015 [24] Pingel 2010 [22]
Type/Topography	↑ plasma IL-10 in the CP group with spastic quadraplegia vs. controls Frequencies of allele and genotype those with spastic quadraplegia vs. controls of *IL-10* polymorphisms: rs1554286, rs151811, rs3024490, rs1800871, and rs1800896	Xia 2018 [25]
Severity	↑ plasma TNF levels correlated with higher GMFCS in spastic diplegia or quadriplegia, and spastic diplegia ↑ whole blood NLR in children with severe motor impairment (GMFCS IV-V) vs. mild motor impairment (GMFCS II-III) living in a rehabilitation centre ↑ whole blood NLR positively correlated with higher GMFCS level	Wu 2015 [24] Riewruja 2020 [23]
Aetiology	4 unique discrete correlations in CSF related to inflammation, specific to preterm birth vs. term and extremely preterm: IL-10 and MIP-1β; IL-12p70 and TNF; IL-1Ra and IL-10; IL-1Ra and MIP-1β. 7 unique discrete correlations in CSF related to inflammation, specific to extreme preterm birth vs. term and preterm birth: IP10 and MIP-1β; IL-1α and IL-6; IL-1α and IL-10; IL-1α and RANTES; IL6 and IL10; IL-6 and RANTES; IL-10 and RANTES	Gorack-Postle 2021 [20]

CP, cerebral palsy; CRP, C-reactive protein; CSF, cerebrospinal fluid; GMFCS, gross motor function classification system; IL, interleukin; MIP-1β, macrophage inflammatory protein; NLR, neutrophil to lymphocyte ratio; Ra, receptor antagonist; RANTES, regulated on activation normal T expressed and secreted; TNF, tumor necrosis factor; vs., versus.

3.2.1. Study Design

Of the 12 included studies, ten were controlled (83%) and two were single arm (17%). All controlled studies compared a CP group to those without CP, however features of the control group were highly variable and many studies had a number of comparator groups. Comparator groups included age-matched controls [6,9,19,24,27], gestational-age matched controls [5], infants, children, adolescents and adults with/without CP [6,18,19,21,22,25,26].

3.2.2. Participant Features

Within the CP group, age was highly variable: one study recruited both infants (<1 year) and children (1–9 years) [25], three studies recruited children [19,21,24], seven studies recruited children and adolescents (10–19 years, [5,6,9,20,22,23,26] and one analyzed adolescents and adults (20–39 years, [18]). Included participants had variable type, topography, severity and etiology of CP (Table 1).

3.2.3. CP Cohort Etiology

Information regarding CP etiology was detailed in five included studies, with information provided in Table 1. One study recruited participants with asphyxia and/or infection [19], one recruited participants with preterm birth and PVL [5], one recruited participants with neonatal encephalopathy [6], and two had mixed participant etiologies (periventricular leukomalacia, birth asphyxia, hypoxia ischemic encephalopathy, neonatal encephalopathy, infection or stroke) [9,25]. All other studies did not provide information relating to CP etiology. A number of studies did specify participant gestational age at birth as a participant demographic. Whilst earlier gestational age (particularly very/extremely preterm) may be a risk factor for CP, it's direct link to CP etiology was not specified. One study did investigate the contribution of gestational age on CSF inflammatory markers in a subgroup analysis [20]. In this study, preterm birth was presented as a CP etiology and details of these findings can be found in Section 3.5.4 below.

3.2.4. Samples Analyzed, Method and Biomarker Details

A range of samples were studied for biomarkers of inflammation including plasma [18,22,24,25,28], serum [6,19], whole blood (including DNA) [6,9,23,25], peripheral blood mononuclear cells (PBMCs) [21], PBMC supernatant or RNA [5], cerebrospinal fluid (CSF) [20] and muscle [26]. Overall, most studies analyzed systemic inflammation from peripheral blood origins (Table 1).

A total of 30 inflammatory analytes were assessed including a variety of cytokines and their receptors. The most common analytes included cytokines such as tumor necrosis factor (TNF) (n = 8 studies), interleukin (IL)-6 (n = 7 studies) and IL-10 (n = 5 studies). Other cytokines, including but not limited to IL-1β, transforming growth factor (TGF)-β1 and IL-8, were less commonly reported, only appearing in three or fewer studies. In addition, a variety of genes were investigated as well as lymphocyte populations (Table 1).

The most common method of analyte analysis was enzyme-linked immunosorbent assay (ELISA, n = 8 studies). Other methods included flow cytometry (n = 3 studies), reverse transcription-polymerase chain reaction (RT-PCR, n = 2 studies), complete blood counts with differential pictures of white blood cells (n = 1 study) and genotyping of single nucleotide polymorphisms (SNPs, n = 1 study).

All studies had results that could be categorized as either biomarkers for (1) immune function [5,9,21], (2) inflammatory status via cytokine analysis [5,6,9,18,19,22–25,29] or (3) genetic changes and gene expression [5,25,26].

3.3. Results of Inflammatory Biomarkers in CP

Of the studies with a comparator group and presented in Table 1, n = 9/10 reported significant changes in inflammation (either inflammatory status, gene expression and/or immune response) in one or more findings in CP compared to a relevant comparator. These changes in inflammation were all systemic, except for one study assessing skeletal muscle [26]. It was noted that there was significantly higher systemic inflammation in adolescents with CP compared to relevant controls across four studies [5,6,9,22]. In the study measuring gene expression in skeletal muscle, higher inflammation was found in participants aged up to 18 years [26], with IL-1β, IL-6 and TNF mRNA being significantly higher in CP than controls.

3.3.1. Stimulation Assays of Immune Function from Case-Control Studies

Three studies analyzed systemic immune responses using stimulation of whole blood or PBMCs with LPS, a Toll-like receptor 4 agonist with an important role in regulation of immune responses to infection, or phorbol 12-myristate 13-acetate (PMA) and ionomycin [5,9,21] to induce cytokine responses in T cells. All studies found a significant increase in a range of cytokines in individuals with CP compared to controls. Statistically significant increases in cytokines for each study included TNF [5], granulocyte-colony stimulating factor (GM-CSF), IL-8 [21], and IL-1α, IL-2, IL-6 [9]. However, regulation of IL-1β was variable, with one study [9] reporting a significant increase following simulation in CP versus age-matched controls, whereas another study [21] found that IL-1β was significantly reduced in children with CP compared to adult controls. Together, these findings demonstrate that systemic immune response, whilst variable, is altered in participants with CP compared to individuals without CP.

3.3.2. Cross-Sectional Cytokine Analysis from Case-Control Studies

A total of ten studies reported on the inflammatory status in CP; eight studies used serum and plasma to report on systemic inflammation [5,6,9,18,19,22,24,25], one analyzed CSF [20] and one analyzed skeletal muscle [26]. Overall there was significant heterogeneity in sample readouts measured via ELISA. TNF, IL-6 and IL-10 were most commonly reported and thus are discussed below for case–control studies. Plasma and serum ELISA results from three studies indicated significant increases in TNF in CP compared to a range of controls without CP [5,19,24]. One study reported no differences in serum/plasma TNF levels [9]. IL-6 was reported as being significantly increased in CP compared to controls in one study [19]. However, overall, IL-6 levels were reported to be not significantly different in CP versus controls in four other studies [5,6,9,22]. ELISA analysis of IL-10 indicated no significant differences in two studies [6,9] and significant increase in expression in one study of CP versus controls [25]. All other ELISA analytes varied significantly in frequency of reporting/analyzing and the outcome of the results (i.e., significant and non-significant findings, Table 1). Overall, whilst there is mounting data for differing TNF, IL-6 and IL-10 cytokine levels in CP versus controls, directionality was mixed.

Differential mRNA expression between individuals with CP and their corresponding controls was investigated in two studies [5,26]. Significant increases in *IL-1β*, *IL-6*, *TNF* mRNA expression in skeletal muscle biopsies [26], and >2-fold increases in 10 TNF-related genes were found from unstimulated PBMCs in CP compared to controls [5]. Additionally, two studies reported two results that are not included in Table 1. In Lin et al. [5], RNA from PBMCs was analyzed in RT-PCR alongside protein expression via ELISA. This validated that *TLR-4*, inhibitor of nuclear factor kappa-B kinase subunit gamma, c-Jun N-terminal kinases and *TNF* genes were significantly higher in the CP group compared to controls.

3.3.3. Proportions of Immune Cell Types in Case-Controls

One study investigating cellular immunity from whole blood stimulated ex vivo with PMA and ionomycin or relevant cytokine ligand followed by flow cytometry analysis [6], indicated that T-cells of the adaptive and innate immune system (including overall, Vδ2, and CD4− CD8− subtypes) and invariant natural killer T (iNKT) cell percentage frequency and absolute numbers were elevated in school-aged children with CP compared to age-matched controls. Vδ1 T cells, Mucosal-associated invariant T (MAIT) cells and B-cells were significantly reduced in children with CP compared to age-matched controls. These results point to an altered distribution and frequency of adaptive immune cells and innate lymphocytes in children with CP. Importantly this study also highlighted differences in immune cell types between neonates with brain injury versus age-matched controls and children with CP, concluding that the immune system may be primed after earlier insult and immune cell changes may persist into school-age.

3.3.4. Genetic Changes and Gene Expression in Case-Controls

One study utilized quantitative PCR to define inherited cytokine SNPs in a moderately sized (n = 188) cohort of infants with and without CP under three years of age. *IL-10* SNPs including rs3024490 and rs1800871 were found to be significantly higher in individuals with CP compared to controls [25]. The study concluded that the *IL-10* SNPs are strongly related to CP and can affect the expression and secretion of the IL-10 cytokine.

3.4. Additional Findings from Single Arm Studies

Two single arm studies were not presented in Table 1 as they did not have a control group [20,23]. Both studies indicated significant differences/associations in inflammatory biomarkers within their CP cohort. One report [23] identified that total white blood cell counts, neutrophil counts and neutrophil-to-lymphocyte ratio were significantly higher in those with CP living in a rehabilitation center setting than those living at home. The other study [20] also showed that inflammatory analytes such as TNF, IL-6 and IL-10 are positively associated with neurotransmitters and neuropeptides (including agoutirelated peptide and Substance P) within a CP cohort via ELISA analysis of CSF.

3.5. Subgroup Findings of Biomakers in CP across Included Studies

Limited data was reported across five studies [20,22–25] that indicated differences in subgroups of those with CP related to age, CP type, severity, topography and etiology (gestational age). A summary of available findings is reported in Table 2.

3.5.1. Participant Age Subgroup Analysis

One study [24] reported that plasma TNF was significantly increased in younger participants with CP aged 1–3 years compared to those aged 4–12 years with CP. Another study [22], however, detected differences between adults with CP versus children without CP: TGFβ1 and CRP were significantly higher in control children compared to adults with CP. These findings may suggest that participant age may influence the degree of inflammation.

3.5.2. Type and Topography of CP Subgroup Analysis

One study [25] reported that a significant increase in anti-inflammatory IL-10 was found in plasma of the CP group with spastic quadriplegia compared to controls, but not for other CP sub-types. This study also found that frequencies of *IL-10* SNPs of those with spastic quadriplegia versus controls were different for rs1554286, rs151811, rs3024490, rs1800871, and rs1800896. These study results may indicate that the differences in type and topography of CP influence *IL-10* SNPs compared to controls and may represent overall differences in IL-10 production.

3.5.3. Severity of CP Subgroup Analysis

One study found no significant correlations between plasma TNF and CP severity level on the Gross Motor Function Classification System (GMFCS) when looking across the whole group of those with CP [24]. However, significantly increased plasma TNF levels correlated with more severe GMFCS levels in the subgroups of patients with spastic diplegia or quadriplegia as well as those just with spastic diplegia. Moreover, in children with CP in a single arm study [23], neutrophil-to-lymphocyte ratio was significantly increased in children with severe motor impairment (GMFCS IV–V) compared to milder motor impairment (GMFCS II–III). Whilst results are variable, these findings suggest CP severity may be associated with altered inflammatory TNF and neutrophil-to-lymphocyte ratio, particularly in those with more severe CP.

3.5.4. Etiology of CP Subgroup Analysis

One single-arm study [20] specifically aimed to elucidate the relationship between CSF inflammatory markers and CP etiology, specifically in relation to gestational age. When comparing those with CP born preterm and extremely preterm, there was a significant difference in the correlations of expression between TNF and substance P. Overall, there were 14 unique positive analyte correlations within the preterm birth subgroup that were not found in other term and extremely preterm gestational age subgroups, however only four of these were related to inflammation. Additionally, another 24 unique positive analyte correlations were identified for those born extremely preterm compared to term and preterm, with seven directly related to inflammatory analytes. Whilst evidence is limited, these results suggest that gestational age at birth is implicated in greater expression of inflammatory CSF cytokines and neuropeptides.

4. Discussion

4.1. The Evidence of Persistent Inflammation in CP

There is ample evidence to support the role of inflammation in the pathogenesis of brain injury and its detrimental role in neurodevelopment. Preclinical and clinical research has demonstrated that inflammation prevents endogenous brain repair and regeneration following injury [9,30] and persistent inflammation has been postulated to predispose people with CP to further cognitive dysfunction and brain injury [10]. Specifically, published research supports that aberrant glial activation contributes to ongoing injurious brain processes, with advances in neuroimaging supporting this hypothesis [10]. Our findings from this scoping review indicate that some biomarkers of inflammation are altered in people with CP. This has been investigated mostly via alterations in systemic inflammation, commonly assayed from peripheral blood serum and plasma. Changes were detected across markers of inflammatory status measured via cytokine analysis, immune function or genetic changes. Twelve published studies (10 controlled) demonstrate significant changes or associations in one or more inflammatory biomarkers compared to a relevant comparator or within subgroups of those with CP. The most commonly reported changes in inflammation in CP were noted for IL-6, TNF and IL-10. This is consistent with the current literature in infants, with previous systematic reviews indicating that higher circulating levels of cytokines including TNF and IL-6 are associated with abnormal neurological findings, including CP [4].

Importantly, our scoping review highlights that inflammation can persist in CP well beyond the acute brain injury period, with significantly higher systemic inflammation from childhood, through to adolescence compared to relevant controls. Some differences in gene function were found in participant groups aged up to 18 years. We also note that some studies report differences in inflammatory status related to age; two studies showed that younger children have greater systemic inflammation compared to older children and adults. Interestingly, in the one study that identified no significant inflammatory differences in plasma CRP between those with CP and controls, all participants were adults. This may indicate that inflammatory status and immune function change over time and may become less pronounced with increasing age, however more research is required to elucidate this hypothesis.

Whilst there are several common biomarkers under investigation including IL-6, TNF and IL-10, there remains high heterogeneity between studies. A total of 30 biomarkers of inflammation as well as a number of additional genes were examined and studies included varied sample types, analysis methods, controls, and age ranges and presentations of participants. Even across the most commonly investigated cytokines of IL-6, TNF and IL-10, studies reported mixed significant and non-significant findings. Remarkably, the majority of studies conclude that there are differences in inflammation in CP, spanning more than

38 significant findings. These primarily include alterations in systemic inflammatory and immune function, and more research should be prioritized to investigate these changes in more detail and in larger cohorts with harmonized biomarker panels.

4.2. Differences in Persistent Inflammation in CP and within Subgroups

CP is a multifactorial and heterogeneous condition, stemming from diverse etiologies and patterns of brain injury, with varied severity and subtype [31]. As such, we cannot assume that inflammation between two individuals with CP will be the same. Whilst data in this area is still emerging, the findings of our scoping review suggest that the variability between and within studies might be explained by subgroups of people with CP. Specifically, we note that participant age, severity of CP, type/topography and etiology may be important to consider when assessing inflammation. We present that those with more severe CP may have higher levels of inflammation, as well as those with spastic quadriplegia. One included study also supports that those with CP born preterm have distinct inflammatory biomarkers, complementing the previously established literature showing unique biomarker profiles in those born preterm and the risk of developing CP [4]. Whilst this data may indicate that there are differences in inflammation both in CP and within subgroups, there may also be contributing factors to persistent inflammation that are not controlled for. For instance, in more severe CP, individuals may have reoccurring infections, micro-aspirations and more extensive muscle contractures [32]. These factors could ultimately explain the higher levels of systemic inflammation observed in both inflammatory and anti-inflammatory cytokines [24,25]. Moreover, the one study that found higher plasma IL-10 in those with spastic quadriplegia may suggest that increased muscle tone alters inflammation [25]. However, interpretation of this finding is limited as other types of CP are not commonly studied. There remains a notable bias towards participants with spastic CP, likely due to prevalence of spastic CP over other CP types. Additionally, we noted that most included studies of this review had a modest sample size (n $\leq$ 150 total) with a mixed participant demographic. Only one study had a large sample size of n = 479 [25] in order to analyze genetic polymorphisms with subgroup analyses of CP subtypes. Future studies will require larger sample sizes to ensure that further subgroup analyses can be conducted, are adequately powered to detect differences and control for subgroup and comorbidity diversity, especially in this heterogenous and complex condition.

4.3. Targeting Inflammation as a Comorbidity of CP

It has been previously proposed that understanding "persistent inflammatory mechanism could lead to safe and effective therapies to treat brains that have experienced developmental disruption long after the initial insult" [9]. This is an interesting concept, and our scoping review demonstrates that inflammation should be recognized as a comorbidity of CP, that is, a factor that coexists alongside the movement and postural impairments experienced by people with CP. Given the remaining uncertainties highlighted above, more research to improve our understanding of the extent of inflammation, its mechanisms in CP, as well as who are most likely to have inflammation and require treatment, will be important next-steps.

Importantly, whilst this review has highlighted a number of inflammatory biomarkers of interest (e.g., IL-6, TNF and IL-10), it is unlikely that any one given cytokine alone will be implicated in the pathogenesis and long-term inflammatory status associated with CP. Instead, a broad immunomodulatory and anti-inflammatory strategy may have its place and are now under investigation in CP. For instance, cell therapies including umbilical cord blood have been demonstrated to improve motor function in children with CP [33,34] primarily working via immunomodulation. Results from this scoping review support the hypothesis that there is persistent inflammation to be targeted. Uncovering the role, extent and impact of this inflammation may also enable research into more treatments that target inflammation.

Alternatively, given the variability in inflammatory biomarkers and likely heterogeneity in any given person with CP, personalized medicine may also be appropriate approach for targeting inflammation in this condition. For instance, we have demonstrated that levels of systemic inflammatory TNF are higher in three studies with a CP sample of n = 117. If this finding is confirmed in more participants with CP compared to controls, TNF may prove a future target for personalized medicine. There are now success stories from clinical translation of inflammatory cytokine drug targets for neonatal conditions including white matter injury and bronchopulmonary dysplasia. These include the use of IL-1 receptor antagonist (anakinra) [35,36] and IL-37 as an endogenous regulator of inflammation that broadly suppresses innate and adaptive immunity [37,38]. A similar approach may be developed in CP if researchers can establish the importance of any one given cytokine for the condition. Additionally, identifying those with persistent inflammation may also help us to understand responders and non-responders to treatments with an inflammatory mechanism of action.

4.4. Outstanding Unknowns of Inflammation in CP

This review highlights that inflammation has a number of dimensions; there are multiple contributors to inflammation spanning the transcriptome that contains the genome, proteome, metabolome, leading to phenotypic changes [39]. However, the majority of results in this scoping review are only reflective of changes at the protein level mainly from peripheral blood serum and plasma. To continue establishing inflammation as a comorbidity of CP, more research should be done to elucidate the contribution of upstream and downstream inflammatory factors. This may also help to uncover novel targets. Additionally, the origins of inflammation associated with early brain injury and resulting CP are yet to be fully understood. For instance, *is inflammation programmed during the brain injury? If this inflammation remains sustained, why and how*? The causes of inflammation may be cellular or from epigenetic programming from the initiating insult [13]. Not to mention, the confounding role of aberrant inflammation following perinatal infection and neonatal sepsis in CP [40,41], as well as maternal immune activation [42] and congenital abnormalities [43]. Current evidence also suggests that more than 30% of all CP may have a genetic cause, with four main types of DNA variations contributing to the pathogenesis of the condition [7]. Genetic and epigenetic changes may not only increase the risk of developing CP, but may also have a role in ongoing signaling pathway dysregulation like Wnt and glycogen synthase kinase-3. These signaling pathways are critical for brain development and neurogenesis in early life but also support regeneration, synaptic plasticity and homeostasis in adults. Information regarding these changes in CP, such as how inflammation is sustained and the implications of persistent inflammation are only just becoming apparent from research findings.

As we work to comprehend how inflammation is sustained, it is also important to understand whether blood biomarkers of systemic inflammation (as commonly reported in this scoping review), remain a direct indicator of central nervous system inflammation in established CP. Whilst we saw one study that analyzed CSF, more should be done to contrast and compare systemic and central inflammation. Research into neurological conditions including stroke has demonstrated that there is strong peripheral immune-brain crosstalk following injury [44,45]. This crosstalk can be bidirectional and therefore systemic immune responses to stimuli may exacerbate brain inflammation, and vice versa. Not to mention, this review has primarily focused on the detrimental effects of inflammation, however the protective and reparative functions of inflammation in the setting of CP have yet to be considered.

This review also highlights that different causal pathways and etiologies of CP, as well as subtypes, may contribute to persistent inflammation. However, evidence is still emerging and most studies did not provide details of CP etiology or investigate subgroup analyses of participants in relation to inflammation. As stated above, powering for this type of investigation is necessary but will be challenging.

4.5. Limitations

We acknowledge some limitations of this study, primarily the heterogeneity of inflammatory biomarkers that restricted synthesis as well as prevented clear directionality findings of any one given cytokine. This limits the clinical utility of the results and we cannot conclude with certainty what inflammatory biomarkers may contribute as a pathogenic mediator or comorbidity of CP. Inflammatory biomarker heterogeneity also meant that analytes were not discussed in the context of pro- and anti-inflammation. The scoping review was also limited by the ability to adequately define the CP cohort, with only five studies reporting CP etiology and most not reporting all participant features like type, topography and severity of CP. As different causal pathways and presentations of CP may influence inflammatory burden and persistence, adequate reporting of participant demographics remains imperative. Additionally, a number of studies included in this scoping review present results in reference to a range of different comparators. In one instance, children with CP were compared to adult controls and this may have influenced results. Overall, the heterogeneity of the participants, biomarkers studied and methodologies employed, in addition to failures in controlling for factors that may influence results (adequate controls, subgroups of CP), limits the scoping review findings and generalizability to people with CP.

5. Conclusions

This scoping review is the first to present the summarized research to date on inflammation in CP. The available evidence indicates that inflammation is pathogenic in CP and may persist in various forms including immune and genetic changes, years after the original injury. Given that persistent inflammation in CP may have deleterious effects across development and into adulthood, inflammation should be recognised as a comorbidity of CP. Whilst there are a number of common cytokines under investigation including IL-6, TNF and IL-10, there remains high heterogeneity between studies and more research is required to improve the strength of the evidence. It is still unclear why inflammation persists, how it persists and if there are subgroups of people with CP who may have more extensive inflammation. Efforts should be made to investigate inflammation in CP in well-controlled, larger studies that adequately address population heterogeneity, which may in turn help support future research into novel treatment options.

Supplementary Materials: The following supporting information can be downloaded at: https://www.mdpi.com/article/10.3390/jcm11247368/s1, File S1: Preferred Reporting Items for Systematic reviews and Meta-Analyses extension for Scoping Reviews (PRISMA-ScR) Checklist [46].

Author Contributions: Conceptualization: M.C.B.P., I.N., M.F.-E. and R.C.D.; literature search: M.C.B.P.; paper screening, extraction and data synthesis: M.C.B.P. and M.F.-E.; interpretation, manuscript writing and editing: M.C.B.P., M.F.-E., I.N., A.R.G., M.F.-E., M.C.F., R.C.D., C.A.N.-P. and M.F.N. All authors have read and agreed to the published version of the manuscript.

Funding: Authors of this research were supported by NHMRC Investigator Grant 1173584 (CAN-P), the Fielding Foundation Fellowship 2017 (MN).

Institutional Review Board Statement: Not applicable.

Informed Consent Statement: Not applicable.

Data Availability Statement: Data is contained within the article or supplementary material.

Conflicts of Interest: The authors declare no conflict of interest.

References

1. Rosenbaum, P.; Paneth, N.; Leviton, A.; Goldstein, M.; Bax, M.; Damiano, D.; Dan, B.; Jacobsson, B. A report: The definition and classification of cerebral palsy April 2006. *Dev. Med. Child Neurol. Suppl.* **2007**, *109*, 8–14. [PubMed]
2. Girard, S.; Kadhim, H.; Roy, M.; Lavoie, K.; Brochu, M.E.; Larouche, A.; Sébire, G. Role of perinatal inflammation in cerebral palsy. *Pediatr. Neurol.* **2009**, *40*, 168–174. [CrossRef] [PubMed]

3. Hagberg, H.; Gressens, P.; Mallard, C. Inflammation during fetal and neonatal life: Implications for neurologic and neuropsychiatric disease in children and adults. *Ann. Neurol.* **2012**, *71*, 444–457. [CrossRef] [PubMed]
4. Magalhães, R.C.; Moreira, J.M.; Lauar, A.O.; da Silva, A.A.S.; Teixeira, A.L.; ACS, E.S. Inflammatory biomarkers in children with cerebral palsy: A systematic review. *Res. Dev. Disabil.* **2019**, *95*, 103508. [CrossRef] [PubMed]
5. Lin, C.Y.; Chang, Y.C.; Wang, S.T.; Lee, T.Y.; Lin, C.F.; Huang, C.C. Altered inflammatory responses in preterm children with cerebral palsy. *Ann. Neurol.* **2010**, *68*, 204–212. [CrossRef]
6. Taher, N.A.B.; Kelly, L.A.; Al-Harbi, A.I.; O'Dea, M.I.; Zareen, Z.; Ryan, E.; Molloy, E.J.; Doherty, D.G. Altered distributions and functions of natural killer T cells and $\gamma\delta$ T cells in neonates with neonatal encephalopathy, in school-age children at follow-up, and in children with cerebral palsy. *J. Neuroimmunol.* **2021**, *356*, 577597. [CrossRef]
7. Upadhyay, J.; Ansari, M.N.; Samad, A.; Sayana, A. Dysregulation of multiple signaling pathways: A possible cause of cerebral palsy. *Exp. Biol. Med.* **2022**, *247*, 779–787. [CrossRef]
8. Hagberg, H.; Mallard, C.; Ferriero, D.M.; Vannucci, S.J.; Levison, S.W.; Vexler, Z.S.; Gressens, P. The role of inflammation in perinatal brain injury. *Nat. Rev. Neurol.* **2015**, *11*, 192–208. [CrossRef]
9. Zareen, Z.; Strickland, T.; Fallah, L.; McEneaney, V.; Kelly, L.; McDonald, D.; Molloy, E.J. Cytokine dysregulation in children with cerebral palsy. *Dev. Med. Child. Neurol.* **2021**, *63*, 407–412. [CrossRef]
10. Fleiss, B.; Gressens, P. Tertiary mechanisms of brain damage: A new hope for treatment of cerebral palsy? *Lancet Neurol.* **2012**, *11*, 556–566. [CrossRef]
11. Schleiss, M.R. Altered cytokine responses in children with cerebral palsy: Pathogenesis and novel therapies. *Dev. Med. Child Neurol.* **2021**, *63*, 365–366. [CrossRef] [PubMed]
12. Sankowski, R.; Mader, S.; Valdés-Ferrer, S.I. Systemic inflammation and the brain: Novel roles of genetic, molecular, and environmental cues as drivers of neurodegeneration. *Front. Cell. Neurosci.* **2015**, *9*, 28. [CrossRef] [PubMed]
13. Romero, B.; Robinson, K.G.; Batish, M.; Akins, R.E. An Emerging Role for Epigenetics in Cerebral Palsy. *J. Pers. Med.* **2021**, *11*, 1187. [CrossRef] [PubMed]
14. Nelson, K.B.; Grether, J.K.; Dambrosia, J.M.; Walsh, E.; Kohler, S.; Satyanarayana, G.; Nelson, P.G.; Dickens, B.F.; Phillips, T.M. Neonatal cytokines and cerebral palsy in very preterm infants. *Pediatr. Res.* **2003**, *53*, 600–607. [CrossRef]
15. Wang, B.; Wang, F.; Wu, D.; Xu, X.; Yang, L.; Zhu, J.; Yuan, J.; Tang, J. Relationship Between TNF-alpha and the Risk of Cerebral Palsy: A Systematic Review and Meta-Analysis. *Front. Neurol.* **2022**, *13*, 929280. [CrossRef]
16. Peters, M.D.; Godfrey, C.; McInerney, P.; Munn, Z.; Tricco, A.C.; Khalil, H. Chapter 11: Scoping Reviews (2020 Version). Available online: https://doi.org/10.46658/JBIMES-20-12 (accessed on 1 December 2022). [CrossRef]
17. Page, M.J.; McKenzie, J.E.; Bossuyt, P.M.; Boutron, I.; Hoffmann, T.C.; Mulrow, C.D. The PRISMA 2020 statement: An updated guideline for reporting systematic reviews. *BMJ* **2021**, *372*, n71. [CrossRef]
18. Ng, T.K.S.; Coughlan, C.; Heyn, P.C.; Tagawa, A.; Carollo, J.J.; Kua, E.H.; Mahendran, R. Increased plasma brain-derived neurotrophic factor (BDNF) as a potential biomarker for and compensatory mechanism in mild cognitive impairment: A case-control study. *Aging* **2021**, *13*, 22666–22689. [CrossRef]
19. Tao, W.; Wen, F.; Yao, H.; Sun, Y. The Influence of Erythropoietin and Proinflammatory Cytokines in the Development of Cerebral Palsy. *Vasc. Dis. Prev.* **2008**, *5*, 29–32.
20. Goracke-Postle, C.J.; Burkitt, C.C.; Panoskaltsis-Mortari, A.; Ehrhardt, M.; Wilcox, G.L.; Graupman, P.; Partington, M.; Symons, F.J. Expression of and correlational patterns among neuroinflammatory, neuropeptide, and neuroendocrine molecules from cerebrospinal fluid in cerebral palsy. *BMC Neurol.* **2021**, *21*, 384. [CrossRef]
21. Koh, H.; Hwang, K.; Lim, H.Y.; Kim, Y.J.; Lee, Y.H. Mononuclear cells from the cord blood and granulocytecolony stimulating factor-mobilized peripheral blood: Is there a potential for treatment of cerebral palsy? *Neural. Regen. Res.* **2015**, *10*, 2018–2024. [CrossRef]
22. Pingel, J.; Barber, L.; Andersen, I.T.; Walden, F.V.; Wong, C.; Døssing, S.; Nielsen, J.B. Systemic inflammatory markers in individuals with cerebral palsy. *Eur. J. Inflamm.* **2019**, *17*, 2058739218823474. [CrossRef]
23. Riewruja, K.; Amarase, C.; Osateerakun, P.; Weerasopone, S.; Limpaphayom, N.; Honsawek, S. Neutrophil-to-lymphocyte ratio predicts the severity of motor impairment in cerebral palsy children living at home and the rehabilitation center: A comparative study. *Biomed. Rep.* **2020**, *13*, 63. [CrossRef] [PubMed]
24. Wu, J.; Li, X. Plasma Tumor Necrosis Factor-alpha (TNF-alpha) Levels Correlate with Disease Severity in Spastic Diplegia, Triplegia, and Quadriplegia in Children with Cerebral Palsy. *Med. Sci. Monit.* **2015**, *21*, 3868–3874. [CrossRef] [PubMed]
25. Xia, L.; Chen, M.; Bi, D.; Song, J.; Zhang, X.; Wang, Y.; Zhu, D.; Shang, Q.; Xu, F.; Wang, X.; et al. Combined Analysis of Interleukin-10 Gene Polymorphisms and Protein Expression in Children With Cerebral Palsy. *Front. Neurol.* **2018**, *9*, 182. [CrossRef]
26. Von Walden, F.; Gantelius, S.; Liu, C.; Borgstrom, H.; Bjork, L.; Gremark, O.; Stal, P.; Nader, G.A.; Ponte, N.E. Muscle contractures in patients with cerebral palsy and acquired brain injury are associated with extracellular matrix expansion, pro-inflammatory gene expression, and reduced rRNA synthesis. *Muscle Nerve* **2018**, *58*, 277–285. [CrossRef] [PubMed]
27. Lee, Y.-H.; Koh, H.; Hwang, K. Intracellular Expression of Neurotrophic Factors in Mononuclear Cells of Cord Blood and G-CSF-Mobilized Peripheral Blood As a Potential Source for Cellular Therapy. *Blood* **2014**, *124*, 5121. [CrossRef]
28. Kadhim, H.; Sebire, G. Immune mechanisms in the pathogenesis of cerebral palsy: Implication of proinflammatory cytokines and T lymphocytes. *Eur. J. Paediatr. Neurol.* **2002**, *6*, 139–142. [CrossRef]

29. Djukic, M.; Gibson, C.S.; Maclennan, A.H.; Goldwater, P.N.; Haan, E.A.; McMichael, G.; Priest, K.; Dekker, G.A.; Hague, W.M.; Chan, A.; et al. Genetic susceptibility to viral exposure may increase the risk of cerebral palsy. *Aust. N. Z. J. Obstet. Gynaecol.* **2009**, *49*, 247–253. [CrossRef]
30. Kitase, Y.; Chin, E.M.; Ramachandra, S.; Burkhardt, C.; Madurai, N.K.; Lenz, C.; Hoon, A.H., Jr.; Robinson, S.; Jantzie, L.L. Sustained peripheral immune hyper-reactivity (SPIHR): An enduring biomarker of altered inflammatory responses in adult rats after perinatal brain injury. *J. Neuroinflammation* **2021**, *18*, 242. [CrossRef]
31. Sadowska, M.; Sarecka-Hujar, B.; Kopyta, I. Cerebral Palsy: Current Opinions on Definition, Epidemiology, Risk Factors, Classification and Treatment Options. *Neuropsychiatr Dis. Treat.* **2020**, *16*, 1505–1518. [CrossRef]
32. Hollung, S.J.; Bakken, I.J.; Vik, T.; Lydersen, S.; Wiik, R.; Aaberg, K.M.; Andersen, G.L. Comorbidities in cerebral palsy: A patient registry study. *Dev. Med. Child. Neurol.* **2020**, *62*, 97–103. [CrossRef] [PubMed]
33. Novak, I.; Badawi, N.; Hunt, R.; Wallace, E.; Walker, K.; Fahey, M. Stem cell intervention for cerebral palsy: Systematic review with meta-analysis. *Dev. Med. Child Neurol.* **2016**, *58* (Suppl. S3), 40. [CrossRef]
34. Sun, J.M.; Case, L.E.; McLaughlin, C.; Burgess, A.; Skergan, N.; Crane, S.; Jasien, J.M.; Mikati, M.A.; Troy, J.; Kurtzberg, J. Motor function and safety after allogeneic cord blood and cord tissue-derived mesenchymal stromal cells in cerebral palsy: An open-label, randomized trial. *Dev. Med. Child Neurol.* **2022**, *64*, 1477–1486. [CrossRef] [PubMed]
35. Stockx, E.M.; Camilleri, P.; Skuza, E.M.; Churchward, T.; Howes, J.M.; Ho, M.; McDonald, T.; Freezer, N.; Hamilton, G.; Wilkinson, M.H.; et al. New acoustic method for detecting upper airway obstruction in patients with sleep apnoea. *Respirology* **2010**, *15*, 326–335. [CrossRef] [PubMed]
36. McGrath-Morrow, S.A.; Ryan, T.; Riekert, K.; Lefton-Greif, M.A.; Eakin, M.; Collaco, J.M. The impact of bronchopulmonary dysplasia on caregiver health related quality of life during the first 2 years of life. *Pediatr. Pulmonol.* **2013**, *48*, 579–586. [CrossRef]
37. Luo, Y.; Cai, X.; Liu, S.; Wang, S.; Nold-Petry, C.A.; Nold, M.F.; Bufler, P.; Norris, D.; Dinarello, C.A.; Fujita, M. Suppression of antigen-specific adaptive immunity by IL-37 via induction of tolerogenic dendritic cells. *Proc. Natl. Acad. Sci. USA* **2014**, *111*, 15178–15183. [CrossRef]
38. Nold, M.F.; Nold-Petry, C.A.; Zepp, J.A.; Palmer, B.E.; Bufler, P.; Dinarello, C.A. IL-37 is a fundamental inhibitor of innate immunity. *Nat. Immunol.* **2010**, *11*, 1014–1022. [CrossRef]
39. Woolfenden, S.; Farrar, M.A.; Eapen, V.; Masi, A.; Wakefield, C.E.; Badawi, N.; Novak, I.; Nassar, N.; Lingam, R.; Dale, R.C. Delivering paediatric precision medicine: Genomic and environmental considerations along the causal pathway of childhood neurodevelopmental disorders. *Dev. Med. Child Neurol.* **2022**, *64*, 1077–1084. [CrossRef]
40. Sewell, E.; Roberts, J.; Mukhopadhyay, S. Association of Infection in Neonates and Long-Term Neurodevelopmental Outcome. *Clin. Perinatol.* **2021**, *48*, 251–261. [CrossRef]
41. Jain, V.G.; Kline, J.E.; He, L.; Kline-Fath, B.M.; Altaye, M.; Muglia, L.J.; DeFranco, E.A.; Ambalavanan, N.; Parikh, N.A.; Cincinnati Infant Neurodevelopment Early Prediction Study Investigators. Acute histologic chorioamnionitis independently and directly increases the risk for brain abnormalities seen on magnetic resonance imaging in very preterm infants. *Am. J. Obstet. Gynecol.* **2022**, *227*. [CrossRef]
42. Estes, M.L.; McAllister, A.K. Maternal immune activation: Implications for neuropsychiatric disorders. *Science* **2016**, *353*, 772–777. [CrossRef] [PubMed]
43. Wienecke, L.M.; Cohen, S.; Bauersachs, J.; Mebazaa, A.; Chousterman, B.G. Immunity and inflammation: The neglected key players in congenital heart disease? *Heart Fail. Rev.* **2022**, *27*, 1957–1971. [CrossRef] [PubMed]
44. Saand, A.R.; Yu, F.; Chen, J.; Chou, S.H. Systemic inflammation in hemorrhagic strokes—A novel neurological sign and therapeutic target? *J. Cereb. Blood Flow Metab.* **2019**, *39*, 959–988. [CrossRef] [PubMed]
45. Stamatovic, S.M.; Phillips, C.M.; Martinez-Revollar, G.; Keep, R.F.; Andjelkovic, A.V. Involvement of Epigenetic Mechanisms and Non-coding RNAs in Blood-Brain Barrier and Neurovascular Unit Injury and Recovery After Stroke. *Front. Neurosci.* **2019**, *13*, 864. [CrossRef]
46. Tricco, A.C.; Lillie, E.; Zarin, W.; O'Brien, K.K.; Colquhoun, H.; Levac, D.; Moher, D.; Peters, M.D.; Horsley, T.; Weeks, L.; et al. PRISMA Extension for Scoping Reviews (PRISMAScR): Checklist and Explanation. *Ann. Intern. Med.* **2018**, *169*, 467–473. [CrossRef]

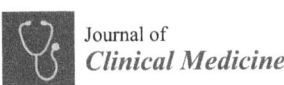

Journal of Clinical Medicine

Article

Correlates of Mental Health in Adolescents and Young Adults with Cerebral Palsy: A Cross-Sectional Analysis of the MyStory Project

Jan Willem Gorter [1,2,*], Darcy Fehlings [2,3], Mark A. Ferro [2,4], Andrea Gonzalez [5], Amanda D. Green [1,2], Sarah N. Hopmans [1,2], Dayle McCauley [2], Robert J. Palisano [2], Peter Rosenbaum [1,2], Brittany Speller [1,2] and on behalf of the MyStory Study Group [†]

[1] Department of Pediatrics, McMaster University, Hamilton, ON L8S 1C7, Canada; amanda.green@communitech.ca (A.D.G.); hopmansn@mcmaster.ca (S.N.H.); rosenbau@mcmaster.ca (P.R.); brittany.speller@mail.utoronto.ca (B.S.)
[2] CanChild Centre for Childhood Disability Research, McMaster University, Hamilton, ON L8S 1C7, Canada; dfehlings@hollandbloorview.ca (D.F.); mark.ferro@uwaterloo.ca (M.A.F.); dmccaul@mcmaster.ca (D.M.); rjp33@drexel.edu (R.J.P.)
[3] Department of Paediatrics, Holland Bloorview Kids Rehabilitation Hospital, University of Toronto, Toronto, ON M4G 1R8, Canada
[4] School of Public Health Sciences, University of Waterloo, Waterloo, ON N2L 3G1, Canada
[5] Department of Psychiatry and Behavioural Neurosciences, McMaster University, Hamilton, ON L8S 1C7, Canada; gonzal@mcmaster.ca
* Correspondence: gorter@mcmaster.ca
[†] Membership of the MyStory Study Group is mentioned in the Acknowledgments.

Abstract: Background: It is important to gain a better understanding of mental health issues in adolescents and young adults (AYA) with cerebral palsy (CP). In this cross-sectional study, we explore if demographics, social and clinical questionnaire scores, and cortisol levels in hair samples from AYA with CP are associated with higher scores on anxiety and/or depression questionnaires. Methods: Data from a community-based sample of 63 AYA with CP (30 females; ages 16 to 30 (median age of 25)) were analyzed. Forty-one (65%) participants (20 females) provided a hair sample. Outcomes were assessed using bivariate linear regression analyses and hierarchical regression analyses. Results: Clinical depressive and anxiety symptoms were present in 33% and 31% of participants, respectively. Family functioning, B = 9.62 (95%CI: 5.49–13.74), fatigue, B = 0.15 (95%CI: 0.05–0.25), and pain, B = 1.53 (95%CI: 0.48–2.58) were statistically significant predictors of depressive symptoms. Fatigue, B = 0.24 (95%CI: 0.12–0.35) and pain, B = 1.63 (95%CI: 0.33–2.94) were statistically significant predictors of anxiety. Cortisol levels from hair samples were not found to be associated with depressive symptoms or anxiety. Conclusions: A high prevalence of mental health problems and co-occurring physical problems was found in AYA with CP. Integrating mental support into regular care for AYA with CP is recommended.

Keywords: mental health; anxiety; depression; cerebral palsy; adolescence; young adults

1. Introduction

There is an increasing movement in the clinical community to re-frame our understanding of disabilities, such as cerebral palsy (CP), as childhood-onset disorders rather than disorders of childhood. Children with CP can expect a longer life span due to medical advances, but they are also more likely to require ongoing supports and services as they age beyond what is required for their typically developing peers [1–5]. Young adults with CP can face challenges with aspects of health and wellness, education, employment, accessible housing, and social relationships. Compared to peers without disabilities, adolescents and young adults (AYA) with CP often report lower employment rates, are less likely to participate in leisure/social activities or pursue post-secondary education, and often are more dependent on their families for living arrangements [3,6–8]. Additional challenges include a lack of access to health care; professionals' lack of knowledge of CP; and lack of information and uncertainty regarding the transition to adulthood process [3,7,9,10].

Chronic health conditions (CHC), including CP, can increase the risk of developing problems related to mental health, chronic pain, and fatigue [9,11–18]. Further, stress, chronic pain, and mental health issues are highly comorbid in patients with CHCs [11,15,19], and this co-morbidity may worsen an individual's outcomes [20]. Most youth mental health studies include a range of CHCs, including epilepsy and juvenile diabetes. However, young adults with physical disabilities have higher scores on depression and anxiety symptoms than those with other CHCs [16,21,22]. Most relevant for the current purpose, one study observed a four-fold increase in the prevalence of emotional disorders in children with CP between seven and eleven-years of age [23] and a systematic review has suggested that children and adolescents with CP may be at an increased risk of developing mental health problems [24]. Indeed, mental illness was the third most common reason for hospital admissions in young adults with CP [21], and recent large database studies have elucidated both a higher prevalence and risk of mental health disorders among adults with CP compared to the general population [17,18]. Given the high prevalence of mental health disorders and comparatively lower frequency of check-ups in this population, many AYA who would benefit from interventions may go unnoticed or treated.

The review [24] further highlights many gaps in the literature, including a reliance on parent-reports for mental health symptoms and an under-reporting of rates of mental health issues in older-adolescent or young adult age groups [24]. CP is one of the most common neurodevelopmental disorders (2 in 1000 live births) and can occur alongside other cognitive and behavioural issues, including autism spectrum disorder, attention deficit hyperactivity disorder (ADHD), and anxiety disorders [8,19,25]. This highlights a need for more targeted research into the mental health of these AYA [24,26]. In this spirit, the current study was conducted to examine the psychosocial and biological correlates of mental health in AYA with CP.

To ease the transition from adolescence into adulthood for AYA with CP, it is important to gain a better understanding of the self-reported prevalence of mental health issues, including symptoms of anxiety and depression. Further, there are important gaps in our understanding of physical and psychosocial factors that might contribute to the development of mental health issues in AYA with CP, either as markers of vulnerability or as co-morbid issues that might aggravate symptoms. The "MyStory" project is a study within the Childhood Cerebral Palsy Integrated Neuroscience Discovery Network (CP-NET) coordinated by CanChild, McMaster University. The project is a longitudinal study investigating the course of physical health, mental health and well-being in AYA with CP. This project includes yearly screening questionnaires on fatigue, pain, anxiety, depression, family functioning, quality of life, and also investigates neurophysiological factors, including changes in stress hormones (cortisol levels). Hair cortisol has been used as a biomarker of hypothalamic–pituitary–adrenal axis activity, and exposure to systemic cortisol over time. It has been associated with a variety of conditions, including changes in mental and physical health, early life trauma, ADHD, worker burnout, and anxiety or depression in different age groups [27–34]. To date, however, no research has explored the use of hair cortisol as a biomarker for mental or physical health in AYA with CP. In this study, we explore cross-sectionally some of the initial relationships discovered in the Year 1 data, including prevalence rates of anxiety and depressive symptoms, and association of demographics (age, gender, gross motor function level), social (family functioning) and clinical (pain, fatigue) questionnaire scores, on anxiety and depression questionnaire scores. We will also begin to investigate relationships between anxiety and depression questionnaire scores and hair cortisol levels.

2. Materials and Methods

2.1. Study Design, Setting and Participants

A sample of AYA (ages 16 to 30) was recruited through CanChild at McMaster University using a variety of methods (posters, recruitment letters, emails). Recruitment strategies included mailing or emailing recruitment letters to individuals who previously participated in CanChild research projects, mailing recruitment letters to eligible participants through a Children's Treatment Centre in Windsor, Ontario, in clinic recruitment at hospitals across Ontario (St. Catharines, Toronto, London, and Hamilton), and organizations supporting people with disabilities sharing the recruitment poster to their communities.

The MyStory project is designed as a quantitative, longitudinal study (though the data subset for this study design is cross-sectional), where participants complete a series of questionnaires and provide hair samples at the same time. All participants completed the Year 1 questionnaires between 2014–2018. Participants participated in the study voluntarily and had the option to complete as many Year 1 questionnaires as desired. Participants were still eligible to participate and complete questionnaires if they declined to provide a hair sample. Participants needed to meet the following criteria to be included in the study: (1) be between the ages of 16 and 30; (2) have a confirmed diagnosis of CP in childhood; (3) reside in Ontario, Canada at registration; (4) be capable of consenting to participation; (5) be able to complete online questionnaires (alone or with assistance); and (6) be able to follow simple instructions.

All aspects of this study were approved by the Hamilton Integrated Research Ethics Board, and recruitment materials at external sites were approved by their relevant ethics boards. All study personnel who had contact with any participants received suicide risk assessment training via the Columbia Suicide Severity Scale (C-SSRS) training module [35]. Should a participant report thoughts of death or suicide, a standardized follow-up protocol was observed including provision of and/or contacting resources and caregivers.

2.2. Patient and Public Involvement

We designed the study based on clinical experiences and the needs expressed by AYA with CP and their families. The Ontario Federation for Cerebral Palsy, a non-profit organization in Ontario that supports people with CP, has been involved since study conception and are key partners in the MyStory study. During the data collection of the MyStory study, participants expressed a desire to share their experiences more broadly and participated in knowledge dissemination activities such as webinars (www.cp-net.org, accessed on 1 April 2022.

2.3. Data Collection and Instruments

Demographic characteristics, including age and gender, and gross motor function were collected from participants. Participants completed the self-reported questionnaires online or by paper and pencil at their homes, by themselves or with the assistance of a family member or peer. Participants' functional capabilities were determined using decision-making questions around major life issues (who decides daily activities and how spending money is used) and daily routine issues (who decides what is eaten, what is done for fun, and the time for bed).

The description of questionnaires are as follows (See Table 1 for summary).

2.3.1. State-Trait Anxiety Inventory (STAI

A 40-item questionnaire based on a 1 to 4 Likert scale. The STAI measures two types of anxiety: state anxiety (S-Anxiety), or anxiety about an event, and trait anxiety (T-Anxiety), or anxiety level as a personal characteristic [36]. The MyStory study asked participants the S-Anxiety questions allowing for understanding on how participants were feeling at the time they completed the questionnaire across time points to better detect longitudinal change [37]. An overall score for S-Anxiety is calculated as a total sum, ranging from 20 to 80, with a higher score indicating greater anxiety. Scores equaling or higher than 40 are thought to suggest possible clinical anxiety [36]. We did not score the S-Anxiety scale if more than 10% of data were missing [38]. The S-Anxiety scale has high internal consistency (α = 0.86–0.95) [36].

2.3.2. Center for Epidemiological Studies Depression Scale (CES-D)

A 20-item self-report instrument that evaluates depressive symptoms defined by the American Psychiatric Association Diagnostic and Statistical Manual (DSM-IV) for a major depressive episode [39]. Participants respond on a 4-point Likert scale, where higher scores indicate higher levels of depression. The overall score for the CES-D is calculated as a total sum, ranging from 0 to 60. Individuals with questionnaire scores equaling 16 or higher are considered to be demonstrating possible clinical depressive symptoms [40,41]. We did not score the CES-D scale when more than four questions were missing following developer guidelines. The CES-D scale has adequate test–retest reliability (0.45–0.70) and high internal consistency (α = 0.85–0.90) [39].

2.3.3. McMaster Family Assessment Device (FAD)

The updated 60-item questionnaire evaluates families on the dimensions of the McMaster Model of Family Functioning [42]. Following the instructions of the questionnaire, youth defined what family meant to them. The questionnaire includes sub-scales on problem solving, communication, roles, affective response, affective involvement, behaviour control and general functioning. This study used the 'general functioning' sub-scale to capture the overall level of family functioning. The general functioning sub-scale contains 12 items to assess overall family health, such as making decisions and feelings of acceptance within the family [42]. Responses are measured on a 4-point Likert scale from 1, indicating strongly agree, to 4, indicating strongly disagree. Total scores are calculated as an average of the 12 items ranging from 1, indicating "best functioning", and 4, indicating "worse functioning" of the family [42,43]. Problematic family functioning is present when individuals score 2.00 or higher in the general functioning sub-scale. We did not score the sub-scale if more than 40% of responses were missing [42]. The FAD general functioning sub-scale has adequate test–retest reliability (0.71) and high internal consistency (α = 0.92) [43].

2.3.4. Fatigue Impact and Severity Self-Assessment (FISSA)

This 37-item fatigue questionnaire allows participants to respond to 30 questions on a 5-point Likert scale (higher scores indicate greater fatigue) and 6 open-ended questions on the impact, severity, and management of experienced fatigue [44]. One question allows participants to respond to a 7-point Likert scale to account for the number of days each week fatigue is experienced. This study used the score for the 31 questions using Likert scale responses, which are used to index the level of fatigue in terms of impact and severity, calculated as a total sum for the fatigue level, with scores ranging from 31 (less fatigue) to 157 (more fatigue). The FISSA was not scored if more than 10% of data were missing [38]. This questionnaire was designed specifically for individuals with CP and has high internal consistency (α = 0.95) and adequate test–retest reliability (0.75) [44].

2.3.5. Pain

This scale, developed by researchers at CanChild, evaluates pain severity and location [45]. It initially asked participants if they had experienced physical pain in the past month. If they responded 'yes', then they were asked the severity of pain and if the pain got in the way of their daily activities on a 10-point Likert scale. The scale then asked participants to indicate the body regions where they had experienced pain. For this study, we calculated the number of painful sites reported by participants as a total sum, as this was the critical measure used in the study that developed this scale [45]. Scores ranged from 0 to 10, with higher scores indicating more painful body sites. We excluded any questionnaires with missing data.

2.3.6. Gross Motor Function Classification System (GMFCS)

Participants functional status was collected using the Gross Motor Function Classification System that categorizes physical abilities on a 5-level scale: Level I—walks without restrictions; Level II—walks without assistive devices but has limitations walking in community and outdoors; Level III—walks with assistive mobility devices and has limitations walking in community and outdoors; Level IV—self-mobility with limitations, may use power mobility devices in the community and outdoors; and Level V—self-mobility with severe limitations even when using assistive technology [46].

2.4. Hair Samples

Participants provided hair samples to assess cortisol levels. Hair cortisol analysis is an emerging biomarker for chronic stress, as systemic cortisol is understood to be incorporated into the hair shaft during hair growth [47]. Participants, with the assistance of a researcher or a family member/friend, provided a hair sample (approx. 3 mm in diameter—50 to 80 strands) from the posterior vertex of the head, and cut as close to the scalp as possible. Studies have demonstrated that hair cortisol levels are positively correlated with measures of perceived stress [30,32,47,48] and permit the retroactive assessment of cortisol for at least three months [49–51]. Along with the hair samples, participants completed a biological questionnaire to collect information on current medications, chemical treatments to hair, smoke exposure, and ethnicity, among other factors. Hair samples were assayed using a validated ELISA protocol to determine concentrations of cortisol in the sample (picogram (pg)/milligram (mg)). The ELISA protocol is outlined in Appendix A.

Table 1. Variables included in the dataset.

Measure	Type	Number of Items	Constructs Examined
Age (years)	Continuous	1	Demographics
Gender (male, female)	Binary	1	Demographics
Gross Motor Functional Classification System (GMFCS)	Ordinal	1	Gross motor function level
State-Trait Anxiety Inventory (STAI), State Anxiety (S-Anxiety)	Continuous *	20	State Anxiety Present; State Anxiety Absent
Center for Epidemiological Studies Depression Scale (CES-D)	Continuous *	20	Negative Affect; Positive Affect; Anhedonia; Somatic Symptoms
McMaster Family Assessment Device (FAD), General Functioning Sub-Scale	Continuous *	12	General Functioning; Overall Level of Family Functioning
Fatigue Impact and Severity Self-Assessment Tool (FISSA)	Continuous *	31	Impact of Fatigue on Daily Living; Fatigue Management and Activity Modification
Pain	Continuous	10	Number of Painful Body Sites

* Classifying scores on Likert-scale questionnaires as continuous is somewhat disputed, but variables will be treated as continuous for this project [52].

2.5. Statistical Analyses

All of the surveys were scored according to the individual survey instructions, including instruction around missing data. Descriptive statistics are reported based on the spread and central tendencies of variables. For each outcome (depression and anxiety, respectively) we completed bivariate linear regression analyses to determine if one or more of our demographic variables (age, gender, GMFCS), scores on questionnaires (FAD, FISSA, pain), or cortisol levels were associated with higher scores on either (A) the CES-D depression scale, or (B) the S-Anxiety scale. We also completed hierarchical regression analyses with CES-D and S-Anxiety and included predictor variables in four blocks: (1) Demographics—age, gender (reference is female), GMFCS (reference is Level 1); (2) Social—FAD; (3) Clinical—

FISSA, pain; and (4) Biological—cortisol levels. All dependent variables were assessed for normality and linearity. All statistical tests were performed as two-tailed, and a statistically significant effect was observed at a $p \leq 0.05$ with 95% confidence intervals. All statistical analyses were performed using SPSS 25.

3. Results

Of the 70 AYA with CP that provided consent to participate in this study, 63 (90%) participants completed at least one questionnaire (FAD, FISSA, CES-D, S-Anxiety, or pain) in Year 1. Of the 37 participants (58%) who completed the GMFCS questionnaire, 14 (38%) identified as Level I; 6 (16%) identified as Level II; 6 (16%) identified as Level III; 10 (27%) identified as Level IV; and 1 (3%) identified as Level V. Most participants decided major life issues and their daily routine alone or in partnership with someone else (Table 2).

Table 2. Participant functional capabilities.

Variable	n	Decides Alone (%)	Decides with Someone Else (%)	Someone Else Decides (%)
Daily activity	53	36 (68%)	16 (30%)	1 (2%)
Use of spending money	53	34 (64%)	17 (32%)	2 (4%)
What is eaten	52	30 (58%)	19 (36%)	3 (6%)
What is done for fun	52	39 (75%)	13 (25%)	0 (0%)
Time for bed	52	43 (83%)	8 (15%)	1 (2%)

Participants who completed at least one questionnaire included 30 (48%) females and 33 (52%) males with a median age of 25 (IQR 23.00–27.00). Among those who completed questionnaires, 51 participants (81%) completed five questionnaires (FAD, FISSA, CES-D, S-Anxiety, pain). Baseline descriptive characteristics, including median questionnaire scores, and the number of participants who completed each questionnaire, are provided in Table 3. We collected 47 hair samples from individuals at the first time point. One individual provided a hair sample, but did not complete any of the questionnaires included in this analysis. Three hair samples could not be processed due to insufficient weight, and two hair samples were removed from our analysis as outliers, resulting in 41/63 (65%) hair samples available (20 females, 21 males).

Table 3. Descriptive characteristics of baseline variables.

Variable	n	Data Missing (n)	Median (1st Quartile, 3rd Quartile)	Mean	Standard Deviation	Min, Max
Age (years)	63	-	25.00 (23.00, 27.00)	24.46	3.30	16.00, 29.00
STAI	58	5	32.00 (25.00, 43.00)	34.96	12.09	20.00, 64.00
CESD	61	2	9.00 (4.00, 17.50)	12.54	10.67	0.00, 46.00
FAD	61	2	1.82 (1.45, 2.45)	1.89	0.58	1.00, 3.27
FISSA	59	4	88.00 (67.00, 105.00)	85.69	24.61	33.00, 141.00
Pain	57	6	2.00 (1.00, 5.00)	2.89	2.389	0.00, 9.00
Cortisol (ng/mL)	41	22	4.22 (2.89, 5.88)	5.09	3.87	0.33, 20.19

Note: As variables were not normally distributed, the median, 1st quartile, and 3rd quartile were reported. The FISSA was normally distributed and Mean and SD (Standard Deviation) were reported. FISSA = Fatigue Impact and Severity Self-Assessment, Pain = Painful Body Sites, FAD = Family Assessment Device, General Functioning Sub-Scale, CESD = Center for Epidemiological Studies Depression Scale, STAI = State-Trait Anxiety Inventory, State Anxiety Scale, Cortisol = Hair cortisol concentration (pg/mg). Data missing = number of data points excluded from analysis due to missing data.

In our samples, 20/61 (33%) of participants had CES-D questionnaire scores equal to or higher than 16, indicative of possible clinical depressive symptoms. Similarly, among participants who completed the S-Anxiety Scale, 18/58 (31%) of participants had a score higher than 40, suggesting possible clinical anxiety. Among the 56 participants who completed both the CES-D and S-Anxiety Scale, 10 participants (18%) scored higher than the cut-offs on both measures, indicating possible clinical depressive symptoms and anxiety. Additionally, among participants who completed the FAD 'general functioning' sub-scale, 25/61 (41%) scored 2.00 or above suggesting unhealthy overall level of family functioning.

3.1. Correlates of Depression

3.1.1. Bivariate Regression Analysis: CES-D

Bivariate regression analyses examined the relationship between age, gender, GMFCS, family functioning (FAD) scores, fatigue (FISSA), pain, and cortisol as predictors of CES-D score. Using regression diagnostics for each analyses, we removed one data point from all analyses that had high residuals. Removal of these data points did not influence the significance of the independent variables.

FAD was statistically significant, $R^2 = 0.28$, $F(1, 56) = 21.80$, $p < 0.001$, Adj $R^2 = 0.27$, indicating around 27% of CES-D variation was predicted by family functioning. FISSA was statistically significant, $R^2 = 0.15$, $F(1, 54) = 9.63$, $p = 0.003$, Adj $R^2 = 0.14$, indicating around 14% of CES-D variation was predicted by FISSA scores. Pain was also statistically significant, $R^2 = 0.14$, $F(1, 53) = 8.575$, $p = 0.005$, Adj $R^2 = 0.12$, indicating around 12% of CES-D variation was predicted by total number of painful body sites. All effect sizes are small according to Cohen's d [53]. Regression coefficients and standard errors are in Table 4.

Table 4. Summary of regression models—predictors of CES-D scores.

Variable	n	B	SE$_b$	ß	95%CI
Age	60	−0.12	0.39	−0.04	−0.90–0.66
Male	60	−3.10	2.53	−0.16	−8.16–1.96
GMFCS Level 2	35	7.21	4.04	0.31	−1.04–15.47
GMFCS Level 3	35	7.41	4.32	0.29	−1.40–16.23
GMFCS Level 4	35	−1.68	3.54	−0.08	−8.90–5.55
GMFCS Level 5	35	15.21	8.57	0.29	−2.30–32.72
FAD	58	9.62	2.06	0.53	5.49–13.74
FISSA	56	0.15	0.05	0.39	0.05–0.25
Pain	55	1.53	0.52	0.37	0.48–2.58
Cortisol	39	−0.18	0.40	−0.71	−1.00–0.64

Note: B = unstandardized regression coefficient, SE$_b$ = Standard Error of the coefficient; ß = standardized coefficient, CES-D = Center for Epidemiological Studies Depression Scale, FAD = Family Assessment Device, General Functioning Sub-Scale, FISSA = Fatigue Impact and Severity Self-Assessment, Pain = Painful Body Sites, GMFCS = Gross Motor Function Classification System, Cortisol = Hair cortisol.

3.1.2. Hierarchical Regression Analysis: CES-D

We examined the relationship between demographic (age, gender, GMFCS), social (FAD), clinical (FISSA, pain), and biological (cortisol levels) predictors of CES-D using a hierarchical regression. Using regression diagnostics, we identified one data point that had high leverage and residual, and it was removed from the model.

The first two models that added demographic and social variables were not statistically significant. The addition of clinical variables made the model statistically significant with the predictor variables accounting for around 41.6% variation in CES-D. The final model with all variables including cortisol was statistically significant accounting for approximately 62.9% variation in CES-D scores. This is a medium effect size according to Cohen's d [53]. Regression coefficients and standard errors are presented in Table 5.

Table 5. Hierarchical regression model summary—CES-D.

Characteristics	Step 1	Step 2	Step 3	Step 4
Demographics				
Age	−0.07 (−1.25, 1.11)	−0.01 (−1.21, 1.19)	−0.22 (−1.31, 0.88)	−1.20 (−2.40, −0.00)
Male Gender	−3.48 (−11.47, 4.51)	−2.21 (−10.84, 6.42)	−10.24 (−19.36, −1.12)	−6.16 (−14.25, 1.93)
GMFCS 2	0.70 (−17.09, 18.48)	1.09 (−16.94, 19.13)	−10.09 (−26.90, 6.72)	−12.13 (−25.80, 1.54)
GMFCS 3	7.59 (−2.99, 18.16)	7.91 (−2.83, 18.64)	0.90 (−12.22, 14.03)	4.81 (−6.26, 15.89)
GMFCS 4	0.23 (−8.47, 8.94)	2.21 (−7.76, 12.19)	−6.20 (−17.19, 4.79)	−2.80 (−12.11, 6.51)
GMFCS 5	17.63 (−0.19, 35.46)	17.69 (−0.37, 35.75)	8.06 (−8.22, 24.33)	19.21 (3.17, 35.24)
Social				
FAD		3.34 (−4.51, 11.19)	−7.78 (−18.05, 2.50)	−9.78 (−18.24, −1.33)
Clinical				
FISSA			0.34 (0.10, 0.593)	0.44 (0.22–0.66)
Pain			−1.82 (−4.14, 0.51)	−3.34 (−5.59, −1.08)
Biological				
Cortisol				−1.30 (−2.37, −0.23)
Model Fit				
R^2	0.37	0.84	0.68	0.81

Note: Results are presented as unstandardized regression coefficients and associated 95% confidence intervals. CES-D = Center for Epidemiological Studies Depression Scale, FAD = Family Assessment Device, General Functioning Sub-Scale, FISSA = Fatigue Impact and Severity Self-Assessment, Pain = Painful Body Sites, GMFCS = Gross Motor Function Classification System, Cortisol = Hair cortisol.

3.2. Correlates of Anxiety

3.2.1. Bivariate Regression Analysis: S-Anxiety

Bivariate regression analyses examined the relationship between age, gender, GMFCS, family functioning (FAD) scores, fatigue (FISSA), pain, and cortisol as predictors of S-Anxiety score. FISSA was statistically significant, $R^2 = 0.23$, $F(1, 55) = 16.74$, $p < 0.001$, Adj $R^2 = 0.22$, indicating around 22% of S-Anxiety variation was predicted by FISSA scores. Pain was statistically significant, $R^2 = 0.10$, $F(1, 55) = 6.26$, $p = 0.015$, Adj $R^2 = 0.09$, indicating around 9% of S-Anxiety variation was predicted by total number of painful body sites. All effect sizes are small according to Cohen's d [53]. When compared to GMFCS Level 1, participants with GMFCS Level 3 were statistically significant, $p = 0.033$. Regression coefficients and standard errors are in Table 6. As seen in Table 6, all statistically significant variables had positive regression weights.

3.2.2. Hierarchical Regression Analysis: S-Anxiety

We examined the relationship between demographic (age, gender, GMFCS), social (FAD), clinical (FISSA, pain), and biological (cortisol levels) predictors of S-Anxiety using a hierarchical regression. Using regression diagnostics, we identified one data point that had high residual, and it was removed from the model.

The second model that included demographic and social predictor variables was statistically significant accounting for around 38.7% of variation in S-Anxiety scores. No other models were statistically significant. Regression coefficients and standard errors are in Table 7.

Table 6. Summary of regression models—predictors of S-Anxiety scores.

Variable	n	B	SE$_b$	ß	95%CI
Age	58	−0.26	0.49	−0.07	−1.25–0.73
Male	58	−2.87	3.19	−0.12	−9.26–3.52
GMFCS Level 2	36	4.80	5.62	0.15	−6.65–16.25
GMFCS Level 3	36	11.83	5.26	0.41	1.11–22.56
GMFCS Level 4	36	4.00	4.46	0.17	−5.10–13.10
GMFCS Level 5	36	3.00	11.16	0.05	−19.76–25.76
FAD	58	4.60	2.72	0.22	−0.84–10.05
FISSA	57	0.24	0.06	0.48	0.12–0.35
Pain	57	1.63	0.65	0.32	0.33–2.94
Cortisol	38	0.04	0.53	0.01	−1.03–1.12

Note: B = unstandardized regression coefficient, SE$_b$ = Standard Error of the coefficient; ß = standardized coefficient, CES-D = Center for Epidemiological Studies Depression Scale, FAD = Family Assessment Device, General Functioning Sub-Scale, FISSA = Fatigue Impact and Severity Self-Assessment, Pain = Painful Body Sites, GMFCS = Gross Motor Function Classification System, Cortisol = Hair cortisol.

Table 7. Hierarchical regression model summary—S-Anxiety.

Characteristics	Step 1	Step 2	Step 3	Step 4
Demographics				
Age	−0.67 (−1.98, 0.64)	−0.63 (−1.77, 0.52)	−0.64 (−1.85, 0.56)	−0.62 (−2.29, 1.06)
Male Gender	3.44 (−5.58, 12.46)	4.67 (−3.28, 12.61)	1.34 (−6.97, 9.64)	1.17 (−9.82, 12.16)
GMFCS 2	−1.41 (−21.18, 18.36)	−0.05 (−17.35, 17.24)	−6.91 (−24.76, 10.95)	−6.89 (−25.85, 12.07)
GMFCS 3	15.17 (2.94, 27.40)	15.52 (4.84, 26.20)	10.55 (−2.67, 23.77)	10.39 (−4.99, 25.77)
GMFCS 4	10.35 (0.66, 20.04)	12.45 (3.78, 21.12)	9.47 (0.58, 18.37)	9.30 (−2.24, 20.84)
GMFCS 5	6.92 (−12.91, 26.75)	7.58 (−9.73, 24.90)	1.26 (−16.15, 18.67)	0.91 (−22.15, 23.96)
Social				
FAD		6.231 (0.57, 11.89)	2.60 (−4.05, 9.25)	2.57 (−4.55, 9.70)
Clinical				
FISSA			0.20 (−0.02, 0.43)	0.2 (−0.04, 0.44)
Pain			−0.92 (−3.51, 1.66)	−0.88 (−4.05, 2.28)
Biological				
Cortisol				0.04 (−1.41, 1.48)
Model Fit				
R^2	0.43	0.60	0.72	0.72

Note: Results are presented as unstandardized regression coefficients and associated 95% confidence intervals. CES-D = Center for Epidemiological Studies Depression Scale, FAD = Family Assessment Device, General Functioning Sub-Scale, FISSA = Fatigue Impact and Severity Self-Assessment, Pain = Painful Body Sites, GMFCS = Gross Motor Function Classification System, Cortisol = Hair cortisol.

4. Discussion and Conclusions

The cross-sectional (Year 1) data in the MyStory project indicates that family functioning (FAD), fatigue, and pain are statistically significant predictors of higher CES-D scores, suggesting that poorer overall family functioning, fatigue, and more painful body sites play a role in increased depressive symptoms in AYA with CP. Similarly, for the S-Anxiety, fatigue (FISSA) and pain were statistically significant positive predictors of anxiety scores, suggesting that fatigue and more painful body sites plays a role in increased anxiety symptoms. However, the effect sizes were small. The hierarchical regression analyses indicate that demographic, social, clinical, and biological factors influence depressive symptoms in AYA with CP.

4.1. Mental Health and Cerebral Palsy

This study further substantiates that anxiety and depression are a substantial problem in AYA with CP [16–18]. The high prevalence of AYA with CP who scored above the cut-offs indicating possible clinical anxiety (31%) and depressive symptoms (33%) in this study is similar to findings in recent database studies from the United States and United Kingdom that used diagnostic codes to identify AYA with CP with formally diagnosed mental health disorders. Whitney et al. [17] found that 28.6% of women 19.5% of men with CP had anxiety related or mood disorders. Smith et al. [18] found those with CP had an increased risk of developing anxiety (hazard ratio, 1.40; 95%CI, 1.21–1.63) and depression (hazard ratio, 1.43; 95%CI, 1.24–1.64) when compared to those without CP. This study included self-reported anxiety and depressive symptoms, which may account for the slightly higher prevalence when compared to studies using diagnostic codes. AYA with CP often do not receive a formal diagnosis of anxiety and/or depression or are considered to not have symptoms severe enough to receive a formal diagnosis. Those experiencing barriers to accessing mental health services describe losing hope as they have inadequate support and funding to assist them with their symptoms [54]. While the median age of participants in our study was 25 years of age, studies focusing on children and adolescents with CP have shown similar prevalence in anxiety and depression [16,19]. The accumulation of this research indicates that mental health issues, such as anxiety and depression, are present throughout the life course of individuals with CP.

A recent review highlighted that aging with CP can be accompanied by a myriad of new and changing neurologic symptoms including pain and fatigue, which are related to mental health conditions such as depression and anxiety [55]. Indeed, pain and fatigue are commonly reported in AYA with CP [56–59] and have been shown to be associated with depressive symptoms and mood (affective) disorders in adults with CP [60] and groups with other conditions [15,61]. This study supports these findings and finds those with more painful body sites also have higher depression scores. Pain can be debilitating and have a substantial impact on individuals' daily functioning, ability to sleep, and quality of life [54,58]. Stress and anxiety has also been reported by AYA with CP as a contributing factor to fatigue [62].

Furthermore, positive family functioning and peer support are key factors that impact mental health [63]. This study found that over 40% of participants reported unhealthy overall family functioning and lower family functioning was a statistically significant predictor of higher depressive scores. We considered physical health (fatigue and pain) and social relationships (family functioning) in this study, but our models could only account for a small portion of the variation in anxiety and depressive scores. Other factors that could be considered in the future to explain the variation include measuring if AYA with CP have meaningful participation at work and in recreation activities, social isolation, and stress associated with school, work, peer relationships, managing finances, and making health care decisions [54]. A decline in social participation can also contribute to a decline in mental health [64].

This is the first study, to our knowledge, that explores the relationship between cortisol from hair samples and anxiety and depression symptoms in AYA with CP. While cortisol was not found to be a predictor of anxiety or depression, the sample size for the cortisol regression analyses only included 38 participants. Cortisol was a statistically significant unique predictor of depressive symptoms in the hierarchical regression model, however the model only included 21 participants with seven possible predictors, suggesting that we may have been nearing the limits of the predictive power of this model given our sample size. A larger sample size with additional hair samples would help us to address some of these shortcomings, and better address the question of whether cortisol is a useful biomarker for mental health in AYA with CP.

4.2. Recommendations for Healthcare System and Providers

Based on the findings from this study, clinicians may benefit from noting that AYA with CP who are reporting high levels of fatigue, more sites of pain, or appear to be having difficulties with their families, may be at a higher risk of developing a clinical anxiety or depressive disorder. Given our finding that around 30% of our sample experience clinically relevant levels of anxiety or depressive symptoms, this area of research is clearly deserving of more focus from the medical community. Integrating mental health services, such as screening tools [65] and timely referrals to mental health professionals, into regular follow up of AYA with CP is recommended due to this high prevalence.

Any mental health services should be sustained when adolescents with CP transition into adult care services (around the age of 18 in Ontario, Canada) well into young adulthood (age 30).

Indeed, a life course approach to care—which highlights the role of person-environment interactions as a key process by which health development occurs—encourages coordination and continuity of healthcare between family-centered service in pediatrics to an individual-centered environment in adult care [66]. This is especially important considering the added challenges surrounding lack of support, access and knowledge reported by AYA with CP during their transition between these two systems, and in turn the potential impact of these challenges on long-term health trajectory [67]. Further, this approach broadens the scope of environmental factors that contribute to health and encourages interventions that alleviate barriers to life experiences and social participation [66]. Indeed, initiatives including mindfulness-based stress reduction programs delivered virtually show promising benefits by educating and enhancing individuals ability to cope with their CP-related symptoms, such as pain and fatigue [68]. Social connectedness, acupuncture, massage, and leisure activities have also been reported to be helpful coping strategies for physical and mental health symptoms [54,69]. Additional strategies to manage family functioning, pain, and fatigue in AYA with CP tailored to the needs of the specific individual and utilizing different delivery methods may help mitigate some of their mental health issues.

4.3. Limitations and Future Directions

The subjective nature of the questionnaire responses allowed us to understand feelings and experiences directly from AYA with CP themselves. However, participants who were more open to sharing their experiences may have opted to participate in the study, thus introducing volunteer bias. Alternative approaches to creating our models may have included reducing our CES-D and S-Anxiety scores to dichotomous variables using the clinical cut-off points ("risk of clinical depression" vs. "lower risk of clinical depression" for example) and performing logistic regression analyses. In addition, though we removed outliers that were statistically different from the rest of our sample, we did not necessarily have a good 'clinical' reason to remove them, and they may have been valid data points. During Year 1 of the MyStory study, we did not collect the Trait Anxiety in the STAI. However, these data are being collected for participants continuing their involvement in the study to allow for further understanding of anxiety in AYA with CP. Future longitudinal analyses are planned for the MyStory study data (data collection is still ongoing) and will include a larger sample size across time points, allowing us to explore how levels of anxiety, fatigue, depression, family functioning, participation, self-management, and quality of life change across time. We also aim to understand if there are age effects to these changes across times to better identify the appropriate timing of strategy and resource implementation for AYA with CP.

Author Contributions: J.W.G. is the guarantor for the study. Conceptualization, J.W.G., D.F., M.A.F., D.M., R.J.P. and P.R.; data curation, A.G., S.N.H. and B.S.; formal analysis, A.G. and B.S.; funding acquisition, J.W.G.; methodology, J.W.G., D.F., M.A.F., D.M., R.J.P. and P.R.; project administration, S.N.H.; resources, A.D.G.; supervision, J.W.G. and D.M.; visualization, A.G., S.N.H. and B.S.; writing—original draft, J.W.G., A.G., D.M. and B.S.; writing—review and editing, D.F., M.A.F., S.N.H., R.J.P. and P.R. All authors participated in the interpretation of data, provided their final approval, and contributed equally to this work. J.W.G. led the writing of the manuscript and is the lead author, and the other authors are listed in alphabetical order. All authors have read and agreed to the published version of the manuscript.

Funding: This research was conducted with the support of the Ontario Brain Institute, an independent nonprofit corporation, funded partially by the Ontario government. The opinions, results and conclusions are those of the authors and no endorsement by the Ontario Brain Institute is intended or should be inferred. This research also received partner contribution by the Scotiabank Chair in Child Health Research held by Jan Willem Gorter. The funders did not have any role in the study design, data collection, analyses, or manuscript preparation.

Institutional Review Board Statement: The study was conducted according to the guidelines of the Declaration of Helsinki and approved by the Hamilton Integrated Research Ethics Board (protocol code 13-840, 17 December 2013).

Informed Consent Statement: Informed consent was obtained from all subjects involved in the study.

Data Availability Statement: The Childhood Cerebral Palsy Integrated Neuroscience Discovery Network (CP-NET) is one Integrated Discovery Program funded by the Ontario Brain Institute. Data collected for studies within CP-NET, including the MyStory study, are added to Brain-CODE and will be accessible to external researchers through data access requests. Data specifically used in this study are available from the corresponding author upon reasonable request.

Acknowledgments: We gratefully acknowledge the adolescents and young adults with cerebral palsy who participated in the MyStory study (The following are members of the MyStory Study: Jan Willem Gorter (principal investigator); Geoff Hall, Peter Rosenbaum, Darcy Fehlings, Caitlin Cassidy, Mark Ferro, Andrea Gonzalez, Sidney Segalowitz, Anna McCormick, Robert Palisano, Leslie Atkinson (co-investigators); Christine Lackner, Diana Tajik-Parvinchi, Amanda Green (post-doctoral fellows); Sarah Hopmans, Dayle McCauley, Brittany Speller, Aya Dudin, Julie Wilson, Helena Viveiros, John Secen (research and project staff members); Andrew Davis (students)). The authors thank Samantha Dong and Randi Mao for updating the literature for this study. We also acknowledge and thank the recruiting clinicians: Paul Stacey, at Niagara Children's Centre in St. Catharines, Caitlin Cassidy at St. Joseph's London in London, and Andrea Lauzon and Mark Bailey at Toronto Rehabilitation Institute in Toronto. We acknowledge the contributions of Jessica Geboers, a Stakeholder Advisory Group member, for presenting and sharing the MyStory research study design and findings. We appreciate the continued partnership with the Ontario Federation of Cerebral Palsy in the MyStory study to recruit participants, plan, and support knowledge translation activities to the CP community.

Conflicts of Interest: The authors declare no conflict of interest.

Appendix A

Cortisol ELISA Protocol: After collection, samples were placed in sealed plastic bags and stored at room temperature until they were assayed. A standardized protocol was used to process hair samples. The first 3 cm of each hair sample (proximal to the scalp) was cut with scissors and placed into a Falcon 50 mL Conical Centrifuge Tube. Hair samples were washed twice with 12 mL of isopropanol while gently shaking samples by hand and then the isopropanol was discarded. Tubes were left open to air dry over 48 h. Using a Retsch CryoMill, dried samples were pulverized at 25 Hz for three minutes. Next, 30–35 mg of ground hair powder was measured and transferred to a 2 mL Eppendorf tube where 1 mL of 100% ethanol was added and shaken at 22 rpm on the RPI Mix-All Laboratory Tube Mixer for 24–72 h at room temperature. Samples were then vortexed for five seconds and centrifuged at 2800 rpm for 15 min after which, 0.8 mL of supernatant was aliquoted into a new 2 mL Eppendorf tube (supernatant tube). The supernatant was left to air dry for 48 h to ensure complete evaporation of the ethanol. Another 1 mL of 100% ethanol was added to the sample tube, and it was rotated at 22 rpm on the RPI Mix-All Laboratory Tube Mixer for 24–72 h at room temperature. Samples were vortexed for five seconds and centrifuged at 2800 rpm for 15 min. During this final extraction stage, 1 mL of the supernatant was aliquoted into the supernatant tube, and it was left to air dry for 48 h. The supernatant was reconstituted with 150 μL of Salimetrics Salivary Cortisol Assay Diluent, vortexed for five seconds, and centrifuged for 10 min. Samples were then assayed in duplicate by ELISA using the High Sensitivity Salivary Cortisol Immunoassay Kit (Cat# 1-3002, Salimetrics, State College, PA, USA), as per manufacturer instructions. Cortisol levels are expressed as pg/mg hair. Intra- and inter-assay coefficients of variance were below 10% in the present study.

References

1. Usuba, K.; Oddson, B.; Gauthier, A.; Young, N.L. Changes in gross motor function and health-related quality of life in adults with cerebral palsy: An 8-year follow-up study. *Arch. Phys. Med. Rehabil.* **2014**, *95*, 2071–2077.e1. [CrossRef] [PubMed]
2. Sienko, S.E. An exploratory study investigating the multidimensional factors impacting the health and well-being of young adults with cerebral palsy. *Disabil. Rehabil.* **2018**, *40*, 660–666. [CrossRef] [PubMed]
3. Oskoui, M.; Shevell, M.I. Cerebral palsy and the transition from pediatric to adult care. *Contin. Lifelong Learn. Neurol.* **2009**, *15*, 64–77. [CrossRef]
4. Bolger, A.; Vargus-Adams, J.; McMahon, M. Transition of care in adolescents with cerebral palsy: A survey of current practices. *PM R* **2017**, *9*, 258–264. [CrossRef] [PubMed]
5. Nguyen, T.; Henderson, D.; Stewart, D.; Hlyva, O.; Punthakee, Z.; Gorter, J. You never transition alone! Exploring the experiences of youth with chronic health conditions, parents and healthcare providers on self-management. *Child Care Health Dev.* **2016**, *42*, 464–472. [CrossRef]
6. Andersson, C.; Mattsson, E. Adults with cerebral palsy: A survey describing problems, needs, and resources, with special emphasis on locomotion. *Dev. Med. Child Neurol.* **2001**, *43*, 76–82. [CrossRef]
7. Nieuwenhuijsen, C.; Donkervoort, M.; Nieuwstraten, W.; Stam, H.J.; Roebroeck, M.E.; Netherlands, T.R.G.S.W. Experienced problems of young adults with cerebral palsy: Targets for rehabilitation care. *Arch. Phys. Med. Rehabil.* **2009**, *90*, 1891–1897. [CrossRef]
8. Weber, P.; Bolli, P.; Heimgartner, N.; Merlo, P.; Zehnder, T.; Kätterer, C. Behavioral and emotional problems in children and adults with cerebral palsy. *Eur. J. Paediatr. Neurol.* **2016**, *20*, 270–274. [CrossRef]
9. Björquist, E.; Nordmark, E.; Hallström, I. Parents' experiences of health and needs when supporting their adolescents with cerebral palsy during transition to adulthood. *Phys. Occup. Ther. Pediatr.* **2016**, *36*, 204–216. [CrossRef]
10. Freeman, M.; Stewart, D.; Cunningham, C.E.; Gorter, J.W. Information needs of young people with cerebral palsy and their families during the transition to adulthood: A scoping review. *J. Transit. Med.* **2018**, *1*, 20180003. [CrossRef]
11. Qadeer, R.A.; Shanahan, L.; Ferro, M.A. Chronic disruptive pain in emerging adults with and without chronic health conditions and the moderating role of psychiatric disorders: Evidence from a population-based cross-sectional survey in Canada. *Scand. J. Pain* **2017**, *17*, 30–36. [CrossRef] [PubMed]
12. Ferro, M.A. Mediated moderation of the relation between maternal and adolescent depressive symptoms: Role of adolescent physical health. *Soc. Psychiatry Psychiatr. Epidemiol.* **2015**, *50*, 1743–1751. [CrossRef] [PubMed]
13. Ferro, M.A.; Gorter, J.W.; Boyle, M.H. Trajectories of depressive symptoms during the transition to young adulthood: The role of chronic illness. *J. Affect. Disord.* **2015**, *174*, 594–601. [CrossRef] [PubMed]
14. Kingsnorth, S.; Orava, T.; Provvidenza, C.; Adler, E.; Ami, N.; Gresley-Jones, T.; Mankad, D.; Slonim, N.; Fay, L.; Joachimides, N. Chronic pain assessment tools for cerebral palsy: A systematic review. *Pediatrics* **2015**, *136*, e947–e960. [CrossRef] [PubMed]
15. Van Der Slot, W.M.; Nieuwenhuijsen, C.; Van Den Berg-Emons, R.J.; Bergen, M.P.; Hilberink, S.R.; Stam, H.J.; Roebroeck, M.E. Chronic pain, fatigue, and depressive symptoms in adults with spastic bilateral cerebral palsy. *Dev. Med. Child Neurol.* **2012**, *54*, 836–842. [CrossRef]
16. McMahon, J.; Harvey, A.; Reid, S.M.; May, T.; Antolovich, G. Anxiety in children and adolescents with cerebral palsy. *J. Paediatr. Child Health* **2020**, *56*, 1194–1200. [CrossRef] [PubMed]
17. Whitney, D.G.; Warschausky, S.A.; Ng, S.; Hurvitz, E.A.; Kamdar, N.S.; Peterson, M.D. Prevalence of Mental Health Disorders Among Adults With Cerebral Palsy: A Cross-sectional Analysis. *Ann. Intern. Med.* **2019**, *171*, 328–333. [CrossRef]
18. Smith, K.J.; Peterson, M.D.; O'Connell, N.E.; Victor, C.; Liverani, S.; Anokye, N.; Ryan, J.M. Risk of Depression and Anxiety in Adults With Cerebral Palsy. *JAMA Neurol.* **2019**, *76*, 294–300. [CrossRef]
19. Rackauskaite, G.; Bilenbergw, N.; Uldall, P.; Bech, B.H.; Ostergaard, J. Prevalence of mental disorders in children and adolescents with cerebral palsy: Danish nationwide follow-up study. *Eur. J. Paediatr. Neurol.* **2020**, *27*, 98–103. [CrossRef]
20. Rayner, L.; Hotopf, M.; Petkova, H.; Matcham, F.; Simpson, A.; McCracken, L.M. Depression in patients with chronic pain attending a specialised pain treatment centre: Prevalence and impact on health care costs. *Pain* **2016**, *157*, 1472. [CrossRef]
21. Young, N.L.; McCormick, A.M.; Gilbert, T.; Ayling-Campos, A.; Burke, T.; Fehlings, D.; Wedge, J. Reasons for hospital admissions among youth and young adults with cerebral palsy. *Arch. Phys. Med. Rehabil.* **2011**, *92*, 46–50. [CrossRef] [PubMed]
22. Helseth, S.; Abebe, D.S.; Andenæs, R. Mental health problems among individuals with persistent health challenges from adolescence to young adulthood: A population-based longitudinal study in Norway. *BMC Public Health* **2016**, *16*, 983. [CrossRef] [PubMed]
23. Bjorgaas, H.M.; Elgen, I.B.; Hysing, M. Trajectories of psychiatric disorders in a cohort of children with cerebral palsy across four years. *Disabil. Health J.* **2021**, *14*, 100992. [CrossRef] [PubMed]

24. Downs, J.; Blackmore, A.M.; Epstein, A.; Skoss, R.; Langdon, K.; Jacoby, P.; Whitehouse, A.J.; Leonard, H.; Rowe, P.W.; Glasson, E.J. The prevalence of mental health disorders and symptoms in children and adolescents with cerebral palsy: A systematic review and meta-analysis. *Dev. Med. Child Neurol.* **2018**, *60*, 30–38. [CrossRef] [PubMed]
25. Craig, F.; Savino, R.; Trabacca, A. A systematic review of comorbidity between cerebral palsy, autism spectrum disorders and Attention Deficit Hyperactivity Disorder. *Eur. J. Paediatr. Neurol.* **2019**, *23*, 31–42. [CrossRef]
26. Odding, E.; Roebroeck, M.E.; Stam, H.J. The epidemiology of cerebral palsy: Incidence, impairments and risk factors. *Disabil. Rehabil.* **2006**, *28*, 183–191. [CrossRef]
27. Pauli-Pott, U.; Schloß, S.; Ruhl, I.; Skoluda, N.; Nater, U.M.; Becker, K. Hair cortisol concentration in preschoolers with attention-deficit/hyperactivity symptoms—Roles of gender and family adversity. *Psychoneuroendocrinology* **2017**, *86*, 25–33. [CrossRef]
28. Chen, X.; Gelaye, B.; Velez, J.C.; Barbosa, C.; Pepper, M.; Andrade, A.; Gao, W.; Kirschbaum, C.; Williams, M.A. Caregivers' hair cortisol: A possible biomarker of chronic stress is associated with obesity measures among children with disabilities. *BMC Pediatr.* **2015**, *15*, 9. [CrossRef]
29. Vives, A.H.; De Angel, V.; Papadopoulos, A.; Barbosa, C.; Pepper, M.; Andrade, A.; Gao, W.; Kirschbaum, C.; Williams, M.A. The relationship between cortisol, stress and psychiatric illness: New insights using hair analysis. *J. Psychiatr. Res.* **2015**, *70*, 38–49. [CrossRef]
30. Wells, S.; Tremblay, P.F.; Flynn, A.; Russell, E.; Kennedy, J.; Rehm, J.; Van Uum, S.; Koren, G.; Graham, K. Associations of hair cortisol concentration with self-reported measures of stress and mental health-related factors in a pooled database of diverse community samples. *Stress* **2014**, *17*, 334–342. [CrossRef]
31. Pochigaeva, K.; Druzhkova, T.; Yakovlev, A.; Onufriev, M.; Grishkina, M.; Chepelev, A.; Guekht, A.; Gulyaeva, N. Hair cortisol as a marker of hypothalamic-pituitary-adrenal Axis activity in female patients with major depressive disorder. *Metab. Brain Dis.* **2017**, *32*, 577–583. [CrossRef]
32. Abell, J.G.; Stalder, T.; Ferrie, J.E.; Shipley, M.J.; Kirschbaum, C.; Kivimäki, M.; Kumari, M. Assessing cortisol from hair samples in a large observational cohort: The Whitehall II study. *Psychoneuroendocrinology* **2016**, *73*, 148–156. [CrossRef] [PubMed]
33. Stalder, T.; Steudte-Schmiedgen, S.; Alexander, N.; Klucken, T.; Vater, A.; Wichmann, S.; Kirschbaum, C.; Miller, R. Stress-related and basic determinants of hair cortisol in humans: A meta-analysis. *Psychoneuroendocrinology* **2017**, *77*, 261–274. [CrossRef] [PubMed]
34. Kornelsen, E.; Buchan, M.C.; Gonzalez, A.; Ferro, M.A. Hair cortisol concentration and mental disorder in children with chronic physical illness. *Chronic Stress* **2019**, *3*, 2470547019875116. [CrossRef] [PubMed]
35. Posner, K.; Brown, G.K.; Stanley, B.; Brent, D.A.; Yershova, K.V.; Oquendo, M.A.; Currier, G.W.; Melvin, G.A.; Greenhill, L.; Shen, S. The Columbia–Suicide Severity Rating Scale: Initial validity and internal consistency findings from three multisite studies with adolescents and adults. *Am. J. Psychiatry* **2011**, *168*, 1266–1277. [CrossRef] [PubMed]
36. Spielberger, C.D. *Manual for the State-Trait Anxiety Inventory*; Consulting Psychologists Press: Palo Alto, CA, USA, 1983.
37. Julian, L.J. Measures of anxiety: State-Trait Anxiety Inventory (STAI), Beck Anxiety Inventory (BAI), and Hospital Anxiety and Depression Scale-Anxiety (HADS-A). *Arthritis Care Res.* **2011**, *63*, S467–S472. [CrossRef] [PubMed]
38. Bennett, D.A. How can I deal with missing data in my study? *Aust. N. Z. J. Public Health* **2001**, *25*, 464–469. [CrossRef] [PubMed]
39. Radloff, L.S. The CES-D Scale:A Self-Report Depression Scale for Research in the General Population. *Appl. Psychol. Meas.* **1977**, *1*, 385–401. [CrossRef]
40. Miller, W.; Anton, H.; Townson, A. Measurement properties of the CESD scale among individuals with spinal cord injury. *Spin. Cord.* **2008**, *46*, 287–292. [CrossRef]
41. Ferro, M.A.; Gorter, J.W.; Boyle, M.H. Trajectories of depressive symptoms in Canadian emerging adults. *Am. J. Public Health* **2015**, *105*, 2322–2327. [CrossRef]
42. Ryan, C.E.; Epstein, N.B.; Keitner, G.I.; Bishop, D.S.; Miller, I.W. *Evaluating and Treating Families: The McMaster Approach*; Taylor & Francis: Oxfordshire, UK, 2005.
43. Byles, J.; Byrne, C.; Boyle, M.H.; Offord, D.R. Ontario Child Health Study: Reliability and validity of the general functioning subscale of the McMaster Family Assessment Device. *Fam. Process.* **1988**, *27*, 97–104. [CrossRef] [PubMed]
44. Brunton, L.K.; Bartlett, D.J. Construction and validation of the fatigue impact and severity self-assessment for youth and young adults with cerebral palsy. *Dev. Neurorehabil.* **2017**, *20*, 274–279. [CrossRef] [PubMed]
45. Bartlett, D.J.; Hanna, S.E.; Avery, L.; Stevenson, R.D.; Galuppi, B. Correlates of decline in gross motor capacity in adolescents with cerebral palsy in Gross Motor Function Classification System levels III to V: An exploratory study. *Dev. Med. Child Neurol.* **2010**, *52*, e155–e160. [CrossRef] [PubMed]
46. Palisano, R.J.; Rosenbaum, P.; Bartlett, D.; Livingston, M.H. Content validity of the expanded and revised Gross Motor Function Classification System. *Dev. Med. Child Neurol.* **2008**, *50*, 744–750. [CrossRef]
47. Stalder, T.; Steudte, S.; Miller, R.; Skoluda, N.; Dettenborn, L.; Kirschbaum, C. Intraindividual stability of hair cortisol concentrations. *Psychoneuroendocrinology* **2012**, *37*, 602–610. [CrossRef]
48. Zhang, Q.; Chen, Z.; Chen, S.; Yu, T.; Wang, J.; Wang, W.; Deng, H. Correlations of hair level with salivary level in cortisol and cortisone. *Life Sci.* **2018**, *193*, 57–63. [CrossRef]
49. Kirschbaum, C.; Tietze, A.; Skoluda, N.; Dettenborn, L. Hair as a retrospective calendar of cortisol production-Increased cortisol incorporation into hair in the third trimester of pregnancy. *Psychoneuroendocrinology* **2009**, *34*, 32–37. [CrossRef]

50. Thomson, S.; Koren, G.; Fraser, L.-A.; Rieder, M.; Friedman, T.; Van Uum, S. Hair analysis provides a historical record of cortisol levels in Cushing's syndrome. *Exp. Clin. Endocrinol. Diabetes* **2009**, *118*, 133–138. [CrossRef]
51. Wosu, A.C.; Valdimarsdóttir, U.; Shields, A.E.; Williams, D.R.; Williams, M.A. Correlates of cortisol in human hair: Implications for epidemiologic studies on health effects of chronic stress. *Ann. Epidemiol.* **2013**, *23*, 797–811.e2. [CrossRef]
52. Carifio, J.; Perla, R. Ten Common Misunderstandings, Misconceptions, Persistent Myths and Urban Legends about Likert Scales and Likert Response Formats and their Antidotes. *J. Soc. Sci.* **2007**, *3*, 106–116. [CrossRef]
53. Lakens, D. Calculating and reporting effect sizes to facilitate cumulative science: A practical primer for t-tests and ANOVAs. *Front. Psychol.* **2013**, *4*, 863. [CrossRef] [PubMed]
54. Hanes, J.E.; Hlyva, O.; Rosenbaum, P.; Freeman, M.; Nguyen, T.; Palisano, R.J.; Gorter, J.W. Beyond stereotypes of cerebral palsy: Exploring the lived experiences of young Canadians. *Child Care Health Dev.* **2019**, *45*, 613–622. [CrossRef] [PubMed]
55. Smith, S.E.; Gannotti, M.; Hurvitz, E.A.; Jensen, F.E.; Krach, L.E.; Kruer, M.C.; Msall, M.E.; Noritz, G.; Rajan, D.S.; Aravamuthan, B.R. Adults with cerebral palsy require ongoing neurologic care: A systematic review. *Ann. Neurol.* **2021**, *89*, 860–871. [CrossRef] [PubMed]
56. Lundh, S.; Nasic, S.; Riad, J. Fatigue, quality of life and walking ability in adults with cerebral palsy. *Gait Posture* **2018**, *61*, 1–6. [CrossRef]
57. van der Slot, W.M.A.; Benner, J.L.; Brunton, L.; Engel, J.M.; Gallien, P.; Hilberink, S.R.; Månum, G.; Morgan, P.; Opheim, A.; Riquelme, I.; et al. Pain in adults with cerebral palsy: A systematic review and meta-analysis of individual participant data. *Ann. Phys. Rehabil. Med.* **2021**, *64*, 101359. [CrossRef]
58. Mckinnon, C.T.; Meehan, E.M.; Harvey, A.R.; Antolovich, G.C.; Morgan, P.E. Prevalence and characteristics of pain in children and young adults with cerebral palsy: A systematic review. *Dev. Med. Child Neurol.* **2019**, *61*, 305–314. [CrossRef]
59. van Gorp, M.; Hilberink, S.R.; Noten, S.; Benner, J.L.; Stam, H.J.; van der Slot, W.M.; Roebroeck, M.E. Epidemiology of Cerebral Palsy in Adulthood: A Systematic Review and Meta-analysis of the Most Frequently Studied Outcomes. *Arch. Phys. Med. Rehabil.* **2020**, *101*, 1041–1052. [CrossRef]
60. Whitney, D.G.; Bell, S.; Whibley, D.; Van der Slot, W.M.; Hurvitz, E.A.; Haapala, H.J.; Peterson, M.D.; Warschausky, S.A. Effect of pain on mood affective disorders in adults with cerebral palsy. *Dev. Med. Child Neurol.* **2020**, *62*, 926–932. [CrossRef]
61. Whitney, D.G.; Warschausky, S.A.; Whibley, D.; Kratz, A.; Murphy, S.L.; Hurvitz, E.A.; Peterson, M.D. Clinical factors associated with mood affective disorders among adults with cerebral palsy. *Neurol. Clin. Pract.* **2020**, *10*, 206–213. [CrossRef]
62. Brunton, L.K.; McPhee, P.G.; Gorter, J.W. Self-reported factors contributing to fatigue and its management in adolescents and adults with cerebral palsy. *Disabil. Rehabil.* **2021**, *43*, 929–935. [CrossRef]
63. McDougall, J.; DeWit, D.J.; Wright, F.V. Social anxiety symptoms among youth with chronic health conditions: Trajectories and related factors. *Disabil. Rehabil.* **2020**, *42*, 3293–3305. [CrossRef] [PubMed]
64. Asano, D.; Takeda, M.; Nobusako, S.; Morioka, S. Self-Rated Depressive Symptoms in Children and Youth with and without Cerebral Palsy: A Pilot Study. *Behav. Sci.* **2020**, *10*, 167. [CrossRef] [PubMed]
65. Bjorgaas, H.M.; Elgen, I.; Boe, T.; Rosenbaum, P.; Hlyva, O.; Freeman, M.; Nguyen, T.; Gorter, J. Mental health in children with cerebral palsy: Does screening capture the complexity? *Sci. World J.* **2013**, *2013*, 468402-02. [CrossRef]
66. Palisano, R.; Rezze, B.D.; Stewart, D.; Rosenbaum, P.; Hlyva, O.; Freeman, M.; Nguyen, T.; Gorter, J. Life course health development of individuals with neurodevelopmental conditions. *Dev. Med. Child Neurol.* **2017**, *59*, 470–476. [CrossRef] [PubMed]
67. Gorter, J.W. Transition to Adult-Oriented Health Care: Perspectives of Youth and Adults with Complex Physical Disabilities. *Phys. Occup. Ther. Pediatr.* **2009**, *29*, 362–366. [CrossRef]
68. Høye, H.; Jahnsen, R.B.; Løvstad, M.; Hartveit, J.F.; Sørli, H.; Tornås, S.; Månum, G. A Mindfulness-Based Stress Reduction Program via Group Video Conferencing for Adults With Cerebral Palsy—A Pilot Study. *Front. Neurol.* **2020**, *11*, 195. [CrossRef] [PubMed]
69. Schwartz, A.E.; Young Adult Mental Health/Peer Mentoring Research Team; Kramer, J.M.; Rogers, E.S.; McDonald, K.E.; Cohn, E.S. Stakeholder-driven approach to developing a peer-mentoring intervention for young adults with intellectual/developmental disabilities and co-occurring mental health conditions. *J. Appl. Res. Intellect. Disabil.* **2020**, *33*, 992–1004. [CrossRef]

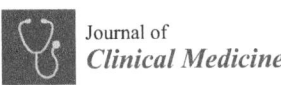

Article

Unmet Health Needs among Young Adults with Cerebral Palsy in Ireland: A Cross-Sectional Study

Jennifer M. Ryan [1,*], Michael Walsh [2], Mary Owens [3], Michael Byrne [4], Thilo Kroll [5], Owen Hensey [3], Claire Kerr [6], Meriel Norris [7], Aisling Walsh [1], Grace Lavelle [8] and Jennifer Fortune [1]

1. Department of Public Health and Epidemiology, RCSI University of Medicine and Health Sciences, D02 DH60 Dublin, Ireland
2. Office of the Chief Clinical Officer, Health Service Executive, D20 HY57 Dublin, Ireland
3. Central Remedial Clinic, D03 R973 Dublin, Ireland
4. National Disability Children & Families Team, Social Care Division, Health Service Executive, D20 HY57 Dublin, Ireland
5. School of Nursing, Midwifery and Health Systems, University College Dublin, D04 V1W8 Dublin, Ireland
6. School of Nursing and Midwifery, Queen's University Belfast, Belfast BT7 1NN, UK
7. College of Health, Medicine and Life Sciences, Brunel University London, London UB8 3PH, UK
8. Institute of Psychiatry, Psychology & Neuroscience, King's College London, London SE5 8AF, UK
* Correspondence: jenniferryan@rcsi.com

Abstract: Data describing the unmet health needs of young adults with cerebral palsy (CP) may support the development of appropriate health services. This study aimed to describe unmet health needs among young adults with CP in Ireland and examine if these differed between young adults who were and were not yet discharged from children's services. In this cross-sectional study, young adults with CP aged 16–22 years completed a questionnaire assessing unmet health needs. Logistic regression was used to examine the association between discharge status and unmet health needs. Seventy-five young adults (mean age 18.4 yr; 41% female; 60% in GMFCS levels I–III) were included in the study. Forty (53%) had been discharged from children's services. Unmet health need, as a proportion of those with needs, was highest for speech (0.64), followed by epilepsy (0.50) and equipment, mobility, control of movement and bone or joint problems (0.39 or 0.38). After adjusting for ambulatory status, unmet health needs did not differ according to discharge status. The proportion of young adults with unmet health needs highlights the importance of taking a life-course approach to CP and providing appropriate services to people with CP regardless of age.

Keywords: cerebral palsy; young people; adolescents; unmet need; health services

1. Introduction

Cerebral palsy (CP) is a lifelong condition that primarily affects movement and function [1]. People with CP commonly experience associated conditions including sensory impairment, intellectual disability and epilepsy [1]. They may also experience complications such as pain and fatigue [2], and have a higher risk of developing chronic conditions such as cardiovascular disease and depression [3,4]. People with CP are frequent users of medical and rehabilitation services [5–7]. However, adults are less likely to use health services than children with CP [8–10].

Adults with CP report challenges accessing health services once discharged from children's services and describe a lack of services to meet their needs [7]. A decline in service use from childhood to adulthood may therefore reflect challenges with accessing health services, rather than reduced health needs in adulthood. Indeed, the combination of a lack of services for adults with CP, challenges accessing appropriate services where they exist, and the development of complications in adulthood, may lead to increases in unmet health needs among young adults with CP. While unmet needs in areas relating to health

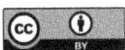

services, education, training and social needs have previously been reported among young adults with CP [11], few studies specifically describe unmet health needs in this population.

Solanke et al. developed an unmet health needs questionnaire specifically for people with CP [12]. They defined a health need as requiring "a health service to minimise the impact of their condition or manage their functional disability" [12]. A need was considered an unmet health need if the individual reported that "the service is not provided or is not adequate" [12]. Solanke identified that adolescents with CP in the United Kingdom had significant unmet health needs in several areas; unmet needs were highest for bone and joint problems, speech and pain [12]. However, unmet health needs did not change significantly when assessed over the subsequent three years. This may be because unmet health needs were initially assessed on adolescents aged between 14 and 18 years, and the secondary effects of ageing with CP did not impact this group enough in the subsequent 3 years to cause an increase in unmet health needs.

Despite the challenges that young adults with CP experience trying to access health services once they have been discharged from children's services [7], there is limited data describing their unmet health needs. Studies describing the unmet health needs of young adults with CP in different contexts are required to support the development of health services to meet their needs. This study aimed to describe unmet health needs among young adults with CP in Ireland and examine if these differed between young adults who were and were not discharged from children's services. We hypothesised that young adults who were discharged from children's services would be more likely to have unmet health needs. A secondary objective of this study was to describe health services accessed by young adults with CP in Ireland.

2. Materials and Methods

2.1. Design and Participants

We used a cross-sectional design. Young adults with CP aged 16–22 years residing in the Republic of Ireland were eligible to participate. In Ireland, people with CP typically receive healthcare from children's services up to age 18, after which they are discharged to adult services. However, age at discharge may vary between individuals and there is no standard age, even within the same service, at which young people are discharged. We included people aged 16–22 years to capture young adults who were pre- and post-discharge. We included young adults in all Gross Motor Function Classification System (GMFCS) levels. We shared information about the study through three national organisations that provide health and social care services to people with CP; in two of these organisatons, five gatekeepers distributed 371 study invites to young people with CP living throughout Ireland. These young people received a paper version of the survey and a stamped, addressed envelope to return the survey. We also shared information about the study through disability officers in higher education, special education needs schools, professional bodies, and social media. We additionally used snowball sampling. Ethical approval was provided by Research Ethics Committees in RCSI, the Central Remedial Clinic and Enable Ireland.

2.2. Data Collection

We collected data using a survey. It was available online and in paper form. The survey was piloted by a person with CP and a parent. Young adults were encouraged to complete the survey alone but could complete it with support from a parent/family member/carer. Alternatively, a parent/family member/carer (hereafter referred to as parent) could complete it on behalf of the person with CP. The survey included questions relating to 1. sociodemographic and CP-related characteristics; 2. use of 11 pre-defined services; 3. use of and needs relating to assistive technology; 4. discharge from children's services (yes/no) and if applicable, age at discharge. The survey also included a validated questionnaire that assessed unmet health needs [12]. The questionnaire asked about the following ten aspects of health care needs of people with CP: speech, mobility, positioning, equipment, pain, epilepsy, control of movement, bone or joint problems, curvature of back and eyesight. The possible responses to questions relating to speech, mobility, positioning and equipment were "help not needed", "need more help" or "getting enough help". Responses from questions relating to the remaining aspects were coded into the same three categories. Those reporting "getting enough help" and "need more help" were identified as having a need, and those reporting "need more help" were identified as having unmet need. As described in a previous study, the proportion of unmet needs to total needs was calculated [12].

2.3. Data Analysis

The distribution of data was explored using Q-Q plots for continuous data, and cross-tabulations for categorical data. Descriptive statistics (e.g., mean, frequency) were used to describe data as appropriate. Age was compared between participants who were pre-and post-discharge using an independent t-test. Remaining participant characteristics were compared between those pre- and post-discharge using Chi-squared tests. The number of services used by people who were pre-and post-discharge was compared using a linear regression adjusting for ambulatory status (i.e., GMFCS levels I–III or I–V). Assumptions of linear regression were assessed using a Q-Q plot of residuals and a scatter plot of residuals against fitted values. Logistic regression was used to compare the odds of currently accessing each service and being able to see a variety of professionals on the same day or place between those pre-and post-discharge, after adjusting for ambulatory status.

Logistic regression was used to examine associations between unmet need for each item (e.g., speech, mobility) as the dependent variable, and discharge status, GMFCS level (level I–III vs. level IV–V) and intellectual disability as independent variables. Only people with reported need for the item were included in the regression model. Unadjusted analyses were firstly conducted, with each independent variable entered separately. If more than 30 people reported need for the item, adjusted analyses were then conducted by entering independent variables into the same model.

3. Results

Seventy-five young adults were included. Nineteen (25.3%) questionnaires were completed by the person with CP alone, 26 (34.7%) were completed with support from a parent, and 29 (38.7%) were completed by a parent on behalf of the person with CP. Forty young adults (53.3%) had been discharged from children's services. The mean (SD) age at discharge was 17.8 (1.2) years (range 15–20 years). Among those who were discharged, there was a mean (SD) of 2.0 (1.7) yr (range 0–6 yr) between the young person's age at discharge and their age when they completed the survey.

Young adults are described in Table 1. The majority were male with a mean (SD) age of 18.4 (2.2) yr (range 16–22 yr). Approximately 84% had spastic CP and 60% were in GMFCS levels I–III. Type of motor abnormality differed between those who were pre- and post-discharge ($p = 0.033$); people post-discharge were more likely to have spastic diplegia or spastic quadriplegia. There was no difference in the proportion of people in GMFCS levels I–III between those pre- and post-discharge. Approximately 28% had intellectual disability, 15% had communication impairment, 15% had feeding impairment, 8% had hearing impairment and 1% had autism spectrum disorder.

Table 1. Description of young adults.

	Pre-Discharge (n = 35)		Post-Discharge (n = 40)			Total (n = 75)	
	Mean	SD	Mean	SD	p Value	Mean	SD
Age	16.7	0.8	19.9	1.9	<0.001	18.4	2.2
	n	(%)	n	(%)		n	(%)
Female	12	34.3	19	47.5	0.246	31	41.3
Currently in education	35	100.0	28	70.0	<0.001	63	84.0
Currently in employment	2	5.7	3	7.5	0.606	5	6.7
Type of motor abnormality							
Spastic hemiplegia	16	45.7	5	12.5	0.033	21	28.0
Spastic diplegia	6	17.1	15	37.5		21	28.0
Spastic quadriplegia	7	20.0	14	35.0		21	28.0
Dyskinetic	1	2.9	2	5.0		3	4.0
Ataxic	1	2.9	1	2.5		2	2.7
Don't know or other	4	11.4	3	7.5		7	9.3
GMFCS level [a]							
I	15	42.9	12	30.0	0.301	27	36.0
II	7	20.0	3	7.5		10	13.3
III	3	8.6	5	12.5		8	10.7
IV	2	5.7	5	12.5		7	9.3
V	8	22.9	14	35.0		22	29.3
Associated impairments							
Intellectual disability	10	28.6	11	27.5	0.918	21	28.0
Communication impairment	7	20.0	4	10.0	0.222	11	14.7
Feeding impairment	5	14.3	6	15.0	0.930	11	14.7
Hearing impairment	3	8.6	3	7.5	0.865	6	8.0
ASD	0	0	1	2.5	0.346	1	1.3
ADHD	0	0	0	0	-	0	0

[a] n = 74.

All young adults lived with parents or family members. Most young adults (84%) were currently in education. Of these, 46% were in a mainstream school, 21% were in a special education needs school, 16% were in university, 8% were in a college of further education and the remainder were in other forms of education such as home schooling or vocational training. Five people were currently in employment, of which 3 were in regular part-time paid work. The five people in employment were also in education. All people pre-discharge were in education compared to 70% of people post-discharge ($p < 0.001$). Twelve people (16%) were in neither education nor employment.

Young adults resided in all regions of Ireland (Table 2). Although only 49% resided in Dublin, 80% of young adults accessed services in Dublin (Table 2).

Table 2. Regions of Ireland in which young people resided and accessed services.

Region (In Order of Population Density from Lowest to Highest)	Young Person (n = 75)	
	Resident, n (%)	Accessed Services [a], n (%)
West	3 (4.0)	3 (4.0)
Border	6 (8.0)	6 (8.0)
Midland	5 (6.7)	5 (6.7)
Mid-West	8 (10.7)	7 (9.3)
South-West	2 (2.7)	2 (2.7)
South-East	7 (9.3)	9 (12.0)
Mid-East	7 (9.3)	6 (8.0)
Dublin	37 (49.3)	60 (80.0)

[a] Respondents may select more than one response.

Approximately 60% of young adults used aids or assistive technology (Table 3). Of these, the most commonly used was a manual wheelchair or electric wheelchair or scooter. Twenty per cent had an unmet need for an aid/assistive technology. There was no difference in use of or unmet need between those pre-and post-discharge.

Table 3. Use of and unmet need for aids and assistive technology.

	Discharge Status			Total, n (%)
	Pre-Discharge, n (%)	Post-Discharge, n (%)	p Value *	
Using aid/assistive technology [a]	20 (57.1)	26 (65.0)	0.660	46 (61.3)
Type of aid/assistive technology [b]				
Manual or electric wheelchair or scooter	13 (65.0)	18 (69.2)		31 (67.4)
Walking aid(s), e.g., orthopaedic footwear, walking stick, frame, rollator	7 (35.0)	14 (53.9)		21 (45.7)
Other [c]	12 (60.0)	15 (58.0)		27 (59.2)
Unmet need for aid/assistive technology [d]	7 (20.0)	8 (20.0)	0.818	15 (20.0)

[a] n = 74. [b] calculated as a percentage of those using assistive technology. [c] includes magnifiers; large print or Braille reading materials; hearing aid(s); communication board; computer or keyboard for communicating; screen reading software; other. [d] n = 72. * adjusted for GMFCS level.

3.1. Health Services

The services that people accessed are reported in Table 4. Of the 11 services listed, the mean (SD) number of services people accessed was 3.2 (2.1) (median 3; range 0–11). The mean (SD) was 3.7 (2.1) services (median 3; range 0–11) among people pre-discharge and 2.9 (2.0) services (median 2; range 0–8) among people post-discharge. People who were discharged accessed on average 1.10 (95% CI 0.20 to 2.00) fewer services than people who were not discharged after adjusting for ambulatory status ($p = 0.017$).

Table 4. Description of services currently accessed by young people (n = 75).

Health Service	Discharge Status			Total, n (%)
	Pre-Discharge, n (%)	Post-Discharge, n (%)	p Value [a]	
Physiotherapy	26 (74.3)	28 (70.0)	0.820	54 (72.0)
Occupational therapy	28 (80.0)	15 (37.5)	<0.001	43 (57.3)
Medical	19 (54.3)	23 (57.5)	0.873	42 (56.0)
Speech and language therapy	15 (42.9)	5 (12.5)	0.002	20 (26.7)
Assistive technology	12 (34.3)	5 (12.5)	0.028	17 (22.7)
Nursing	3 (8.6)	11 (27.5)	0.145	14 (18.7)
Social work	9 (25.7)	5 (12.5)	0.106	14 (18.7)
Psychology	6 (17.1)	5 (12.5)	0.626	11 (14.7)
Personal assistance [b]	2 (5.7)	9 (22.5)	0.142	11 (14.7)
Personal care [c]	3 (8.6)	7 (17.5)	0.609	10 (13.3)
Dietetics	5 (14.3)	1 (2.5)	0.050	6 (8.0)

[a] adjusted for GMFCS level. [b] refers to assistance provided inside and outside of the home, including personal care, support in the workplace and socialising, to enable people to live as independently as possible. [c] refers to support with activities of daily living (e.g., eating, dressing).

After adjusting for ambulatory status, people who were discharged were less likely to access occupational therapy (OR: 0.11, 95% CI 0.03 to 0.36; $p < 0.001$), speech and language therapy (OR: 0.14, 95% CI 0.04 to 0.49; $p = 0.002$), dietetics (OR: 0.10, 95% CI 0.01 to 1.00; $p = 0.050$), and assistive technology services (OR: 0.26, 95% CI 0.08 to 0.86; $p = 0.028$).

Thirty-four (45.3%) people said they could see a variety of professionals on the same day or in the same place. Pre-discharge, three people (8.6%) said this was not applicable as they were only accessing one professional compared to seven (17.5%) post-discharge. Discharge status and ability to see a variety of professionals on the same day or place were not associated after adjusting for ambulatory status ($p = 0.132$).

3.2. Reported Health Needs and Unmet Health Needs

The percentage of young adults with reported health needs and unmet health needs are described in Table 5. Needs were highest for mobility, equipment and control of movement. Unmet need, as a proportion of those with needs, was highest for speech (0.64) and epilepsy (0.50). Unmet need was similar for equipment, mobility, control of movement, bone or joint problems (0.39 or 0.38). Discharge status was not associated with unmet need in unadjusted or adjusted analyses (Tables S1 and S2). In unadjusted analysis, ambulatory status was associated with unmet need relating to speech (OR: 6.00, 95% CI 1.00 to 35.9, $p = 0.050$) and eyesight (OR 12.9, 95% CI 2.22 to 74.5, $p = 0.004$), with people in GMFCS levels IV-V more likely to report unmet needs than people in levels I-III. Intellectual disability was associated with unmet need relating to mobility (OR: 3.64, 95% CI 1.10 to 12.0, $p = 0.034$). Intellectual disability and ambulatory status were not associated with unmet need in adjusted analyses.

Table 5. Reported needs and unmet needs as a proportion of need.

Item	Pre-Discharge (n = 35)		Post-Discharge (n = 40)		Total (n = 75)	
	Reported Needs, n (%)	Unmet Need	Reported Needs, n (%)	Unmet Need	Reported Needs, n (%)	Unmet Need
Speech [a]	15 (45.5)	0.60	10 (26.3)	0.70	25 (35.2)	0.64
Epilepsy [b]	8 (24.2)	0.50	6 (16.2)	0.50	14 (20.0)	0.50
Equipment [c]	22 (66.7)	0.45	29 (72.5)	0.34	51 (69.9)	0.39
Mobility	29 (82.9)	0.31	27 (67.5)	0.44	56 (74.7)	0.38
Control of movement [d]	21 (61.8)	0.30 *	28 (70.0)	0.43	49 (66.2)	0.38 *
Bone or joint problems [e]	16 (47.1)	0.31	23 (60.5)	0.43	39 (54.2)	0.38
Positioning [a]	18 (54.6)	0.28	19 (50.0)	0.32	37 (52.1)	0.30
Curvature of back [e]	12 (35.3)	0.17	18 (47.4)	0.39	30 (41.7)	0.30
Eyesight [d]	17 (50.0)	0.20 **	23 (57.7)	0.35	40 (54.1)	0.29 **
Pain [d]	17 (48.6)	0.18	18 (46.2)	0.12 *	35 (47.3)	0.15 *

[a] n = 71. [b] n = 70. [c] n = 73. [d] n = 74. [e] n = 72. * denominator is number with reported needs minus one because one person with reported needs did not provide an answer for the related unmet need question. ** denominator is number with reported needs minus two because two people with reported needs did not provide an answer for the related unmet need question.

When respondents were asked if they had any other concerns about their physical health, mental health or emotional wellbeing that their doctors, nurses and therapists had not dealt with, 28 people (39.4%) reported a concern. In response to an open-ended question asking for details about this concern(s) that were not dealt with, 16 (23%) reported a concern about mental health. Of these, 12 stated anxiety and 6 stated depression. Additionally, 6 people (8%) reported a concern relating to dental health. Other concerns reported by 1 to 3 people each were concerns with sleep, hand use, circulation, pressure sores, continence and menstrual periods.

4. Discussion

This study aimed to describe unmet health needs among young adults with CP in Ireland and examine if these differed between young adults who were and were not discharged from children's services. Unmet health need was highest for speech. More than a third of young adults reported unmet health needs in several other health areas. In contrast to our hypothesis, unmet health needs did not differ between those who were and were not discharged from children's services.

Similar to previous reports [6,7], physiotherapy was the most commonly used service among young adults with CP. The percentage of young adults, post-discharge, who accessed occupational therapy and speech and language therapy in this study was also similar to the percentages reported in a meta-analysis of service use [7]. The relatively low percentage of young adults with access to psychology found in this study has also been reported in other studies [6–8]. This is the first study to our knowledge to compare if the proportion of young adults accessing services differs between those who have and have not been discharged from children's services. Studies have compared use of services between adolescents and young adults with CP, and similarly found that non-ambulatory adolescents were less likely to use occupational therapy and speech and language therapy than non-ambulatory young adults [8,9]. However, the variation in the age at discharge found in this study highlights that it is insufficient to use age as a proxy indicator of whether a person has been discharged from children's services if examining health and health service use of people with CP.

In a study of adolescents with CP aged 14–18 years in the UK, parents also reported the highest unmet need for speech [12]. The proportion of parents reporting unmet need for speech (0.60) was similar to the proportion we observed (0.64). Unmet needs for mobility, equipment, epilepsy, control of movement and eyesight reported in this study were higher than that reported by parents and adolescents in the UK [12]. Conversely, unmet need for pain was lower in our sample, despite the prevalence of pain being similar [12]. Unmet needs for positioning, bone or joint problems and curvature of the back reported by young adults in this study were similar to those reported by parents and adolescents in the UK [12]. However, a direct comparison of unmet health needs is challenging because of differences in characteristics of the samples and health systems. Our sample included more people in GMFCS levels IV and V. This may explain higher unmet needs given people with greater functional limitations report greater unmet need in some areas such as equipment or positioning [11,12]. However, they may report lower unmet need for pain because they are more likely to have regular access to a professional to discuss their pain with.

We found no difference in unmet health needs between those pre- and post-discharge. Similarly, no increase in unmet health needs was observed after adolescents in the UK were discharged from children's services [12]. This is in contrast to what we hypothesised. However, it may be because we included people up to age 22 years only or because the average time since discharge was only 2 years among those who were discharged. Adults with CP may not experience an increase in unmet health needs until they are beyond 22 years or until they are several years post-discharge, when they potentially start experiencing secondary effects of ageing with CP and have difficulties accessing appropriate services to mitigate these effects [2,7].

Disability is an evolving concept. As the changing, or simply ongoing, health needs of a person with CP interact with a lack of appropriate health services, they will be hindered from fully and effectively participating in society on an equal basis with others. Our findings highlight areas for service development. Young adults who were pre- and post-discharge had high unmet needs for speech and equipment. However, young adults who were discharged from children's services were less likely to access speech and language therapy, occupational therapy and assistive technology services. These services have an important role in supporting young adults to participate in employment or training and recreational activities, and to develop social relationships and independence. Thus, provision of these services should be enhanced for young adults with CP rather than removed. The need for speech and language assessment, referral to a professional with expertise in vocational skills and independent living is outlined in clinical guidelines for adults with CP in the UK [13]. Further, people with CP living in countries that have ratified the United Nations Convention on the Rights of Person with Disabilities have a human right to services and supports that enable them to maintain full physical, mental, social and vocational ability [14]. This includes access to high-quality, affordable assistive products and professionals with the skills and knowledge to assess their need for and prescribe assistive products [14].

The relatively low percentage of young people accessing psychology in combination with the number of young adults who reported an unmet need relating to mental health also highlights an area for service development. Young adults with CP in Canada have similarly described challenges accessing mental health support [15]. Experiencing a mental disorder in adolescence predicts poor mental health in adulthood and can have a long-term impact on a person's personal and economic life [16,17]. Intervening during adolescence and young adulthood, to reduce risk factors may prevent transition from subthreshold levels of anxiety/depression to comorbid mental health conditions in adulthood [18–20].

In comparison to population-based data on people with CP born in Northern Ireland between 1981 and 2001 and data from a meta-analysis of adults with CP [2,21], we believe our sample is representative of adults with CP in terms of gender, ambulatory status, and type of motor disorder. However, people with spastic unilateral CP, people with intellectual disability and people with communication impairment may be underrepresented in our sample. The cross-sectional design of this study and comparison between young adults who were and were not discharged, rather than following the same cohort over time, is a limitation of this study. However, the findings are still useful for describing unmet health needs in this population, particularly when limited data on this population currently exists in the literature. Our study is also limited by responses being collected from either the person with CP, their parent or both because their perception of unmet needs may differ; parents' reports of unmet health needs are typically higher than adolescents' [12]. The number of people reporting needs in some areas, particularly epilepsy, was small. Thus, the proportion with unmet needs may not be precise. Similarly, when examining associations between unmet need, GMFCS level, ID and discharge status, the small number of people reporting needs resulted in wide confidence intervals for odds ratios. Thus, any associations observed should be interpreted as areas for further exploration only. A further limitation is the lack of data describing socio-economic status of participants, which may contribute to unmet health needs.

5. Conclusions

In conclusion, this study confirms that young adults with CP have unmet needs in several health areas. Findings also indicate that young adults who are discharged from children's services are less likely to access some health services. The presence of unmet health needs among young people who are pre- and post-discharge highlights the importance of taking a life-course approach to CP and providing appropriate services to people with CP regardless of age. Providing appropriate mental and physical health services to young adults with CP is not only essential for promoting health, it is essential for enabling young adults to develop independence and participate in all areas of life as they choose.

Supplementary Materials: The following supporting information can be downloaded at: https://www.mdpi.com/article/10.3390/jcm11164847/s1, Table S1: Associations between intellectual disability, ambulatory status, discharge status and unmet need for speech, epilepsy, equipment, mobility and control of move-ment; Table S2: Associations between intellectual disability, ambulatory status, discharge status and unmet need for bone or joint problems, positioning, curvature of back, eyesight and pain.

Author Contributions: Conceptualization, J.M.R., M.W., T.K., O.H., C.K., M.N., A.W., G.L. and J.F.; investigation, J.F.; methodology, J.F., J.M.R., M.W., M.B., M.O., T.K., O.H., C.K., M.N., A.W. and G.L.; formal analysis, J.M.R. and J.F.; resources, M.W., M.O., M.B. and T.K.; writing—original draft preparation, J.M.R. and J.F.; writing—review and editing, M.W., M.O., M.B., T.K., O.H., C.K., M.N., A.W. and G.L.; project administration, J.M.R. and J.F.; funding acquisition, J.M.R., M.W., M.B., T.K., O.H., C.K., M.N., A.W. and G.L. All authors have read and agreed to the published version of the manuscript.

Funding: This research was funded by the Health Research Board and the Central Remedial Clinic (APA-2019-004).

Institutional Review Board Statement: The study was conducted in accordance with the Declaration of Helsinki, and approved by the Ethics Committees of RCSI (protocol REC201911010, 6 February 2020), Central Remedial Clinic (protocol 73001, 9 July 2020) and Enable Ireland (protocol RA72 JR 2020, 16 September 2020).

Informed Consent Statement: Written informed consent was not obtained from those who completed the online survey as it was anonymous and completion indicated consent. However, prior to completing the anonymous online survey, participants confirmed they had read and understood the information leaflet, knew they could withdraw at any time and were happy to complete the questionnaire. Where a person completed a paper survey, they provided written informed consent. People under the age of 18 years similarly provided written informed consent when completing a paper questionnaire and their parent/guardian additionally provided consent for their child to participate.

Data Availability Statement: The data that support the findings of this study are openly available in Zenodo at http://doi.org/10.5281/zenodo.6968034.

Acknowledgments: We thank the members of the Young Person Advisory Group and the Parent Advisory Group for their work throughout the study and interpretation of study findings. We thank Sebastian Koppe from Enable Ireland for his support with recruitment and interpreting study findings. We thank Amanda Breen from the Central Remedial Clinic for her support with interpreting study findings. We also thank the following people who helped us recruit to this study: Alison McCallion, Rory O'Sullivan and Trish MacKeogh from the Central Remedial Clinic; Helen McDaid from the Health Service Executive.

Conflicts of Interest: The authors declare no conflict of interest. The funders had no role in the design of the study; in the collection, analyses, or interpretation of data; in the writing of the manuscript, or in the decision to publish the results.

References

1. Rosenbaum, P.; Paneth, N.; Leviton, A.; Goldstein, M.; Bax, M.; Damiano, D.; Dan, B.; Jacobsson, B. A report: The definition and classification of cerebral palsy April 2006. *Dev. Med. Child Neurol. Suppl.* **2007**, *109*, 8–14. [PubMed]
2. van Gorp, M.; Hilberink, S.R.; Noten, S.; Benner, J.L.; Stam, H.J.; van der Slot, W.M.; Roebroeck, M.E. Epidemiology of Cerebral Palsy in Adulthood: A Systematic Review and Meta-analysis of the Most Frequently Studied Outcomes. *Arch. Phys. Med. Rehabil.* **2020**, *101*, 1041–1052. [CrossRef] [PubMed]
3. Smith, K.J.; Peterson, M.; O'Connell, N.E.; Victor, C.; Liverani, S.; Anokye, N.; Ryan, J. Risk of Depression and Anxiety in Adults With Cerebral Palsy. *JAMA Neurol.* **2019**, *76*, 294–300. [CrossRef] [PubMed]
4. Ryan, J.M.; Peterson, M.D.; Matthews, A.; Ryan, N.; Smith, K.J.; O'Connell, N.E.; Liverani, S.; Anokye, N.; Victor, C.; Allen, E. Noncommunicable disease among adults with cerebral palsy: A matched cohort study. *Neurology* **2019**, *93*, e1385–e1396. [CrossRef] [PubMed]
5. Carter, B.; Bennett, C.V.; Jones, H.; Bethel, J.; Perra, O.; Wang, T.; Kemp, A. Healthcare use by children and young adults with cerebral palsy. *Dev. Med. Child. Neurol.* **2021**, *63*, 75–80. [CrossRef] [PubMed]
6. Ryan, J.M.; Lavelle, G.; Theis, N.; Kilbride, C.; Noorkoiv, M. Patterns of Health Service Use Among Young People With Cerebral Palsy in England. *Front. Neurol.* **2021**, *12*, 659031. [CrossRef] [PubMed]
7. Manikandan, M.; Kerr, C.; Lavelle, G.; Walsh, M.; Walsh, A.; Ryan, J.M. Health service use among adults with cerebral palsy: A mixed-methods systematic review. *Dev. Med. Child Neurol.* **2022**, *64*, 429–446. [CrossRef] [PubMed]
8. McDowell, B.C.; Duffy, C.; Parkes, J. Service use and family-centred care in young people with severe cerebral palsy: A population-based, cross-sectional clinical survey. *Disabil. Rehabil.* **2015**, *37*, 2324–2329. [CrossRef] [PubMed]
9. Roquet, M.; Garlantezec, R.; Remy-Neris, O.; Sacaze, E.; Gallien, P.; Ropars, J.; Houx, L.; Pons, C.; Brochard, S. From childhood to adulthood: Health care use in individuals with cerebral palsy. *Dev. Med. Child. Neurol.* **2018**, *60*, 1271–1277. [CrossRef] [PubMed]
10. Liljenquist, K.; O'Neil, M.E.; Bjornson, K.F. Utilization of Physical Therapy Services During Transition for Young People With Cerebral Palsy: A Call for Improved Care Into Adulthood. *Phys. Ther.* **2018**, *98*, 796–803. [CrossRef] [PubMed]
11. Nieuwenhuijsen, C.; Van Der Laar, Y.; Donkervoort, M.; Nieuwstraten, W.; Roebroeck, M.E.; Stam, H.J. Unmet needs and health care utilization in young adults with cerebral palsy. *Disabil. Rehabil.* **2008**, *30*, 1254–1262. [CrossRef] [PubMed]
12. Solanke, F.; Colver, A.; McConachie, H. Are the health needs of young people with cerebral palsy met during transition from child to adult health care? *Child Care Health Dev.* **2018**, *44*, 355–363. [CrossRef] [PubMed]
13. NICE. Cerebral Palsy in Adults NICE Guideline [NG119]. 2019. Available online: https://www.nice.org.uk/guidance/ng119 (accessed on 3 August 2022).

14. Khasnabis, C.; Mirza, Z.; MacLachlan, M. Opening the GATE to inclusion for people with disabilities. *Lancet* **2015**, *386*, 2229–2230. [CrossRef]
15. Hanes, J.E.; Hlyva, O.; Rosenbaum, P.; Freeman, M.; Nguyen, T.; Palisano, R.J.; Gorter, J.W. Beyond stereotypes of cerebral palsy: Exploring the lived experiences of young Canadians. *Child. Care Health Dev.* **2019**, *45*, 613–622. [CrossRef] [PubMed]
16. Philipson, A.; Alaie, I.; Ssegonja, R.; Imberg, H.; Copeland, W.; Möller, M.; Hagberg, L.; Jonsson, U. Adolescent depression and subsequent earnings across early to middle adulthood: A 25-year longitudinal cohort study. *Epidemiol. Psychiatr. Sci.* **2020**, *29*, e123. [CrossRef] [PubMed]
17. Ssegonja, R.; Alaie, I.; Philipson, A.; Hagberg, L.; Sampaio, F.; Möller, M.; von Knorring, L.; Sarkadi, A.; Langenskiöld, S.; von Knorring, A.-L.; et al. Depressive disorders in adolescence, recurrence in early adulthood, and healthcare usage in mid-adulthood: A longitudinal cost-of-illness study. *J. Affect. Disord.* **2019**, *258*, 33–41. [CrossRef] [PubMed]
18. Patton, G.C.; Coffey, C.; Romaniuk, H.; Mackinnon, A.; Carlin, J.B.; Degenhardt, L.; Olsson, C.A.; Moran, P. The prognosis of common mental disorders in adolescents: A 14-year prospective cohort study. *Lancet* **2014**, *383*, 1404–1411. [CrossRef]
19. Konaszewski, K.; Niesiobędzka, M.; Surzykiewicz, J. Resilience and mental health among juveniles: Role of strategies for coping with stress. *Health Qual Life Outcomes* **2021**, *19*, 58. [CrossRef] [PubMed]
20. Wille, N.; The BELLA Study Group; Bettge, S.; Ravens-Sieberer, U. Risk and protective factors for children's and adolescents' mental health: Results of the BELLA study. *Eur. Child. Adolesc. Psychiatry* **2008**, *17*, 133–147. [CrossRef] [PubMed]
21. McConnell, K.; Livingstone, E.; Perra, O.; Kerr, C. Population-based study on the prevalence and clinical profile of adults with cerebral palsy in Northern Ireland. *BMJ Open* **2021**, *11*, e044614. [CrossRef] [PubMed]

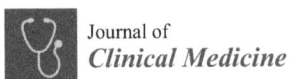

Journal of
Clinical Medicine

Article

Post-Fracture Inpatient and Outpatient Physical/Occupational Therapy and Its Association with Survival among Adults with Cerebral Palsy

Daniel G. Whitney [1,2,*], Tao Xu [3], Daniel Whibley [1,2], Dayna Ryan [1], Michelle S. Caird [4], Edward A. Hurvitz [1] and Heidi Haapala [1]

1. Department of Physical Medicine and Rehabilitation, University of Michigan, Ann Arbor, MI 48109, USA
2. Institute for Healthcare Policy and Innovation, University of Michigan, Ann Arbor, MI 48109, USA
3. Kidney Epidemiology and Cost Center, School of Public Health, University of Michigan, Ann Arbor, MI 48109, USA
4. Department of Orthopaedic Surgery, University of Michigan, Ann Arbor, MI 48109, USA
* Correspondence: dgwhit@umich.edu

Abstract: Physical and/or occupational therapy (PT/OT) may improve post-fracture health and survival among adults with cerebral palsy (CP), but this has not been studied in the inpatient setting. The objective was to quantify the association between acute inpatient and outpatient PT/OT use with 1-year mortality among adults with CP. This was a retrospective cohort study of adults with CP with an incident fragility fracture admitted to an acute care or rehabilitation facility using a random 20% Medicare fee-for-service dataset. Acute care/rehabilitation PT/OT was measured as the average PT/OT cost/day for the length of stay (LOS). Weekly exposure to outpatient PT/OT was examined up to 6 months post-fracture. Cox regression examined the adjusted association between the interaction of acute care/rehabilitation average PT/OT cost/day and LOS with 1-year mortality. A separate Cox model added time-varying outpatient PT/OT. Of 649 adults with CP, average PT/OT cost/day was associated with lower mortality rate for LOS < 17 days (HR range = 0.78–0.93), and increased mortality rate for LOS > 27 days (HR $\geq$ 1.08) (all, $p < 0.05$). After acute care/rehabilitation, 44.5% initiated outpatient PT/OT, which was associated with lower mortality rate (HR = 0.52; 95% CI = 0.27–1.01). Post-fracture inpatient and outpatient PT/OT were associated with improved 1-year survival among adults with CP admitted to acute care/rehabilitation facilities.

Keywords: cerebral palsy; physical therapy; occupational therapy; fracture; bone fragility; mortality

1. Introduction

Fractures represent a quadruple threat to adults with cerebral palsy (CP) as they are common, begin to accumulate early in life [1], associated with premature morbidity and mortality [2–5], and are economically costly [6]. Clinical rehabilitation, including physical and/or occupational therapy (PT/OT), may be effective at mitigating post-fracture health declines, but this has been seldom studied among adults with CP.

Within the U.S. healthcare system, there are different post-fracture rehabilitation pathways that may improve health outcomes in the general population, particularly if rehabilitation is initiated early [7–10]. We recently characterized post-fracture rehabilitation pathways among a large cohort of adults with CP with an incident fragility fracture to better understand the current fracture care landscape. The majority (>70%) were discharged home without acute care or inpatient rehabilitation, and more than half of this home discharge group did not initiate outpatient PT/OT within 6 months post-fracture, potentially impacting recovery [11]. For example, this study found that PT/OT use within 6 months post-fracture among those with a home discharge (without acute care/rehabilitation) was associated with improved 1-year survival [11]. While the mechanisms were not examined,

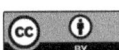

these findings suggest that outpatient PT/OT may improve post-fracture health among adults with CP.

The effectiveness of early rehabilitation applied in acute care and inpatient settings to mitigate post-fracture health declines has not been investigated for adults with CP. In our recent study [11], ~1 in 5 adults with CP with a fragility fracture were admitted to acute care/rehabilitation facilities, but the effect of post-fracture rehabilitation on outcomes was not examined in this cohort (only in the home discharge cohort). The goal of these facilities is to restore enough function through early and/or intensive rehabilitation, predominately PT/OT, in a short time span and address adaptive equipment needs (e.g., assistive mobility devices) to enable safe home discharge of the patient as quickly as possible. The design and implementation of acute care/rehabilitation PT/OT depends in part on several patient-level factors, such as issues with fracture healing, pain, and the ability to perform and tolerate therapies. Adults with CP have long-standing issues with pain, function, and medical complexity, which may be exacerbated by a fracture [12–18]. These factors may alter the initiation and volume of PT/OT sessions and the duration (i.e., number of days) that inpatient PT/OT services are applied in the acute care/rehabilitation setting. Taken together, there may be a spectrum of acute care/rehabilitation PT/OT use patterns that may differently associate with post-fracture outcomes.

A better understanding of how acute care/rehabilitation PT/OT use associates with post-fracture outcomes among adults with CP admitted to acute care/rehabilitation facilities could inform post-fracture care. Further, determining if outpatient PT/OT after acute care/rehabilitation improves post-fracture outcomes may identify additional opportunities to improve post-fracture care for this population. Accordingly, the primary objective of this study was to determine the association between acute care/rehabilitation PT/OT use with 1-year mortality among adults with CP that sustained an incident fragility fracture. We hypothesized that higher acute care/rehabilitation PT/OT volume would be associated with improved 1-year survival conditional on shorter acute care/rehabilitation lengths of stay (i.e., interaction between PT/OT volume and length of stay). The secondary objective was to determine if initiating outpatient PT/OT within 6 months post-fracture was associated with 1-year survival. We hypothesized that initiating outpatient PT/OT within 6 months post-fracture would be associated with improved 1-year survival even after accounting for acute care/rehabilitation PT/OT.

2. Materials and Methods

2.1. Data Source

This retrospective cohort study used claims data from a random 20% sample of the Medicare fee-for-service database (Centers for Medicare & Medicaid Services, Baltimore, MD, USA) Part A (hospital insurance) and Part B (medical insurance. This study did not have access to Part C (Medicare Advantage Plan) or Part D (medication prescription coverage). Medicare is a federal program in the U.S. providing health insurance to adults ≥65 years of age, individuals with certain disabilities including CP at any age, or individuals with end-stage renal disease. Individuals that are enrolled in Medicare can have dual enrollment with Medicaid. Medicare pays first for Medicare-covered services that are also covered by Medicaid, including the diagnostic and rehabilitation-based services needed to conduct this study without bias from missing information from those with dual enrollment in Medicare and Medicaid.

Claims data are primarily used for billing reimbursement of healthcare services, but can be used for research purposes to identify medical conditions and healthcare service use based on unique codes attached to claims. The codes used to identify the variables in this study are presented in Table S1. The data for this study are de-identified prior to the researcher access. Therefore, patient consent was not required and the University's Institutional Review Board approved this study as non-regulated (HUM00158800).

2.2. Cohort Selection

A flow chart to derive the final sample is presented in Figure S1. This study included adults ≥18 years with CP that had an incident fragility fracture (index data = fracture date) at an identifiable site between 1 January 2014–31 December 2017 with an admission to an acute care and/or an Inpatient Rehabilitation Facility. This study combined acute care and acute inpatient rehabilitation services because PT/OT is often applied early in the acute care setting, which can inform admission decisions to an Inpatient Rehabilitation Facility. Thus, combining services provides a more comprehensive assessment of the extent and timing of acute PT/OT.

To be included in the analysis, adults with ≥12 months of continuous enrollment in Part A and B prior to the fracture date (for baseline data) and with ≥30 days of continuous enrollment in Part A and B after the fracture date were included. This study excluded adults that died within 30 days post-fracture as they may represent excessively frail individuals that may not benefit from post-fracture rehabilitation [19]. This study excluded adults that were admitted to a Skilled Nursing Facility because these patients and the rehabilitation treatment are fundamentally different. Finally, adults with a combined acute care/rehabilitation length of stay >31 days were excluded ($n = 22$, ~3%) as this length of stay is atypical and may represent more complex cases presenting with a constellation of complications unrelated to the fracture.

Adults with CP were identified by ≥1 inpatient or ≥2 outpatient claims (with a pertinent code for CP) on separate days within 12 months of one another. A fragility fracture was identified as a ≥1 inpatient or outpatient claim (with a pertinent code for fracture) without a trauma code (e.g., car accident) 7 days before to 7 days after the index fracture date [2,20].

2.3. Acute Care/Rehabilitation PT/OT

This study had access to the Medicare Provider Analysis and Review (MEDPAR) file, which aggregates entire inpatient stays into a single claim. The single claim provides a length of stay and total charges for PT and OT services provided during the acute care/rehabilitation stay, but it does not provide dates of PT or OT services, number of PT or OT sessions, or any details of the PT or OT sessions (e.g., activities). We developed a "volume" measure of inpatient PT/OT as the average cost/day: after standardizing the PT and OT costs to 2017 U.S. dollars, the standardized cost was divided by the acute care/rehabilitation length of stay for each person, e.g., USD 10,000 for PT/OT services during a 10-day stay in the acute care/rehabilitation setting = USD 1000/day. The assumption is that higher average cost/day reflects a greater volume of therapy during the inpatient stay. This study examined PT/OT and not PT and OT separately to capture physical-based rehabilitation that is more inclusive of the varied functional abilities of the population with CP, and to be consistent with how outpatient PT/OT was captured in this study, as described below.

To assess if the average PT/OT cost/day measure was driven by geographical differences in therapy service costs, we developed a generalized linear model with gamma distribution and log-link function, which is appropriate for analyzing healthcare cost data [21–23]. This model estimated the marginal means and cost ratio of average PT/OT cost/day for two geographical variables (in separate models) after adjusting for age, gender, race, dual eligibility with Medicaid, comorbidities, acute care/rehabilitation length of stay, and fracture site. The results of the models suggest that the average PT/OT cost/day did not differ across the 4 U.S. regions or 9 U.S. Divisions (Table S2) (findings were similar when PT and OT cost/day were examined separately).

2.4. Outpatient PT/OT

"Initiation" of outpatient PT/OT is defined in this study as attending the first PT/OT session post-fracture, as opposed to scheduling a PT/OT appointment. Outpatient PT/OT was identified from outpatient files (i.e., Outpatient, Part B, Home Health Agency) using a comprehensive list of codes for physical, occupational, and other therapies of a physical nature (excludes PT/OT evaluations) [24]. Some of these codes cannot distinguish between therapy types or can be used interchangeably for outpatient and home settings. To avoid misclassification, codes were combined into a single indicator of any outpatient PT/OT use.

While the MedPar file (to capture inpatient PT/OT) aggregates all services into a single claim for the entire inpatient stay, outpatient files contain individual claims for each service provided based on the date of service, allowing for a more granular assessment of the date of services. For the post-fracture period, dichotomous variables were created to indicate outpatient PT/OT use per week (starting at week 1) through 6 months post-fracture based on the date of the service claim. A 6-month period was selected to capture an early post-fracture period that may be crucial to implement therapies to improve long-term outcomes, while allowing sufficient time to capture those that may have delayed initiation of PT/OT use, such as from fracture healing [25].

2.5. Mortality

All-cause mortality from 31 days to 1-year post-fracture was identified by the date of death. More than 99% of Medicare recorded deaths have been validated [26].

2.6. Descriptive Characteristics

Information on age, gender (female, male), race, U.S. region of residence, the original reason for Medicare entitlement, and dual eligibility with Medicaid was retrieved. Epilepsy and intellectual disabilities were identified in the same manner as CP and mutually exclusive subgroups were created. The Whitney Comorbidity Index (WCI) was used to characterize (multi-)morbidity profiles using the data from the 1-year baseline period. The WCI was developed [27] and validated [28] specifically for adults with CP. For this study, to avoid overlap with the design, the WCI was modified (WCImod) by removing bone fragility, summing the presence of 26 morbidities relevant to aging with CP.

2.7. Statistical Analysis

Baseline descriptive characteristics, acute care/rehabilitation variables (i.e., length of stay, average PT/OT cost/day), and outpatient PT/OT variables (i.e., proportion that initiated within 6 months post-fracture, time to first use) were summarized. The crude mortality rate with 95% confidence intervals (CI) was estimated for the entire cohort, then by fracture site, as the number of deaths per 100 person years. To visualize the time-varying mortality rate, the cumulative incidence of mortality was plotted for the entire cohort, then by fracture site, using the Fine-Gray approach [29].

For the primary objective, we developed Cox proportional hazards regression models where the outcome was mortality and the primary exposure was the interaction between average PT/OT cost/day and acute care/rehabilitation length of stay, before and after adjusting for possible confounders. To visualize the interaction, we estimated the hazard ratio (HR) of average PT/OT cost/day for length of stays at 1, 3, and every other day until 31 days. Individuals were examined until death, loss to follow-up, or end of the follow-up period, whichever came first. There were a limited number of outcome events for modelling. Confounder selection for adjustment was considered by harmonizing the "disjunctive cause criterion" [30] and data-driven approaches, including univariate associations with possible confounders and variable selection using the regularization technique, Least Absolute Shrinkage and Selection Operator (data not shown) [31,32]. When all approaches were taken together, the final model adjusted for age and WCImod as all other variables (e.g., gender, race, U.S. region of residence, epilepsy and/or intellectual disabilities, fracture site) were found to have little-to-no effect on associations, and some additional confounder-adjusted models increased model over-fitting.

For the secondary objective, time-varying outpatient PT/OT use was added to the fully adjusted Cox regression model from above to determine its adjusted association with 1-year mortality. Outpatient PT/OT was treated as a time-updated exposure from time 0 (fracture date) to the first indication of outpatient PT/OT use up to 6 months post-fracture.

Adults that initiated outpatient PT/OT contributed time to the non-exposed PT/OT group from time 0 to their first week of PT/OT exposure, and then contributed time to the exposed PT/OT group thereafter.

The proportional hazards assumption was tested in all models based on the weighted Schoenfeld residuals.

2.8. Sensitivity Analysis

Data-driven variable selection techniques did not identify fracture site as statistically important in the studied associations. We therefore performed a sensitivity analysis that included fracture site to test for moderating effects on associations between inpatient and outpatient PT/OT use (in separate models) with mortality.

There is potential for survival bias in the model assessing the adjusted association between time-varying outpatient PT/OT use within 6 months post-fracture with 1-year mortality. Therefore, a sensitivity analysis was performed with the mortality risk window moved to 6 months to 1-year post-fracture and individuals were excluded who died or were lost to follow-up <6 months post-fracture.

Analyses were performed using SAS version 9.4 (Cary, NC, USA) and $p < 0.05$ (two-tailed) was considered statistically significant.

3. Results

Baseline descriptive characteristics of the 649 adults with CP with an incident fragility fracture that were admitted to acute care/rehabilitation are presented in Table 1. The prevalence of each comorbidity from the WCI is presented in Table S3.

Table 1. Baseline characteristics of adults with cerebral palsy with a fragility fracture that were admitted to an acute care/rehabilitation setting (n = 649).

Age, mean (SD)	59.8 (15.3)
18–40 years, % (n)	13.3 (86)
41–64 years, % (n)	48.1 (312)
65 years, % (n)	38.7 (251)
Gender, % (n)	
Female	53.0 (344)
Male	47.0 (305)
Race, % (n)	
Black	9.9 (64)
Hispanic	2.0 (13)
White	85.2 (553)
Other	2.9 (19)
U.S. region of residence, % (n)	
Northeast	22.8 (148)
Midwest	24.2 (157)
South	32.5 (211)
West	20.5 (133)
Original reason for Medicare entitlement, % (n)	
Old age and survivor's insurance	18.8 (122)
Disability insurance benefits (DIB)	80.6 (523)
End-stage renal disease (ESRD)	*
Both DIB and ESRD	*
Dual eligibility with Medicaid, % (n)	
Full	65.2 (423)
Partial	4.3 (28)
None	30.5 (198)
Co-occurring neurological conditions, % (n)	
None	59.3 (385)
Epilepsy	12.2 (79)
Intellectual disabilities	10.6 (69)
Epilepsy + intellectual disabilities	17.9 (116)

Table 1. *Cont.*

Whitney Comorbidity Index, median (IQR)	3 (1–6)
Fracture site, % (n)	
Vertebral column	14.0 (91)
Hip	32.4 (210)
Non-proximal femur	9.7 (63)
Leg/ankle	18.2 (118)
Humerus	6.0 (39)
Forearm	2.5 (16)
Multiple sites	17.3 (112)

SD, standard deviation; IQR, interquartile range. * Values suppressed as $n < 11$ to maintain patient de-identification.

3.1. Acute Care/Rehabilitation PT/OT Use

The median and interquartile range (IQR) for acute care/rehabilitation length of stay and average PT/OT cost/day for the stay is presented in Table 2. The length of stay was similar across fracture sites with a median of 5 days except for forearm fractures (2 days). Median average PT/OT cost/day ranged by fracture site from USD 40/day (non-proximal femur) to USD 344/day (hip). The majority of the costs came from PT vs. OT services, except the relatively similar PT and OT costs for forearm fractures.

Table 2. Length of stay and average physical therapy (PT) and/or occupational therapy (OT) costs per day in the acute care/rehabilitation setting within 31 days post-fracture for the entire cohort ($n = 649$) and then by fracture site.

	Length of Stay	Average PT/OT Cost/Day	Average PT Cost/Day	Average OT Cost/Day
	Days	USD/Day	USD/Day	USD/Day
Entire cohort	5 (3, 8)	212 (56, 438)	146 (24, 299)	38 (0, 156)
By fracture site				
Vertebral column	5 (3, 8)	119 (0, 354)	77 (0, 224)	0 (0, 97)
Hip	5 (3, 7)	344 (184, 534)	239 (133, 373)	106 (0, 201)
Non-proximal femur	5 (3, 10)	40 (0, 308)	31 (0, 196)	0 (0, 93)
Leg/ankle	5 (3, 8)	183 (84, 413)	153 (47, 295)	0 (0, 122)
Humerus	5 (3, 9)	136 (0, 241)	102 (0, 138)	0 (0, 112)
Forearm	2 (2, 4)	120 (0, 314)	0 (0, 137)	0 (0, 170)
Multiple sites	5 (3, 8)	189 (45, 349)	130 (4, 245)	14 (0, 126)

Values are median (interquartile range).

3.2. Outpatient PT/OT Use

Among the entire cohort, 44.5% ($n = 289$) initiated outpatient PT/OT within 6 months post-fracture and their median (IQR) time to the first outpatient PT/OT use was 10 (6–13) weeks. The proportion that initiated outpatient PT/OT within 6 months post-fracture varied by fracture site from 18.8% (forearm) to 59.8% (multiple simultaneous sites), but median time to first PT/OT use was similar across fracture sites (Table 3).

3.3. One-Year Mortality Rate

During the 1-year follow-up, 1 person (with a hip fracture) was lost to follow-up and 8.9% ($n = 58$) died. The crude mortality rate for the entire cohort was 9.4 per 100 person years (95% CI = 7.0–11.9) and varied based on fracture site from 0 (forearm) to 19.2 (95% CI = 7.9–30.6) (non-proximal femur) (Table 4). The cumulative incidence of 1-year mortality for the entire cohort and by fracture site is shown in Figure 1.

Table 3. Proportion of and median time to first outpatient physical or occupational therapy (PT/OT) service within 6 months post-fracture for the entire cohort (n = 649) and then by fracture site.

	Initiated Outpatient PT/OT within 6 Months Post-Fracture	Time to First PT/OT Use within 6 Months Post-Fracture
	% (n)	Median (IQR) in Weeks
Entire cohort	44.5 (289)	10 (6, 13)
By fracture site		
Vertebral column	53.9 (49)	10 (5, 15)
Hip	40.0 (84)	9 (6, 12)
Non-proximal femur	27.0 (17)	9 (5, 12)
Leg/ankle	44.9 (53)	11 (7, 15)
Humerus *	<45.0 (<20)	10 (6, 13)
Forearm *	<30.0 (<11)	11 (4, 15)
Multiple sites	59.8 (67)	10 (7, 16)

IQR, interquartile range. * Values not provided due to n < 11 to maintain patient de-identification.

Table 4. Mortality rate (MR) within 1-year post-fracture for the entire study cohort and then by fracture site.

	Sample Size (n)	MR Per 100 Person Years (95% CI)
Entire cohort	649	9.4 (7.0, 11.9)
By fracture site		
Vertebral column	91	11.6 (4.4, 18.9)
Hip	210	6.4 (2.9, 10.0)
Non-proximal femur	63	19.2 (7.9, 30.6)
Leg/ankle	118	7.1 (2.2, 12.0)
Humerus	39	17.0 (3.4, 30.6)
Forearm	16	0 (0, 0)
Multiple sites	112	9.4 (3.6, 15.3)

CI, confidence interval.

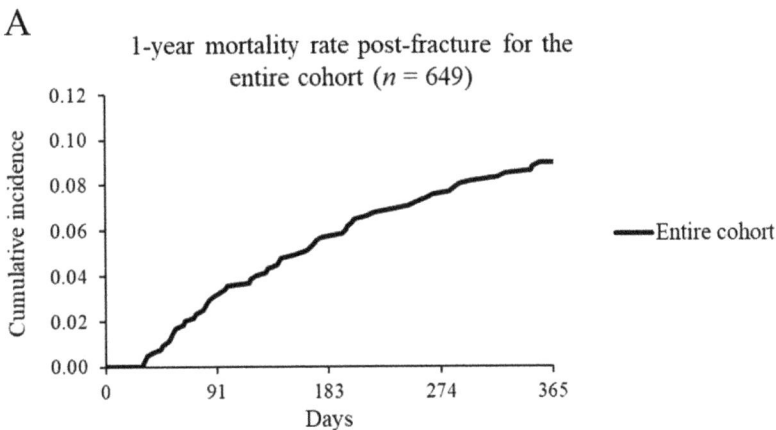

Figure 1. Cont.

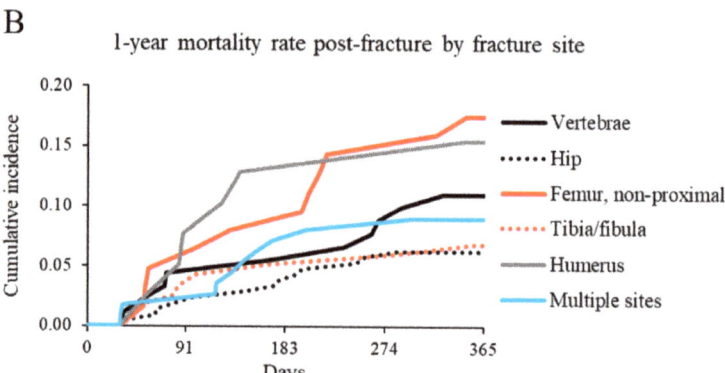

Figure 1. Mortality rate. Cumulative incidence of mortality from 31 days to 1-year post-fracture among (**A**) the entire cohort of adults with cerebral palsy with an incident fragility fracture and (**B**) then by fracture site.

3.4. Association between PT/OT Use and 1-Year Mortality

As hypothesized, there was evidence of an interaction between acute care/rehabilitation average PT/OT cost/day with the length of stay in unadjusted and adjusted models (both p for interaction, ≤0.001). The unit of measurement for the average PT/OT cost/day (continuous variable) was set to USD 60/day. This was done to produce an effect estimate that is more readily interpretable as compared to a much smaller effect estimate when modelling the continuous exposure as USD 1/day. All other model and statistical parameters are unchanged with this transformation. The average PT/OT cost/day was associated with lower mortality rate, but the effect diminished linearly with increasing length of stay until ~17 days, after which the association became non-significant and then significantly associated with increased mortality rate (Figure 2).

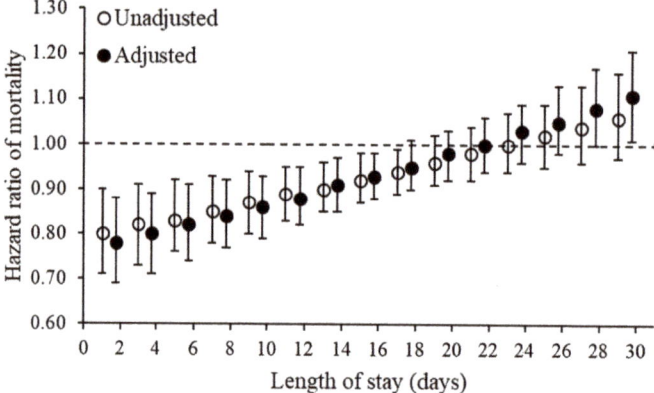

Figure 2. Therapy volume by length of stay effect on mortality. Examining the interaction between the acute care/rehabilitation average physical/occupational therapy cost/day and length of stay for the outcome, 1-year mortality rate, among adults with cerebral palsy with an incident fragility fracture. The open and closed circles represent the hazard ratio (vertical lines are the 95% confidence interval) of mortality (y-axis) for the average physical/occupational therapy cost/day for that length of stay at 1, 3, 5, and every other day until 29 days (x-axis). The same length of stay was estimated for the unadjusted and adjusted models, but positioned next to one another on the graph as opposed to on top of one another to enhance visual interpretation. If the 95% confidence interval (vertical lines extending from the open/closed circles) cross 1.00 (dashed line), the association is not statistically significant at $p < 0.05$. The adjusted model accounted for age and the Whitney Comorbidity Index.

Time-varying outpatient PT/OT use (as time to the first service use) was added to the model and was associated with lower mortality rate (HR = 0.52; 95% CI = 0.27–1.01, p = 0.053). Adding time-varying outpatient PT/OT use did not alter the conclusions drawn about the average PT/OT cost/day conditional on length of stay (Figure S2) or its interaction (p for interaction, <0.001).

There was no statistical evidence that the proportional hazards assumption was violated in any model. Fitted penalized B-spline curves were examined, and there was insufficient evidence to indicate time-varying associations between the exposures of interest with the outcome, to determine if early vs. later initiation had differential effects on mortality rate.

3.5. Sensitivity Analysis

To enhance model parsimony, fracture site was grouped as: vertebral column; hip; lower extremities (non-proximal femur and leg/ankle); upper extremities (humerus and forearm); and multiple simultaneous sites. There was no strong evidence of an interaction between fracture site with the inpatient or outpatient PT/OT variables (both p for interaction, >0.05).

When the mortality risk window was examined from 6 months to 1-year, there were 21 deaths out of 612 (3.4%) adults eligible for this analysis. The effect estimate of time-varying outpatient PT/OT use within 6 months post-fracture was similar to the main analysis (HR = 0.48; 95% CI = 0.17–1.32), suggesting no strong evidence of survival bias.

4. Discussion

This study among 649 adults with CP with an incident fragility fracture found that acute care/rehabilitation PT/OT was associated with improved 1-year survival, but this was conditional on lengths of stay <17 days. Additionally, adults with CP that initiated outpatient PT/OT within 6 months post-fracture had a 48% lower mortality rate, even after accounting for acute care/rehabilitation PT/OT; although, this was not statistically significant (95% CI = 0.27–1.01, p = 0.053). There was no strong evidence to suggest that the timing of inpatient or outpatient PT/OT use appreciably associated with mortality rate. Further, there was no strong evidence to suggest that certain fracture sites were driving the observed associations. However, caution in these interpretations is advised given the relatively small sample and number of outcome events. Taken together, these findings suggest that inpatient and outpatient PT/OT are associated with improved survival up to 1-year following a fragility fracture among adults with CP admitted to an acute care/rehabilitation setting.

The study cohort likely does not represent the broader population of adults with CP that sustain a fragility fracture. Decisions to admit a patient to acute care/rehabilitation post-fracture are typically made on a case-by-case basis using clinical judgement. Allocating adults with CP with a fragility fracture to acute care/rehabilitation or other post-fracture rehabilitation pathways may be subject to greater variability than adults without CP, possibly motivated by the patient characteristics. For example, in a previous study, we found that adults with CP with an incident fragility fracture that were discharged home (without acute care/rehabilitation) were younger, more medically complex, and less likely to have sustained a fracture at the hip, femur, and multiple simultaneous sites compared to those admitted to acute care/rehabilitation [11]. It therefore remains unknown whether acute care/rehabilitation PT/OT has similar effects for all adults with CP that sustain a fragility fracture. Although, we speculate that early and appropriately intensive rehabilitation would likely have a more favorable benefit: risk ratio for all adults with CP that sustain a fragility fracture.

This observational study does not address causality. As anticipated, there was an interaction between the "volume" of acute care/rehabilitation PT/OT (as average PT/OT cost/day) with the length of stay. A higher volume was associated with improved survival for length of stays <17 days, after which the association became non-significant until

27 days. Indeed, after this duration, a higher volume of therapy was significantly associated with increased mortality (Figure 2). There are potential study design and prognostic factors to consider here. For example, confounding by indication is a possibility. The need for more therapy and a longer duration of inpatient stay may be related to greater underlying medical needs or fracture complexity that may itself be associated with a higher mortality risk [33,34]. However, this study accounted for confounding by medical complexity via the WCI (comorbidity index), thus mitigating this potential source of bias. The observational study design is unable to tease out whether outcomes actually improved for individuals relative to not having received (or receiving less) acute care/rehabilitation PT/OT, especially for those with higher mortality rates. For example, the adjusted HR of 1-year mortality was ~1.00 for average PT/OT cost/day for a length of stay of 21 days (Figure 2). For these individuals, the mortality risk may have been even higher if they had not received any PT/OT in the acute care/rehabilitation setting.

In this study, 44.5% of adults with CP with a fragility fracture admitted to an acute care/rehabilitation facility initiated outpatient PT/OT within 6 months post-fracture. This is similar to the 43.1% of adults with CP discharged home without acute care/rehabilitation post-fracture [11]. Consistent with our prior study in the home discharge cohort, the findings of this study suggest an association between outpatient PT/OT use within 6 months post-fracture and improved 1-year survival among those admitted to an acute care/rehabilitation facility. One possible mechanism for these findings is that PT/OT mitigates the decline in function following a fracture, which likely prevents or decelerates the progression of health declines associated with inactivity. Fragility fractures are associated with an increased risk of cardiorespiratory diseases [2,3,5], which in turn mediates [35] a portion of the excess fracture-related mortality [4] among adults with CP. In studies not focused on CP, post-fracture rehabilitation has been reported to mitigate the loss of function and risk of mortality [7,8]. Rehabilitation-based interventions, such as PT/OT, can improve function for individuals with CP [36], which may reduce the risk of cardiorespiratory disease and other health declines and thus improve survival.

The limitations of this study that may directly impact conclusions must be discussed. First, the "volume" measure, average PT/OT cost/day, is not validated and it is unknown how well it captures the full, comprehensive breadth of physical-based rehabilitation post-fracture. Moreover, PT/OT was combined from the acute care and/or an Inpatient Rehabilitation Facility, primarily to begin understanding the timing of PT/OT initiation and its effect on post-fracture outcomes. However, PT/OT applied in the Inpatient Rehabilitation Facility setting is more intensive than in the acute care setting, and can include additional care (e.g., social workers) and therapies (e.g., speech, language, psychology). Therefore, the association between greater inpatient PT/OT use (condition on length of stays <17 days) and lower mortality may be influenced by the more comprehensive rehabilitative care from Inpatient Rehabilitation Facilities as compared to the acute care setting. Unfortunately, the data files we had access to did not allow for the distinction between whether the PT/OT was done in an acute care or Inpatient Rehabilitation Facility. Second, 1-year mortality was the outcome, which is not necessarily highly specific to measuring effectiveness of clinical rehabilitation services. However, improving function post-fracture can increase independence and health, thus having downstream effects on survival [7–9]. Given the scant research attention to date on the topic, these findings should be considered an early step to document high-level associations with the most consequential outcome of post-fracture health declines for adults with CP [4]. Future studies are needed to measure specific outcomes that will allow for a more detailed assessment of PT/OT effectiveness, as well as the mechanisms linking rehabilitation to improved survival to ultimately improve PT/OT services for adults with CP. Third, the type of therapy intervention or focus of the PT/OT services cannot be ascertained from claims. Fourth, bias from unmeasured confounding is possible as claims does not contain information about the severity of CP or other relevant variables; e.g., functional status. However, the analytic plan comprehensively identified relevant confounders available for analysis and adjusted for variables that serve as reasonable proxies for medical complexity.

5. Conclusions

Study findings provide new evidence that acute care/rehabilitation PT/OT is associated with improved 1-year survival among adults with CP with a fragility fracture, conditional on the acute care/rehabilitation length of stay. This study also identified that initiating outpatient PT/OT use within 6 months post-fracture was associated with improved 1-year survival. While more research is needed, there may be great value in improving access to and delivery of inpatient and outpatient PT/OT services post-fracture for adults with CP to mitigate their otherwise rapid post-fracture health declines.

Supplementary Materials: The following supporting information can be downloaded at: https://www.mdpi.com/article/10.3390/jcm11195561/s1, Figure S1: Flow chart; Figure S2: Therapy volume by length of stay effect on mortality; Table S1: International Classification of Diseases, Ninth (ICD-9) and Tenth (ICD-10) Revision, Clinical Modification, Healthcare Common Procedure Coding System (HCPCS), Current Procedural Terminology (CPT), and Revenue codes to identify variables for this study; Table S2: Adjusted marginal means and cost ratio for U.S. region and division of residence with the outcome as average cost per day for physical/occupational therapy* during the post-fracture acute care/rehabilitation stay ($n = 649$); Table S3: Prevalence of Whitney Comorbidity Index comorbidities for adults with cerebral palsy with a fragility fracture that were admitted to an acute care/rehabilitation setting ($n = 649$).

Author Contributions: Conceptualization, D.G.W., D.W., H.H., E.A.H., M.S.C. and D.R.; methodology, D.G.W., D.W., T.Z., H.H.; validation, D.G.W. and T.X.; formal analysis, D.G.W. and T.X.; resources, D.G.W.; data curation, T.X.; writing—original draft preparation, D.G.W.; writing—review and editing, all authors; visualization, D.G.W.; project administration, D.G.W.; funding acquisition, D.G.W. All authors have read and agreed to the published version of the manuscript.

Funding: This research was funded by the National Institutes of Health, grant number R01AR076994, the University of Michigan Office of Health Equity and Inclusion Diversity Fund (no grant number), and The American Occupational Therapy Foundation Health Services Research Grant (no grant number). The APC was funded by The American Occupational Therapy Foundation Health Services Research Grant.

Institutional Review Board Statement: Ethical review and approval were waived for this study because the data were de-identified prior to administration to researchers, and patient consent was not required.

Informed Consent Statement: Patient consent was waived due to de-identification prior to administrating data to researchers.

Data Availability Statement: Data is not available by the research team. Data was obtained from the Centers for Medicare & Medicaid Services under Data Use Agreements.

Conflicts of Interest: The authors declare no conflict of interest. The funders had no role in the design of the study; in the collection, analyses, or interpretation of data; in the writing of the manuscript, or in the decision to publish the results.

References

1. Whitney, D.G.; Hurvitz, E.A.; Caird, M.S. Critical periods of bone health across the lifespan for individuals with cerebral palsy: Informing clinical guidelines for fracture prevention and monitoring. *Bone* **2021**, *150*, 116009. [CrossRef]
2. Etter, J.P.; Kannikeswaran, S.; Hurvitz, E.A.; Peterson, M.D.; Caird, M.S.; Jepsen, K.J.; Whitney, D.G. The respiratory disease burden of non-traumatic fractures for adults with cerebral palsy. *Bone Rep.* **2020**, *13*, 100730. [CrossRef] [PubMed]
3. Whitney, D.G.; Bell, S.; Etter, J.P.; Prisby, R.D. The cardiovascular disease burden of non-traumatic fractures for adults with and without cerebral palsy. *Bone* **2020**, *136*, 115376. [CrossRef]
4. Whitney, D.G.; Bell, S.; Hurvitz, E.A.; Peterson, M.D.; Caird, M.S.; Jepsen, K.J. The mortality burden of non-trauma fracture for adults with cerebral palsy. *Bone Rep.* **2020**, *13*, 100725. [CrossRef] [PubMed]
5. Whitney, D.G.; Xu, T.; Berri, M. Post-fracture pneumonia risk and association with health and survival outcomes for adults with cerebral palsy: A retrospective cohort study. *Bone* **2022**, *159*, 116390. [CrossRef] [PubMed]

6. Whitney, D.G.; Caird, M.S.; Jepsen, K.J.; Hurvitz, E.A.; Hirth, R.A. Excess healthcare spending associated with fractures among adults with cerebral palsy. *Disabil. Health J.* **2022**, *15*, 101315. [CrossRef]
7. Singh, N.A.; Quine, S.; Clemson, L.M.; Williams, E.J.; Williamson, D.A.; Stavrinos, T.M.; Grady, J.N.; Perry, T.J.; Lloyd, B.D.; Smith, E.U.; et al. Effects of high-intensity progressive resistance training and targeted multidisciplinary treatment of frailty on mortality and nursing home admissions after hip fracture: A randomized controlled trial. *J. Am. Med. Dir. Assoc.* **2012**, *13*, 24–30. [CrossRef]
8. Tedesco, D.; Gibertoni, D.; Rucci, P.; Hernandez-Boussard, T.; Rosa, S.; Bianciardi, L.; Rolli, M.; Fantini, M.P. Impact of rehabilitation on mortality and readmissions after surgery for hip fracture. *BMC Health Serv. Res.* **2018**, *18*, 701. [CrossRef]
9. Binder, E.F.; Brown, M.; Sinacore, D.R.; Steger-May, K.; Yarasheski, K.E.; Schechtman, K.B. Effects of extended outpatient rehabilitation after hip fracture: A randomized controlled trial. *JAMA* **2004**, *292*, 837–846. [CrossRef] [PubMed]
10. Albin, S.R.; Koppenhaver, S.L.; Van Boerum, D.H.; McPoil, T.G.; Morgan, J.; Fritz, J.M. Timing of initiating manual therapy and therapeutic exercises in the management of patients after hindfoot fractures: A randomized controlled trial. *J. Man Manip. Ther.* **2018**, *26*, 147–156. [CrossRef] [PubMed]
11. Whitney, D.G.; Xu, T.; Ryan, D.; Whibley, D.; Caird, M.S.; Hurvitz, E.A.; Haapala, H. Post-fracture rehabilitation pathways and association with mortality among adults with cerebral palsy. *Clin. Rehabil.* **2022**, in press. [CrossRef] [PubMed]
12. Whitney, D.G.; Hurvitz, E.A.; Ryan, J.M.; Devlin, M.J.; Caird, M.S.; French, Z.P.; Ellenberg, E.C.; Peterson, M.D. Noncommunicable disease and multimorbidity in young adults with cerebral palsy. *Clin. Epidemiol.* **2018**, *10*, 511–519. [CrossRef]
13. Whitney, D.G.; Schmidt, M.; Haapala, H.; Ryan, D.; Hurvitz, E.A.; Peterson, M.D. Timecourse of Morbidity Onset among Adults Living with Cerebral Palsy. *Am. J. Prev. Med.* **2021**, *61*, 37–43. [CrossRef]
14. O'Connell, N.E.; Smith, K.J.; Peterson, M.D.; Ryan, N.; Liverani, S.; Anokye, N.; Victor, C.; Ryan, J.M. Incidence of osteoarthritis, osteoporosis and inflammatory musculoskeletal diseases in adults with cerebral palsy: A population-based cohort study. *Bone* **2019**, *125*, 30–35. [CrossRef] [PubMed]
15. Ryan, J.M.; Peterson, M.D.; Ryan, N.; Smith, K.J.; O'Connell, N.E.; Liverani, S.; Anokye, N.; Victor, C.; Allen, E. Mortality due to cardiovascular disease, respiratory disease, and cancer in adults with cerebral palsy. *Dev. Med. Child Neurol.* **2019**, *61*, 924–928. [CrossRef] [PubMed]
16. Van Der Slot, W.M.; Nieuwenhuijsen, C.; Van Den Berg-Emons, R.J.; Bergen, M.P.; Hilberink, S.R.; Stam, H.J.; Roebroeck, M.E. Chronic pain, fatigue, and depressive symptoms in adults with spastic bilateral cerebral palsy. *Dev. Med. Child Neurol.* **2012**, *54*, 836–842. [CrossRef]
17. Whitney, D.G.; Schmidt, M.; Hurvitz, E.A. Shared Physiologic Pathways among Comorbidities for Adults with Cerebral Palsy. *Front. Neurol.* **2021**, *12*, 742179. [CrossRef] [PubMed]
18. Hurvitz, E.A.; Whitney, D.G.; Waldron-Perrine, B.; Ryan, D.; Haapala, H.J.; Schmidt, M.; Gray, C.; Peterson, M.D. Navigating the Pathway to Care in Adults With Cerebral Palsy. *Front. Neurol.* **2021**, *12*, 734139. [CrossRef] [PubMed]
19. Lindenauer, P.K.; Stefan, M.S.; Pekow, P.S.; Mazor, K.M.; Priya, A.; Spitzer, K.A.; Lagu, T.C.; Pack, Q.R.; Pinto-Plata, V.M.; ZuWallack, R. Association between Initiation of Pulmonary Rehabilitation after Hospitalization for COPD and 1-Year Survival among Medicare Beneficiaries. *JAMA* **2020**, *323*, 1813–1823. [CrossRef]
20. Keshishian, A.; Boytsov, N.; Burge, R.; Krohn, K.; Lombard, L.; Zhang, X.; Xie, L.; Baser, O. Examining the Effect of Medication Adherence on Risk of Subsequent Fracture among Women with a Fragility Fracture in the U.S. Medicare Population. *J. Manag. Care Spec. Pharm.* **2017**, *23*, 1178–1190. [CrossRef] [PubMed]
21. Barber, J.; Thompson, S. Multiple regression of cost data: Use of generalised linear models. *J. Health Serv. Res. Policy* **2004**, *9*, 197–204. [CrossRef]
22. Diehr, P.; Yanez, D.; Ash, A.; Hornbrook, M.; Lin, D.Y. Methods for analyzing health care utilization and costs. *Annu. Rev. Public Health* **1999**, *20*, 125–144. [CrossRef]
23. Mantopoulos, T.; Mitchell, P.M.; Welton, N.J.; McManus, R.; Andronis, L. Choice of statistical model for cost-effectiveness analysis and covariate adjustment: Empirical application of prominent models and assessment of their results. *Eur. J. Health Econ.* **2016**, *17*, 927–938. [CrossRef]
24. Conner, B.C.; Xu, T.; Kamdar, N.S.; Haapala, H.; Whitney, D.G. Physical and occupational therapy utilization and associated factors among adults with cerebral palsy: Longitudinal modelling to capture distinct utilization groups. *Disabil. Health J.* **2022**, *15*, 101279. [CrossRef]
25. Presedo, A.; Dabney, K.W.; Miller, F. Fractures in patients with cerebral palsy. *J. Pediatric Orthop.* **2007**, *27*, 147–153. [CrossRef]
26. Jarosek, S. Death Information in the Research Identifiable Medicare Data. Available online: https://www.resdac.org/articles/death-information-research-identifiable-medicare-data#:~{}:text=Overall%2C%2099%25%20of%20death%20days%20have%20been%20validated.,-The%20most%20common&text=However%2C%20RRB%20beneficiaries%20comprise%20a,and%2098%25%20are%20SSA%20beneficiaries (accessed on 14 December 2020).
27. Whitney, D.G.; Kamdar, N.S. Development of a new comorbidity index for adults with cerebral palsy and comparative assessment with common comorbidity indices. *Dev. Med. Child Neurol.* **2021**, *63*, 313–319. [CrossRef]
28. Whitney, D.G.; Basu, T. Whitney Comorbidity Index to monitor health status for adults with cerebral palsy: Validation and thresholds to assist clinical decision making. *Dev. Med. Child Neurol.* **2021**, *63*, 853–859. [CrossRef]
29. Fine, J.P.; Gray, R.J. A proportional hazards model for the subdistribution of a competing risk. *J. Am. Stat. Assoc.* **1999**, *94*, 496–509. [CrossRef]

30. VanderWeele, T.J. Principles of confounder selection. *Eur. J. Epidemiol.* **2019**, *34*, 211–219. [CrossRef]
31. Tibshirani, R. Regression shrinkage and selection via the Lasso. *J. Roy. Stat. Soc. B (Methodol.)* **1996**, *58*, 267–288. [CrossRef]
32. Steyerberg, E.W.; Eijkemans, M.J.C.; Habbema, J.D.F. Application of shrinkage techniques in logistic regression analysis: A case study. *Stat. Neerl.* **2001**, *55*, 76–88. [CrossRef]
33. Mubark, I.; Abouelela, A.; Genena, A.; Al Ghunimat, A.; Sarhan, I.; Ashwood, N. Mortality Following Distal Femur Fractures Versus Proximal Femur Fractures in Elderly Population: The Impact of Best Practice Tariff. *Cureus* **2020**, *12*, e10744. [CrossRef]
34. Neuman, M.D.; Silber, J.H.; Magaziner, J.S.; Passarella, M.A.; Mehta, S.; Werner, R.M. Survival and functional outcomes after hip fracture among nursing home residents. *JAMA Intern. Med.* **2014**, *174*, 1273–1280. [CrossRef]
35. Whitney, D.G. Mediating effects of post-fracture cardiorespiratory disease on mortality for adults with cerebral palsy: A cohort study. *Ann. Phys. Rehabil. Med.* **2022**, *65*, 101661. [CrossRef]
36. Ross, S.M.; MacDonald, M.; Bigouette, J.P. Effects of strength training on mobility in adults with cerebral palsy: A systematic review. *Disabil. Health J.* **2016**, *9*, 375–384. [CrossRef]

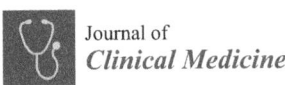

Article

Underlying Causes of Death among Adults with Cerebral Palsy

Mark D. Peterson [1,2,*], Allecia M. Wilson [3] and Edward A. Hurvitz [1]

[1] Department of Physical Medicine and Rehabilitation, Michigan Medicine, University of Michigan, Ann Arbor, MI 48109, USA
[2] Institute for Healthcare Policy and Innovation, Michigan Medicine, University of Michigan, Ann Arbor, MI 48109, USA
[3] Department of Pathology, Michigan Medicine, University of Michigan, Ann Arbor, MI 48109, USA
* Correspondence: mdpeterz@med.umich.edu

Abstract: Background: Adults with cerebral palsy (CP) represent a growing population whose healthcare needs are poorly understood. The purpose of this study was to examine trends in the underlying causes of death (UCOD) among adults with CP in the United States. Methods: A national cohort was created from the Centers for Disease Control and Prevention Wide-ranging Online Data for Epidemiologic Research (WONDER) database from 1999 to 2019. The UCOD was determined using the International Statistical Classification of Diseases and Related Health Problems, Tenth Revision (ICD-10 code G80x, Infantile CP) based on death certificate adjudication. Crude and age-adjusted mortality rates (AAMRs), as well as 95% confidence intervals (CIs) were calculated for adults with CP. Results: There were 25,138 deaths where CP was listed as the UCOD between 1999–2019. There was a steady increase in the UCOD attributable to CP in both crude mortality rates and AAMRs, with the highest rates occurring in 2019. The highest co-occurring secondary causes of death were other diseases of the nervous system (e.g., epilepsy), diseases of the respiratory system (e.g., pneumonia), symptoms, signs, and abnormal clinical and laboratory findings, not elsewhere classified (e.g., dysphagia), and diseases of the circulatory system (e.g., cardiovascular disease). Conclusions: Listing the UCOD as CP should be accompanied by other mechanisms leading to mortality in this population.

Keywords: cerebral palsy; epidemiology; mortality; age-adjusted mortality rates; death certificate; medical education

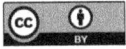

1. Introduction

Cerebral palsy (CP) arises early in life and is viewed as a non-progressive pediatric condition affecting movement, muscle tone, or posture [1]. With improvements in care, individuals with CP live well into late adulthood-prompting a recent paradigm shift to recognize the unique needs of this population across the lifespan [2,3]. Unfortunately, across healthcare systems, adults with CP are often confined to pediatric hospitals and ambulatory care services [4], and they struggle to receive appropriate care, even for the most common disorders such as musculoskeletal comorbidities [5]. As individuals with CP age, they face unique challenges which make their medical care highly complex [6–8] and are at risk for dying at younger ages—often from undiagnosed, preventable, noncommunicable diseases [9], and potentially preventable respiratory causes [10].

Mortality records for CP are prone to errors due to the high prevalence of comorbid physical, cognitive, and mental health issues [6,11,12]; however, CP is not a standalone "underlying cause of death" (UCOD) among adults *with* CP. Previous work has demonstrated that postmortem diagnostic overshadowing is common among deceased adults with CP and other neurodevelopmental and intellectual disabilities [13–15]. This practice prohibits the identification of the actual medical cause of death and does nothing to inform public health or preventive care efforts to reduce premature mortality. Indeed, the accuracy of the death certificate is vital as it provides important information about the decedent, the circumstances of death, and the true underlying cause(s) of death. Individuals with more severe forms of CP may die in long-term care facilities, in hospice, or at home, resulting in inherent challenges with accurate mortality reporting. The purpose of this study was to examine temporal trends in CP as the UCOD overall and across subgroups stratified by rural-urban area designation in the US. Further, we sought to determine secondary causes of death when CP was listed as the UCOD.

2. Methods

We used the US Centers for Disease Control and Prevention Wide-ranging Online Data for Epidemiologic Research (CDC WONDER) database [16]. The Underlying Cause of Death (UCOD) data available on WONDER are county-level national mortality and population data spanning the years 1999–2019. Each death certificate contains a single underlying cause of death, up to 20 additional multiple causes, and demographic data including ethnicity. The number of deaths, crude death rates or age-adjusted death rates, and 95% confidence intervals and standard errors for death rates can be obtained by place of residence (total U.S., region, state, and county), age group (single-year-of age, 5-year age groups, 10-year age groups, and infant age groups), race, Hispanic ethnicity, gender, year, cause-of-death, injury intent, and injury mechanism, drug/alcohol-induced causes, and urbanization categories. Data are also available for the place of death, month and week day of death, and whether an autopsy was performed. For this study, the UCOD was determined using the International Statistical Classification of Diseases and Related Health Problems, Tenth Revision (ICD-10 code G80x, Infantile cerebral palsy) based on death certificate adjudication. Crude mortality rates and 95% confidence intervals were calculated for adults over 20 years of age, and age-adjusted mortality rates (AAMRs) were calculated for adults over 25 years of age between 1999 and 2019. We were limited to doing this because calculations for crude mortality were openly available for all ages, whereas age-adjusted mortality was limited by CDC WONDER to 10-year age bands as follows: (1) <1 year; (2) 1–4 years; (3) 5–14 years; (4) 15–24 years; (5) 25–34 years; (6) 35–44 years; (7) 45–54 years; (8) 55–64 years; (9) 65–74 years; (10) 75–84 years; and (11) 85+ years. The AAMRs were calculated by multiplying the age-specific death rate for each age group by the corresponding weight from the 2000 standard US population, summing across all age groups, and then multiplying by 100,000. Crude mortality and AAMR are expressed per 100,000 population per year.

For the most recent available year (2019), we divided our population using the National Center for Health Statistics urban-rural classification scheme into large metropolitan ($\geq$1 million), medium and small metropolitan (50,000–999,999), and rural (< 50,000) counties per the 2013 US Census classification [17]. Results were further categorized by age (20–34, 35–49, 50–64, and $\geq$ 65 years), sex, race, and ethnicity. We also examined underlying *and* multiple causes of death with a stepwise approach: when CP was determined as the "underlying cause of death" but there were other causes of mortality in the death certificate, we examined crude mortality of those secondary causes across all possible ICD-10 codes. As data were publicly available and deidentified, ethics committee approval was not required.

3. Results

Between 1999 and 2019, there were 25,138 deaths where the UCOD was listed as ICD-10 G80x: Infantile cerebral palsy. There was an increase in deaths attributable to CP in both crude mortality rates and AAMRs from 1999 to 2019, with the highest occurring in 2019 (Table 1).

Most deaths attributed to CP in 2019 occurred in large metropolitan areas (n = 866 [45.8%]) followed by medium and small metropolitan areas (n = 653 [34.5%]), and rural areas (n = 374 [19.7%]); however, the crude mortality rates were significantly higher among lower population areas (Table 2). The majority of deaths attributable to CP occurred among adults that died in a medical facility (n = 633 [33.4]), at home (n = 588 [31.1%]), or in hospice or a long-term care facility (n = 566 [30%]).

Table 1. Trends of "cerebral palsy" (G80x: Infantile cerebral palsy) listed as the underlying cause of death from 1999 to 2019.

Year	Deaths	Population	Crude Rate per 10,000	95% CI	AAMR * per 100,000	95% CI
1999	620	199,000,198	0.3	0.3–0.3	0.3	0.3–0.3
2000	670	200,948,641	0.3	0.3–0.4	0.3	0.3–0.3
2001	727	204,062,414	0.4	0.3–0.4	0.3	0.3–0.3
2002	753	206,451,793	0.4	0.3–0.4	0.3	0.3–0.3
2003	872	208,682,117	0.4	0.4–0.4	0.4	0.4–0.4
2004	936	211,050,944	0.4	0.4–0.5	0.4	0.4–0.5
2005	978	213,511,339	0.5	0.4–0.5	0.4	0.4–0.5
2006	1056	216,055,494	0.5	0.5–0.5	0.4	0.4–0.5
2007	1062	218,481,776	0.5	0.5–0.5	0.5	0.5–0.5
2008	1190	220,975,702	0.5	0.5–0.6	0.5	0.5–0.5
2009	1141	223,491,138	0.5	0.5–0.5	0.5	0.5–0.5
2010	1221	225,477,982	0.5	0.5–0.6	0.5	0.5–0.5
2011	1230	228,746,768	0.5	0.5–0.6	0.5	0.5–0.6
2012	1259	231,409,240	0.5	0.5–0.6	0.5	0.5–0.5
2013	1418	233,880,752	0.6	0.6–0.6	0.6	0.5–0.6
2014	1429	236,721,454	0.6	0.6–0.6	0.6	0.5–0.6
2015	1555	239,293,130	0.6	0.6–0.7	0.6	0.6–0.7
2016	1622	241,022,445	0.7	0.6–0.7	0.7	0.6–0.7
2017	1696	243,565,966	0.7	0.7–0.7	0.7	0.6–0.7
2018	1810	245,184,769	0.7	0.7–0.8	0.7	0.7–0.8
2019	1893	246,614,107	0.8	0.7–0.8	0.8	0.7–0.8
Total	25,138					

* AMMRs—age-adjusted mortality rates; CI—confidence intervals; AMMRs were calculated for adults over 25 years.

Table 2. Adults with cerebral palsy who died in 2019, with the underlying cause of death listed as "cerebral palsy".

	Deaths	Population	Crude Rate per 100,000	95% CI
All Ages	2168	328,239,523	0.7	0.6–0.7
Adults	1893	246,614,107	0.8	0.7–0.8
Age Categories				
20–34 years	479	67,573,261	0.7	0.6–0.8
35–49 years	331	44,168,826	0.7	0.7–0.8
40–49 years	408	62,056,895	0.7	0.6–0.7
50–64 years	498	62,925,688	0.8	0.7–0.9
≥65 years	508	54,058,263	0.9	0.9–1.0
Gender				
Female	849	126,652,620	0.7	0.6–0.7
Male	1044	119,961,487	0.9	0.8–0.9
Race/Ethnicity				
White	1555	193,833,509	0.8	0.8–0.8
Black	301	32,937,597	0.9	0.8–1.0
Asian	26	16,590,321	0.2	0.1–0.2
Hispanic	187	39,870,392	0.5	0.4–0.5
Other	11	3,252,680	n/a	n/a
Urbanization				
Metro (Large)	866	137,873,755	0.6	0.6–0.7
Metro (Medium and Small)	653	73,879,878	0.9	0.8–1.0
Non-Metro (Rural)	374	34,860,474	1.1	1.01–1.2

There were 6443 unique combinations of multiple causes of death, with CP listed as the UCOD (Table 3). The highest co-occurring causes of death were other diseases of the nervous system (36.4%), diseases of the respiratory system (17.2%), symptoms, signs, and abnormal clinical and laboratory findings, not elsewhere classified (15.3%), and diseases of the circulatory system (8.2%) (individual ICD-10 diseases or causes co-occurring with the primary cause of death [CP] can be found in Supplementary Table S1).

Table 3. Adults with cerebral palsy who died in 2019, with the underlying cause of death listed as "cerebral palsy", and other multiple causes of death.

Population n = 246,614,107	Deaths	Crude Rate per 100,000	95% CI
A00-B99 (Certain infectious and parasitic diseases)	205	0.1	0.1-0.1
C00-D48 (Neoplasms)	20	0.0	0.0-0.0
D50-D89 (Diseases of the blood and blood-forming organs and certain disorders involving the immune mechanism)	34	0.0	0.0-0.0
E00-E89 (Endocrine, nutritional, and metabolic diseases)	229	0.1	0.1-0.1
F01-F99 (Mental and behavioral disorders)	154	0.1	0.1-0.1
G00-G98 (Diseases of the nervous system)	2344	1.0	0.9-1.0
H00-H59 (Diseases of the eye and adnexa)	5	n/a	n/a
I00-I99 (Diseases of the circulatory system)	528	0.2	0.2-0.2
J00-J98 (Diseases of the respiratory system)	1110	0.5	0.4-0.5
K00-K92 (Diseases of the digestive system)	154	0.1	0.1-0.1
L00-L98 (Diseases of the skin and subcutaneous tissue)	41	0.0	0.0-0.0
M00-M99 (Diseases of the musculoskeletal system and connective tissue)	58	0.0	0.0-0.0
N00-N99 (Diseases of the genitourinary system)	165	0.1	0.1-0.1
P00-P96 (Certain conditions originating in the perinatal period)	7	n/a	n/a
Q00-Q99 (Congenital malformations, deformations, and chromosomal abnormalities)	29	0.0	0.0-0.0
R00-R99 (Symptoms, signs, and abnormal clinical and laboratory findings, not elsewhere classified)	984	0.4	0.4-0.4
S00-T98 (Injury, poisoning, and certain other consequences of external causes)	170	0.1	0.1-0.1
V01-Y89 (External causes of morbidity and mortality)	202	0.1	0.1-0.1
Y88.3 (Sequelae of surgical and medical procedures as the cause of abnormal reaction of the patient, or of later complication, without mention of misadventure at the time of the procedure)	4	n/a	n/a

4. Discussion

Especially among adults, CP as a standalone UCOD is not sufficient to aid in the understanding of the natural pathophysiology of disease progression. If listed as the UCOD, appropriate mechanisms of death should be listed above it. These other disease mechanisms should clearly represent a causative link directly to CP. If not, CP should not be utilized as the UCOD. Our findings corroborate that of previous studies which have found high rates of mortality attributed to CP, among adults with CP, across developed countries [13,18,19]. According to the current data, the UCOD of more than 25,000 adults with CP were labeled as CP in the US, from 1999 to 2019. While it is certainly understandable that challenges exist with correctly identifying the mechanisms of death in complex medical conditions, labeling a cause of death as CP must be accompanied by other mechanisms leading to death in this population, to bolster our understanding of the natural history of the condition.

Our study also demonstrated numerous secondary/co-occurring causes of death in adults with CP, where CP was listed as the UCOD. The highest co-occurring causes of death were other diseases of the nervous system (e.g., epilepsy), diseases of the respiratory system (e.g., pneumonia), symptoms, signs, and abnormal clinical and laboratory findings, not elsewhere classified (e.g., dysphagia), and diseases of the circulatory system (e.g., cardiovascular disease). By comparison, the most common UCODs for adults without CP in 2019 included (crude mortality rate per 100,000) (#1) diseases of heart (200.8); (#2) malignant neoplasms (182.7); (#3) accidents (52.7); (#4) chronic lower respiratory diseases (47.8); and (#5) cerebrovascular diseases (45.7).

Mortality statistics compiled from death certificates are used to measure health quality, set public health goals and policies, and to direct research and resources. A physician's principal responsibility in death registration is to complete the medical portion of the death certificate, including the cause of death, according to the Physicians' Handbook on Medical Certification of Death (available at www.cdc.gov/nchs/data/misc/hb_cod.pdf). The ICD Tenth Revision expanded these coding guidelines in 1999 to be more inclusive, particularly those from indirect causes. We found that a greater proportion of death certificates with CP as the underlying cause of death came from rural areas, and among adults that died at home, in long-term care, or in hospice care. There are unique challenges that face accurate death registration among these patients; however, efforts are needed to facilitate the development of improved clinical screening and rigorous mortality reporting to complete the medical portion of the death certificate for these patients. Several important clinical reporting strategies need to be adopted when an adult with CP dies, including: (1) CP should never be listed as the only cause of death, and (2) CP should not be utilized as the UCOD without the mechanism of death also listed. Limitations include possible errors in coding the cause of death on death certificates and documentation of race/ethnicity. Further, using the CDC WONDER database, we did not have access to individual-level data, which makes it impossible to compute group-based statistical analyses or comparisons to adults without CP. Future research is needed to understand the disparities in mortality rates for CP as the underlying cause of death, between urban and rural areas.

5. Conclusions

Given the non-progressive nature of CP, adults with CP may experience a myriad of other diseases that more accurately reflect their true cause of death. CP should not be utilized as the primary UCOD as a default in every patient with CP. This hinders our ability to fully understand the conditions that evolve in adult patients with CP. Between 1999 and 2019, there were more than 25,000 deaths attributed to CP as the underlying cause. Most deaths attributed to CP occurred in large metropolitan areas; however, both crude and age-adjusted mortality rates were significantly higher among rural areas. The highest secondary causes of death were other diseases of the nervous system (e.g., epilepsy), diseases of the respiratory system (e.g., pneumonia), symptoms, signs, and abnormal clinical and laboratory findings (e.g., dysphagia), and diseases of the circulatory system (e.g., cardiovascular disease). Labeling a cause of death as CP must be accompanied by other mechanisms leading to death in this population, to bolster our understanding of the natural history of the condition as well as to increase our understanding of preventable causes of death. Efforts are needed to facilitate the development of improved clinical screening and rigorous death registration to complete the medical portion of the death certificate for this population of patients.

Supplementary Materials: The following are available online at https://www.mdpi.com/article/10.3390/jcm11216333/s1, Table S1: Adults that died in 2019, with the underlying cause of death listed as "cerebral palsy", and 6443 unique combinations of multiple causes of death.

Author Contributions: Formal analysis, M.D.P.; investigation, M.D.P. and E.A.H.; data curation, M.D.P.; writing – original draft, M.D.P., A.M.W. and E.A.H.; supervision, M.D.P. All authors have read and agreed to the published version of the manuscript.

Funding: This research received no external funding.

Institutional Review Board Statement: Not applicable.

Informed Consent Statement: Not applicable.

Data Availability Statement: Data are publicly available through the US Centers for Disease Control and Prevention Wide-ranging Online Data for Epidemiologic Research (CDC WONDER) database: https://wonder.cdc.gov/Deaths-by-Underlying-Cause.html.

Conflicts of Interest: The authors declare no conflict of interest.

References

1. Rosenbaum, P.; Paneth, N.; Leviton, A.; Goldstein, M.; Bax, M.; Damiano, D.; Dan, B.; Jacobsson, B. A report: The definition and classification of cerebral palsy April 2006. *Dev. Med. Child Neurol.* **2007**, *109*, 8–14. [CrossRef]
2. Peterson, M.D.; Hurvitz, E.A. Cerebral Palsy Grows Up. *Mayo Clin. Proc.* **2021**, *96*, 1404–1406. [CrossRef] [PubMed]
3. Hurvitz, E.A.; Whitney, D.G.; Waldron-Perrine, B.; Ryan, D.; Haapala, H.J.; Schmidt, M.; Gray, C.; Peterson, M.D. Navigating the Pathway to Care in Adults with Cerebral Palsy. *Front. Neurol.* **2021**, *12*, 734139. [CrossRef] [PubMed]

4. Goodman, D.M.; Hall, M.; Levin, A.; Watson, R.S.; Williams, R.G.; Shah, S.S.; Slonim, A.D. Adults with Chronic Health Conditions Originating in Childhood: Inpatient Experience in Children's Hospitals. *Pediatrics* **2011**, *128*, 5–13. [CrossRef] [PubMed]
5. Thorpe, D.; Gannotti, M.; Peterson, M.D.; Wang, C.-H.; Freburger, J. Musculoskeletal diagnoses, comorbidities, and physical and occupational therapy use among older adults with and without cerebral palsy. *Disabil. Health J.* **2021**, *14*, 101109. [CrossRef] [PubMed]
6. Whitney, D.G.; Warschausky, S.A.; Ng, S.; Hurvitz, E.A.; Kamdar, N.S.; Peterson, M.D. Prevalence of Mental Health Disorders Among Adults with Cerebral Palsy. *Ann. Intern. Med.* **2019**, *171*, 328–333. [CrossRef] [PubMed]
7. Ryan, J.M.; Peterson, M.D.; Matthews, A.; Ryan, N.; Smith, K.J.; O'Connell, N.E.; Liverani, S.; Anokye, N.; Victor, C.; Allen, E. Noncommunicable disease among adults with cerebral palsy. *Neurology* **2019**, *93*, e1385–e1396. [CrossRef] [PubMed]
8. Peterson, M.; Ryan, J.; Hurvitz, E.A.; Mahmoudi, E. Chronic Conditions in Adults with Cerebral Palsy. *JAMA* **2015**, *314*, 2303–2305. [CrossRef] [PubMed]
9. O'Connell, N.E.; Smith, K.J.; Peterson, M.; Ryan, N.; Liverani, S.; Anokye, N.; Victor, C.; Ryan, J. Incidence of osteoarthritis, osteoporosis and inflammatory musculoskeletal diseases in adults with cerebral palsy: A population-based cohort study. *Bone* **2019**, *125*, 30–35. [CrossRef] [PubMed]
10. Stevens, J.; Turk, M.A.; Landes, S.D. Cause of death trends among adults with and without cerebral palsy in the United States, 2013–2017. *Ann. Phys. Rehabilitation Med.* **2021**, *65*, 101553. [CrossRef] [PubMed]
11. Peterson, M.D.; Lin, P.; Kamdar, N.; Mahmoudi, E.; Marsack-Topolewski, C.N.; Haapala, H.; Muraszko, K.; Hurvitz, E.A. Psychological morbidity among adults with cerebral palsy and spina bifida. *Psychol. Med.* **2021**, *51*, 694–701. [CrossRef] [PubMed]
12. Smith, K.J.; Peterson, M.; O'Connell, N.E.; Victor, C.; Liverani, S.; Anokye, N.; Ryan, J. Risk of Depression and Anxiety in Adults with Cerebral Palsy. *JAMA Neurol.* **2018**, *76*, 294–300. [CrossRef] [PubMed]
13. Landes, S.D.; Stevens, J.D.; Turk, M.A. Postmortem Diagnostic Overshadowing: Reporting Cerebral Palsy on Death Certificates. *J. Health Soc. Behav.* **2022**. [CrossRef] [PubMed]
14. Landes, S.D.; Stevens, J.D.; Turk, A.M. Obscuring effect of coding developmental disability as the underlying cause of death on mortality trends for adults with developmental disability: A cross-sectional study using US Mortality Data from 2012 to 2016. *BMJ Open* **2019**, *9*, e026614. [CrossRef] [PubMed]
15. Landes, S.D.; Turk, M.A.; Finan, J.M. Factors associated with the reporting of Down syndrome as the underlying cause of death on US death certificates. *J. Intellect. Disabil. Res.* **2022**, *66*, 454–470. [CrossRef] [PubMed]
16. CDC. Underlying Cause of Death 1999–2019 on CDC WONDER Online Database, Released in 2020. National Center for Health Statistics. 2021. Available online: http://wonder.cdc.gov/ucd-icd10.html (accessed on 9 July 2021).
17. Ingram, D.D.; Franco, S.J. 2013 NCHS Urban-Rural Classification Scheme for Counties. *Vital Health Stat.* **2014**, *166*, 1–73.
18. Duruflé-Tapin, A.; Colin, A.; Nicolas, B.; Lebreton, C.; Dauvergne, F.; Gallien, P. Analysis of the medical causes of death in cerebral palsy. *Ann. Phys. Rehabilitation Med.* **2014**, *57*, 24–37. [CrossRef] [PubMed]
19. Ryan, J.M.; Peterson, M.; Ryan, N.; Smith, K.J.; O'Connell, E.N.; Liverani, S.; Anokye, N.; Victor, C.; Allen, E. Mortality due to cardiovascular disease, respiratory disease, and cancer in adults with cerebral palsy. *Dev. Med. Child Neurol.* **2019**, *61*, 924–928. [CrossRef] [PubMed]

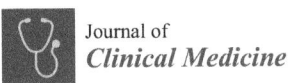

Article

Respiratory Health Inequities among Children and Young Adults with Cerebral Palsy in Aotearoa New Zealand: A Data Linkage Study

Alexandra Sorhage [1,*], Samantha Keenan [2], Jimmy Chong [3], Cass Byrnes [4,5], Amanda Marie Blackmore [6], Anna Mackey [1], Timothy Hill [2], Dug Yeo Han [7] and Ngaire Susan Stott [1,8]

1 Paediatric Orthopaedics, Starship Children's Health, Auckland 1023, New Zealand
2 Kidz First Paediatrics, 100 Hospital Road, Auckland 2025, New Zealand
3 Paediatric Rehabilitation Service, Starship Children's Health, Auckland 1023, New Zealand
4 Paediatric Respiratory Service, Starship Children's Health, Auckland 1023, New Zealand
5 Department of Paediatrics, University of Auckland, Auckland 1010, New Zealand
6 Telethon Kids Institute, 15 Hospital Ave., Perth 6009, Australia
7 Starship Research and Innovation, Starship Children's Health, Auckland 1023, New Zealand
8 Department of Surgery, University of Auckland, Auckland 1023, New Zealand
* Correspondence: nzcpregister@adhb.govt.nz; Tel.: +64-093-074-949 (ext. 21898)

Abstract: (1) Background: Respiratory disease is a leading cause of morbidity, mortality, and poor quality of life in children with cerebral palsy (CP). This study describes the prevalence of CP-related respiratory disease and the non-modifiable risk factors for respiratory-related hospital admissions in the Aotearoa New Zealand population. (2) Methods: New Zealand Cerebral Palsy Register (NZCPR) participant data and de-identified data from the National Minimum Dataset and Pharmaceutical Dispensing Collections were linked to identify all respiratory-related hospital admissions and respiratory illness-related antibiotic exposure over 5 years in individuals with CP (0–26 years). (3) Results: Risk factors for respiratory-related hospital admissions included being classified Gross Motor Function Classification System (GMFCS) IV or V compared to GMFCS I [OR = 4.37 (2.90–6.58), $p < 0.0001$; OR = 11.8 (7.69–18.10), $p < 0.0001$, respectively,]; having ≥2 antibiotics dispensed per year [OR = 4.42 (3.01–6.48), $p < 0.0001$]; and being of Māori ethnicity [OR = 1.47 (1.13–1.93), $p < 0.0047$]. Māori experienced health inequities compared to non-Māori, with greater functional disability, and also experienced greater antibiotic dispensing than the general population. (4) Conclusion: Māori children and young adults have a higher risk of respiratory-related illness. Priority should be given to the screening for potentially modifiable risk factors for all children with CP from diagnosis onwards in a way that ensures Māori health equity.

Keywords: cerebral palsy; respiratory; hospitalisations; antibiotics; Indigenous; inequities

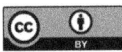

1. Introduction

Cerebral palsy (CP) is the most common childhood physical disability in high income countries, with a prevalence between 1.4 and 2.1 cases per 1000 live births [1]. Respiratory-related illness in CP is the most common cause of mortality, morbidity, and poor quality of life, especially for those living with greater disability [≈26% of the CP population is classified as combined Gross Motor Function Classification System (GMFCS) IV and V] [2,3]. Adults with CP have a 14-fold risk of death from respiratory disease compared to the general population [4], and more severely impaired children with CP have a higher frequency of hospital admissions and a longer length of stay related to respiratory illness, with a greater risk of early mortality [5]. The pathway to respiratory disease in children with CP is complex and multifactorial and impacts all levels of disability, with 45% of all people with CP having respiratory symptoms [6].

In Aotearoa New Zealand (AoNZ), the general paediatric population (<15 years of age) experience the highest respiratory hospitalisation rates (comparable only to adults >65 years of age), with hospital admissions for bronchiolitis, asthma, wheeze and viral pneumonia having increased to over 21,000 annually since 2000 [7]. The rates and severity of bronchiectasis are also higher than documented in other developed countries [8,9].

Significant health inequities for Indigenous NZ Māori compared with NZ European are well-recognised [10,11], with Māori children and young people in particular experiencing adverse health and social outcomes as a result of socio-political and economic environmental drivers [12,13]. The Impact of Respiratory Disease in NZ report (2018) stated that 'All indicators showed inequality in health by ethnic group. Pacific peoples and Māori shared the highest respiratory health burden' [7]. For respiratory infections, the relative risks are 1.7–18.2 for Māori and Pasifika as compared to NZ European, ranging from 2.1 for pneumonia to 3.9 for bronchiolitis between the most and least deprived areas of socioeconomic deprivation [10]. This indicates that NZ Māori living with CP—especially those classified as GMFCS IV and V—are likely to be more vulnerable to respiratory disease.

CP Registry information and hospital admission data have been recently used in Australia to describe the impact of respiratory disease for people with CP, and three non-modifiable predictive risk factors for future respiratory-related hospital admission were identified: (i) GMFCS V; (ii) ≥ 1 respiratory-related hospital admission in the previous year; and (iii) ≥ 2 courses of antibiotics in the previous year [14]. In AoNZ, less is known about the impact of respiratory illness in children with CP, and although hospital admissions have increased over 14 years, the reasons for hospitalisation are not well-documented [15]. Most CP hospitalisations in the 0–24-year age-range have a primary diagnosis of CP (42%), with associated diagnoses including respiratory disease (11%) [16].

The primary aim of this study was to describe the prevalence of respiratory disease and non-modifiable risk factors for hospital admissions for children and young people in AoNZ. In particular, this study aimed to identify any inequities between Indigenous NZ Māori children with CP and other ethnic groups, between the GMFCS levels, and between the different levels of socioeconomic deprivation. The secondary aim of the study was to describe the dispensing of antibiotics for respiratory-related illness in children with CP and to examine the differences between ethnic groups, GMFCS levels, and levels of socioeconomic deprivation.

2. Materials and Methods

2.1. Study Design

A 5-year (2014–2019) retrospective cohort design study used data linkage for all children and young people diagnosed with CP and registered with the NZCPR who met the following criteria: (i) aged 0–26 years, (ii) residing in AoNZ at the time of data extraction and matched to de-identified data on hospitalisations and antibiotic dispensing for respiratory infections.

2.2. Data Sources

The NZCPR is a national register established in 2015 with ethics approval (HDEC 13/NTA/130) in order to collect health data and information relevant to CP (including demographic data and clinical information such as type, topography, and GMFCS). This includes the ability to link to Health New Zealand (previously known as the Ministry of Health) datasets. Data were extracted from the NZCPR and linked to Health New Zealand datasets using the unique electronic National Health Index (NHI) number [17]. The NHI was encrypted, and only de-identified data were used for analysis.

Each hospital is required to code and report hospital admissions (including emergency department admissions >3 h in duration) information to Health New Zealand at monthly intervals. The collective database is called the National Minimum Dataset (also known as Hospital Events data) [18]. Primary and secondary diagnoses at the time of discharge are coded using the International Statistical Classification of Diseases (ICD). The ICD 10th

Revision codes included for analysis were J09-J99 as a primary or secondary diagnosis only (excluding J30-J39 for other diseases of upper respiratory tract) for all hospital admissions years 2014–2019.

In AoNZ, antibiotics for systemic use are only available with a prescription, and, at the time of the study, were dispensed free of charge for children aged 13 years or under and incurred a nominal charge for those aged >14 years. Prescriptions dispensed from a community pharmacy seeking government subsidisation are recorded in the Health New Zealand database known as the Pharmaceutical Collection [19]. This does not include antibiotics dispensed in hospital or by a medical practitioner directly. Data for antibiotics dispensed were classified using the Anatomical Therapeutic Chemical (ATC) classification system under agents "for systemic use" defined as "anti-bacterials". Antibiotics were identified by individual names (e.g., amoxicillin trihydrate). The antibiotics that were more likely to be used in clinical practice to treat respiratory-related infections were identified by one of the authors (Cass Byrnes) who is a Paediatric Respiratory Specialist (Supplementary Table S1). A single course was defined as one course if dispensed on separate days, irrespective of the days separating dispensing events. A single course was also defined as one course, even if multiple antibiotics had been dispensed on the same day.

In Health New Zealand datasets, ethnicity is linked to the NHI and is usually collected at the point of the person's contact with hospital services. Prioritised ethnicity was used for analysis. Prioritisation is a method that assigns people who identify with more than one ethnic group to a single mutually exclusive category based on an established hierarchy, with the aim of giving priority to non-European groups and special priority to Māori and Pacific Island groups [20]. The ethnicity coding used was in line with Statistics New Zealand level 1 categories for national standards reporting [European; NZ Māori; Pasifika (also referred to as Pacific Island Peoples); Asian; and MELAA -Middle Eastern/Latin American/African] [21].

Based on nine Census variables, the NZDep is an area-based measure of socioeconomic deprivation in New Zealand, measuring the level of deprivation for people within a small (10%) geographical area. Each NZDep decile contains 10 deciles, with decile 1 representing the least deprived score and 10 the most deprived [22]. For analysis, the deprivation indices were assigned to quintiles, with quintile 1 representing the 20% least deprived data zone and quintile 5 representing the 20% most deprived zone. Due to the unreliability of the 2018 census data, the NZDep 2013 was used.

2.3. Statistical Analysis

A total of 1286 NZCPR participants met the inclusion criteria. Descriptive statistics were used to summarise the cohort using cross-tabulation and median IQR and range. Chi square and Logistic regression were carried out for binary dependent variables. Multivariate regression was carried out using significant factors from univariate regression where appropriate.

Population data between the 5 yearly censuses were adjusted by linear interpolation to calculate the total population aged under 27 years in each geographical region for 2014–2020 using 2013 and 2018 Census data between ethnic groups (Asian, Māori, Pasifika, European, and MELAA). Since the observed data are the counts of admission and dispensing in each year, the data were analysed using a generalised linear model, modelling the observed counts data as having a Poisson distribution and plotted as a fitted line. A p value of < 0.05 was considered to be statistically significant.

Statistical analyses were carried out using SAS 9.4 (SAS Institute Inc., Cary, NC, USA) and R (R Core Team (2021). R: A language and environment for statistical computing. R Foundation for Statistical Computing, Vienna, Austria [23].

3. Results

3.1. Cohort Description

Full age, gender, and ethnicity data were available for 1286 participants, with missing data for the GMFCS in 73 (6%) and the measure of socioeconomic deprivation in 3 (0.3%). At the time of NZCPR data extraction, the median age of participants was 14 years; IQR = 10–19, of which 28 (2%) were <5 years; 856 (67%) were aged between 5 and 17 years; and 402 (31%) aged between 18 and 26 years. The Auckland metro region is home to 33% of AoNZ's population. Of the present cohort, 542 (42%) were living in this region. Demographic and clinical descriptors are detailed in Table 1. There were 734 (57%) male and 552 (43%) female participants, and 410 (34%) participants were classified as GMFCS IV and V. In terms of ethnicity, the cohort was comparable to the AoNZ general population for this age group [23] with 639 (50%) of the cohort being European, followed by Māori 342 (27%), Pasifika 135 (11%), Asian 137 (11%), and MELAA 32 (2%). Overall, 342 (25%) were living in higher areas of deprivation (quintile 5) compared to 254 (20%) in the least deprived areas (quintile 1); with 177 (28%) of European participants living in quintile 1 compared to 8 (25%) of MELAA, 8 (6%) of Pasifika, and 32 (9%) of Māori participants.

Table 1. Demographics of the Study Participants, including median age and gender distribution, GMFCS, and NZDep quintile distribution by ethnic group.

	Cohort Demographic and Clinical Descriptors					
	European	NZ Māori [1]	Pasifika	Asian	MELAA [2]	Total
Age (n = 1286) Median (range)	15 (2–26)	14 (3–26)	15 (4–26)	13 (2–26)	14 (5–26)	14 (2–26)
Gender (n = 1286) M: F	379: 260	186: 156	76: 59	73: 64	20: 12	734:552
GMFCS [3] levels (n = 1213) I: II: III: IV: V	204: 157: 72: 89: 72	97: 65: 30: 64: 64	30: 31: 7: 35: 30	44: 37: 9: 29: 14	5: 11: 2: 7: 6	381:301:121: 224:186
Unknown GMFCS [2] (n = 73)	45	22	2	4	0	
NZDep [4] Quintiles (n = 1283) 1: 2: 3: 4: 5	177: 139: 131: 109: 82	32: 32: 43: 92: 143	8: 11: 13: 39: 63	28: 34: 25: 22: 27	8: 2: 4: 9: 9	254: 218: 216: 271: 324

[1] Indigenous population in Aotearoa New Zealand, [2] Middle Eastern Latin American African, [3] Gross Motor Function Classification System. [4] NZDep is an area-based measure of socioeconomic deprivation in New Zealand

Differences in the distribution of GMFCS classification were found for Māori participants when compared to non-Māori participants (Table 2). When participants were grouped by GMFCS IV-V as compared to GMFCS I-III, Māori participants were more likely to be classified as GMFCS IV- or V than non-Māori participants ($p = 0.0065$).

Māori were also significantly over-represented in quintile 5 ($p < 0.0001$) compared to their non-Māori counterparts (Table 2). Similar findings are found for Māori in the general AoNZ population [12].

3.2. Respiratory-Related Hospital Admissions

Three hundred and fifty three of the 1286 participants (27%) had 1374 hospital admissions related to respiratory illness, with a median admission rate of 2.0, IQR = 1.0–5.0 over the 5-year period. Of the total admissions, 316/1374 (23%) were following Emergency Department (ED) visits, with no difference found in the proportion of ED presentations between Māori and non-Māori participants ($p = 0.2031$). A significantly higher percentage of participants classified as GMFCS IV- V (201/316, 64%) presented to ED than those classified as GMFCS I–III (102/316, 32%, $p < 0.0001$). A significantly higher percentage of those living in quintiles 4 or 5 (180/301, 57%) presented to ED than those living in quintiles 1 or 2 (81/316, 26%, $p = 0.0009$). Median lengths of stay (LoS), excluding ED admissions, were similar for Māori (Median = 3 days, IQR = 1–6) and non-Māori participants (Median = 3 days, IQR = 2–6).

Table 2. Comparisons of Māori and non-Māori children and young adults with CP by age, gender, GMFCS, and NZDep quintiles.

	Cohort Descriptors for Māori and Non-Māori		
	NZ Māori [1] (N = 320)	Non-Māori (N = 943)	p
Age Median (range)	14 (3–26)	15 (2–26)	
Gender (n = 1286) M: F	186: 156	548: 395	0.2329
GMFCS [2] levels (n = 1213) I: II: III: IV: V	97: 65: 30: 64: 64	283: 236: 91: 160: 122	0.0319
NZDep [3] Quintiles (n = 1286) 1: 2: 3: 4: 5	32: 32: 43: 92: 143	221: 186: 173: 179: 182	<0.0001

[1] Indigenous population in Aotearoa New Zealand. [2] Gross Motor Function Classification System. [3] NZDep is an area-based measure of socioeconomic deprivation in New Zealand.

Following a univariate regression analysis for demographic and clinical variables, participants classified as GMFCS IV or V were found to have higher odds of having a respiratory-related hospital admission than participants classified as GMFCS I (Table 3). Māori participants were more likely to have a respiratory-related hospital admission than non-Māori; participants living in the area of highest deprivation (quintile 5) were 50% more likely to have an admission than those living in low deprivation areas (quintile 1); and the participants who had two or more antibiotics dispensed/year were four times more likely to have a respiratory-related hospital admission (Table 3). Through multivariate analysis within the Māori group, it was determined that the odds of respiratory-related hospital admissions were significantly higher in GMFCS IV- V than GMFCS I- III [OR = 5.55 (2.66–11.6) $p < 0.0001$], whereas there was no association with the level of deprivation (quintile 5 compared with quintile 1) [OR = 0.92 (0.36–2.33), $p = 0.8505$].

Population data for the age group and timeframe of interest showed that European participants experienced significantly lower rates of admission per 100,000 people in overall years than their Māori counterparts ($p < 0.001$). MELAA participants had a much smaller representation in the cohort but the highest overall admissions of 1.8× (84%) higher than the rate of NZ Māori ($p < 0.0001$) (Figure 1). Hospital admission rates for children and young adults with CP remained relatively steady for European and Asian groups over time but declined significantly for Pasifika ($p = 0.0003$). An apparent decline was found not to be significant for MEELA ($p = 0.571$). NZ Māori were the only group who experienced a trend to higher admission rates over this time.

3.3. Antibiotic Dispensing for Respiratory-Related Illness

Overall, a total of 9647 episodes of antibiotics were dispensed for 1170/1286 (91%) of the cohort with a median of 5 episodes, IQR = 3–11 over the 5-year timeframe, with no differences found between GMFCS, ethnicity, or quintiles. Most individuals had none or only one episode per year, but 151/1286 (12%) had ≥2 episodes of antibiotics/year dispensed over the timeframe. No significant differences were found amongst ethnicities (including Māori and non-Māori) or amongst quintiles for ≥2 episodes of antibiotic dispensing per year; however, univariate analysis found that children classified as GMFCS V were almost three times more likely to have ≥2 episodes of antibiotics dispensed per year than those classified as GMFCS I (Table 4).

Table 3. Univariate regression analysis and odds ratio analysis for respiratory-related admissions for children and young adults with CP for gender, GMFCS, ethnicity, NZDep quintile variables, and if ≥2 antibiotics dispensed per year.

	Respiratory-Related Admissions (n = 353)		p
	N (%)	Odds Ratio (95% CI)	
Gender (vs. male)			
Male	201 (57)	1.00	
Female	152 (43)	1.01 (0.79–1.29)	0.9518
GMFCS [1] Level (vs. Level I)			
I	46 (14)	1.00	
II	70 (21)	2.21 (1.47–3.32)	<0.0001
III	17 (5)	1.19 (0.65–2.17)	
IV	84 (25)	4.37 (2.90–6.58)	
V	115 (35)	11.8 (7.69–18.1)	
GMFCS [1] Group (vs. Level I/II/III)			
I/II/III	133 (40)	1.00	
IV/V	199 (60)	4.75 (3.63–6.22)	<0.0001
Ethnicity (vs. NZ Māori [2])			
NZ Māori	114 (32)	1.00	
European	152 (43)	0.62 (0.47–0.83)	0.0004
Pasifika	50 (14)	1.18 (0.78–1.78)	
Asian	27 (8)	0.49 (0.31–0.79)	
MELAA [3]	10 (3)	0.91 (0.42–1.98)	
NZ Māori (vs. non-Māori)			
Non-Māori	239 (68)	1.00	
NZ Māori	114 (32)	1.47 (1.13–1.93)	0.0046
NZDep [4] Quintiles (vs. Q1)			
Q1 (least deprived)	55 (16)	1.00	
Q2	62 (18)	1.44 (0.95–2.19)	0.2506
Q3	61 (17)	1.42 (0.94–2.17)	
Q4	79 (22)	1.49 (1.00–2.21)	
Q5 (most deprived)	95 (27)	1.50 (1.02–2.20)	
Antibiotic Dispensing			
< 2 Episodes/year	34 (11)	1.00	
≥2 Episodes/year	314 (36)	4.42 (3.01–6.28)	<0.0001

[1] Gross Motor Function Classification System. [2] Indigenous population in Aotearoa New Zealand. [3] Middle Eastern Latin American African. [4] NZDep is an area-based measure of socioeconomic deprivation in New Zealand. Q = Quintile.

Using population data for the age group and timeframe of interest, overall rates of total antibiotic dispensing for children and young adults with CP decreased over time for all ethnic groups. When compared to Māori, all other ethnic groups had significantly lower rates of antibiotic dispensing, with Asian participants having the lowest rate (−53%) followed by European (−41%), MELAA (−26%), and Pasifika (−17%) ($p < 0.0001$) (Figure 2).

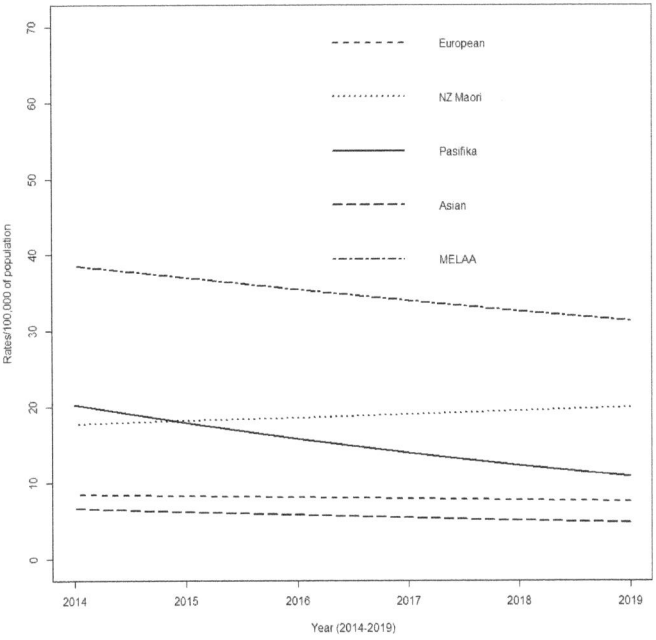

Figure 1. Incidence rates of total hospital admissions for children and young adults with cerebral palsy by ethnicity, Aotearoa New Zealand; 2014–2019.

Table 4. Univariate analysis and odds ratio analysis for ≥2 antibiotic episodes per year for gender, GMFCS, ethnicity, and NZDep quintile.

	≥2 Antibiotic Episodes/Year (*n* = 151) OR		*p*
	N (%)	Odds Ratio (95% CI)	
Gender (vs. male)			
Male	94 (32)	1.00	
Female	57 (38)	0.79 (0.56–1.13)	0.1926
GMFCS [1] Level (vs. Level I)			
I	60 (40)	1.00	
II	30 (20)	1.75 (1.09–2.81)	0.0053
III	15 (10)	1.37 (0.74–2.53)	
IV	21 (14)	1.98 (1.17–3.37)	
V	13 (7)	2.78 (1.48–5.22)	
GMFCS [1] Group (vs. Level I/II/III)			
I/II/III	105 (76)	1.00	
IV/V	34 (25)	1.80 (1.20–2.71)	0.0047
Ethnicity (vs. NZ Māori [2])			
NZ Māori	36 (24)	1.00	
European	85 (56)	1.42 (0.94–2.15)	0.0862
Pasifika	8 (5)	0.55 (0.25–1.21)	
Asian	18 (12)	1.43 (0.78–2.62)	

Table 4. Cont.

	≥2 Antibiotic Episodes/Year (n = 151)	OR	p
MELAA [3]	4 (3)	1.41 (0.46–4.30)	
NZ Māori (vs. non-Māori)			
Non-Māori	115 (76)	1.00	
NZ Māori	36 (24)	0.78 (0.53–1.17)	0.2291
NZDep [4] Quintiles (vs. Q1)			
Q1 (least deprived)	33 (22)	1.00	
Q2	21 (14)	0.68 (0.38–1.22)	0.7604
Q3	27 (18)	0.92 (0.53–1.59)	
Q4	32 (21)	0.83 (0.49–1.39)	
Q5 (most deprived)	38 (25)	0.82 (0.50–1.36)	

[1] Gross Motor Function Classification System; [2] Indigenous population in Aotearoa New Zealand; [3] Middle Eastern Latin American African; [4] NZDep is an area-based measure of socioeconomic deprivation in New Zealand. Q = Quintile.

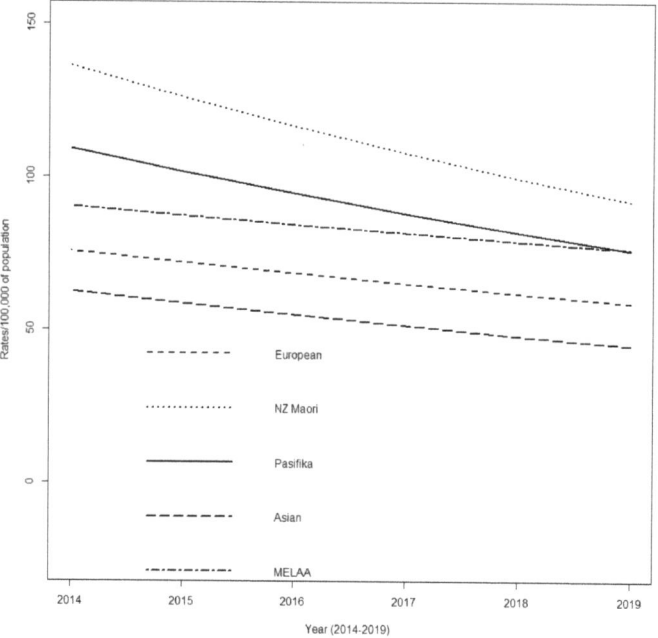

Figure 2. Incidence rates of total antibiotic dispensing for children and young adults with cerebral palsy by ethnicity, Aotearoa New Zealand; 2014–2019.

4. Discussion

This study has shown that almost all children and young adults with CP had antibiotics dispensed for respiratory-related illness in the community over the study time frame, with high rates of ED presentations and hospital admissions for respiratory illness. One in ten children and young adults with CP had >2 courses of antibiotics per year, with children classified as GMFCS V being almost three times more likely to have ≥2 antibiotics dispensed per year than those classified as GMFCS I. One in five children and young adults with CP experienced a respiratory-related hospital admission, with individual risk factors including being classified as GMFCS IV or V compared to GMFCS I; having ≥2 episodes of antibiotics dispensed per year; living in the most deprived quintile (Q5) compared to the least deprived Q1; and being of NZ Māori ethnicity.

There are few international studies of admission rates with respiratory illness in children with CP. However, a comparable Australian study reported that 11% of Western Australian participants with CP experienced a respiratory-related admission over a 3-year timeframe with GMFCS V experiencing admission rates 23 times higher than GMFCS I [14]. Direct comparison of the data shows that in AoNZ, 27% of our participants had 1374 hospital admissions, an average of 3.6 per person over 5 years. In Western Australia, 16% of participants had 332 respiratory hospital admissions, an average of 4.3 per person over 5 years [24]. These data paint a picture of a high overall risk of respiratory-related hospital admissions in children and young adults with CP, a risk which is much higher than the reported risk in the general population for admissions with other respiratory illnesses such as RSV (reported to range from 1.3 to 10.5 hospitalizations per 1000 in the age group 1–2 years) [25].

In the current study, Indigenous NZ Māori children and young adults with CP experienced a higher incidence of respiratory-related hospital admissions over time when compared to non-Māori participants and were more likely to function at GMFCS levels IV or V. Individuals with CP and GMFCS levels IV or V often have associated co-morbidities, such as oropharyngeal motor dysfunction and recurrent seizures [26,27]. Overall, oropharyngeal motor dysfunction is common in people with CP [25] and results in sequential direct aspiration leading to aspiration pneumonia, acute respiratory infections, and chronic airway inflammation [28]. Similarly, seizures can lead to temporary altered muscle tone and reduced consciousness, which may increase the risk of aspiration, leading to aspiration pneumonia. Not surprisingly then, oropharyngeal motor dysfunction and seizures are major risk factors for an increased risk of hospitalization with respiratory-related illness in children with CP [29]. The association between GMFCS levels and potentially modifiable medical risk factors could explain why NZ Māori, who had greater physical disability in this study, also experienced a higher incidence of respiratory-related hospital admissions over time. Further research should help determine the prevalence of oropharyngeal motor dysfunction and seizure disorder in this group and whether the optimisation of medical management could help to reduce their risk of hospitalisation with respiratory disease.

Trend data for the CP population showed that over the 5 years of the study, the rate of admission to hospital with respiratory illnesses either remained stable or dropped for all ethnic groups. From the trend data, NZ Māori had the second highest rate of hospital admission, second only to MELAA participants. Surprisingly, being of MELAA ethnicity did not reach significance as a risk factor in the analysis of individual risk factors, perhaps due to the very small numbers in this group (32 children). Unlike most countries, AoNZ's social policy does not bar refugees or asylum seekers on the grounds of medical conditions or disabilities and allocates over half of its international allocation to MELAA regions [30]. It is unknown if this small group of MELAA participants were predominantly an immigrant population, with health outcomes reflecting prior lack of access to health care in their originating countries, or whether they were born in AoNZ and self-identified as MELAA.

This is the first study to use a pharmaceutical dispensing dataset to identify antibiotic use to treat respiratory-related illness in CP. Antibiotics were widely used, with those classified as GMFCS V having significantly higher chances of receiving ≥ 2 courses/year dispensed. NZ Māori children and young adults with CP consistently had the highest rates of antibiotic episodes per 100,000 of population compared to other ethnicity groups over the 5 years. Hobbs, et al., also reported that Māori children received more antibiotic courses than European children and young adults and suggested that much of this prescription was for self-limiting viral respiratory infections [31]. This suggests that changes in antibiotic prescribing practice for NZ Māori children and young adults may still lag behind changes in prescribing for other ethnic groups.

Limitations

The NZCPR is not a population-based register and is not fully ascertained, but it is representative of 60% of the estimated CP population in AoNZ; ascertainment strategies have been biased towards tertiary care/hospital ascertainment, which could account for a slightly higher proportion of GMCFS IV and V when compared to the Australian Cerebral Palsy Register (ACPR GMFCS IV-V 26% compared to NZCPR GMFCS IV-V 34%) [2].

Hospital admissions data do not include community or primary care presentations for respiratory illness, which would further add to the understanding of respiratory illness in the community. We have used antibiotic prescribing data as a proxy for respiratory infection and have followed guidelines to identify those antibiotics commonly used for respiratory infection. Consistency and regional differences in coding (in particular, for ED admissions) have been questioned in the past; however, processes have been universally implemented to significantly improve reliability and it is less likely to be of concern for our timeframe of interest [32,33]. The Pharmaceutical Collection does not account for hospital or GP dispensing, although the latter, especially for antibiotics, would be rare. Moreover, dispensing medication does not always mean it is taken, or taken as prescribed, and although a financial incentive is in place, not all pharmacies need to partake in contributing data. However, participation is thought to be high. The methodology used for defining an episode could overestimate actual antibiotic dispensing, as some episodes may have been an extension of the preceding course; however, it is thought that, taking into consideration the limitations, antibiotic exposure is likely to be underreported [31]. Therefore, the high rates for antibiotic dispensing found in this study are likely to be, if anything, an underestimate of the true levels of antibiotic dispensing and usage. The antibiotics included for analysis may not be exclusively used for respiratory illness. The Mortality Collection dataset was not used to identify mortality with an underlying cause of respiratory illness, as data were available until only 2017. We did not collect respiratory viral panel results or sputum cultures from hospital admissions as these results are not available through dataset linkage, but recognise that those with specific pathogens, such as Pseudomonas aeruginosa, may have more severe and/or chronic respiratory disease [34]. We also did not look at coding for aspiration, an issue that has been associated with recurrent pneumonia in children generally [35] and with cerebral palsy in particular [36]. It is also associated with more significant pathogenic infection [34], although this is likely to align along the GMFCS levels of disability.

5. Conclusions and Future Directions

While some factors may not be modifiable, to improve morbidity and mortality, modifiable risk factors require management [37] with the aim of moving from a reactive care model to a surveillance, preventative, whānau-centred (family-centred), and child-centred model. The second phase of the project is to test the feasibility of the CP Respiratory Checklist (developed in Western Australia for health professionals and families) in AoNZ for use in clinical practice as the first step in the shift towards the early identification of modifiable risk factors for respiratory illness [38]. Identifying inequities assists in focusing resources that promote equity in the early years of childhood [39]. All health care professionals caring for children with CP can make positive contributions to eliminating health inequities through the re-orientation of systemic and health determinants and the adoption of equity-focused practices [40].

Supplementary Materials: The following supporting information can be downloaded at: https://www.mdpi.com/article/10.3390/jcm11236968/s1, Supplementary Table S1: Antibiotics chosen to represent treatment for respiratory illness by chemical formulation name.

Author Contributions: Conceptualization: A.S., A.M., J.C., C.B., N.S.S., A.M.B. and T.H. Methodology: A.S., A.M., A.M.B., J.C., S.K., T.H., C.B. and N.S.S. Validation: A.M.B., D.Y.H., A.S. and S.K. Formal Analysis: D.Y.H., A.S. and S.K. Investigation: D.Y.H., A.S. and S.K. Resources: D.Y.H. Data curation: D.Y.H., A.S. and S.K. Writing—original draft: A.S., N.S.S. and A.M.B. Writing—review and editing: A.S., A.M., J.C., S.K., C.B., N.S.S., A.M.B., T.H. and D.Y.H. Visualisation: A.S., A.M., J.C., S.K., C.B., N.S.S., A.M.B., T.H. and D.Y.H. Project administration: A.S. and N.S.S. Funding Acquisition: A.M., A.S., J.C., C.B., N.S.S., A.M.B. and T.H. All authors have read and agreed to the published version of the manuscript.

Funding: This research was funded by The Starship Foundation, New Zealand; grant number A+8974.

Institutional Review Board Statement: This de-identified data-linkage study was approved by the Auckland Health Research Ethics Committee AH21942 (expiry 29/01/2024).

Informed Consent Statement: Patient consent was waived because this was a de-identified data linkage study and it was not required by ethics at the time of the study.

Data Availability Statement: In keeping with the Data Management Protocol as part of the Ethics approval, all data is stored securely within the NZCPR folder held within the Health New Zealand IT system. To access de-identified data, please email your request to nzcpregister@adhb.govt.nz.

Conflicts of Interest: We have no conflict of interest to declare.

References

1. McIntyre, S.; Goldsmith, S.; Webb, A.; Ehlinger, V.; Hollung, S.J.; McConnell, K.; Arnaud, C.; Smithers-Sheedy, H.; Oskoui, M.; Khandaker, G.; et al. Global prevalence of cerebral palsy: A systematic analysis. *Dev. Med. Child Neurol.* **2022**, *64*, 1494–1506. [CrossRef] [PubMed]
2. Smithers-Sheedy, H.; McIntyre, S.; Badawi, N.; Goldsmith, S.; Balde, I.; Gibson, C.; Reid, S.; Reddihough, D.; Maloney, E.; Khandaker, G.; et al. *Australian Cerebral Palsy Register Report*; Cerebral Palsy Alliance: Sydney, NSW, Australia, 2018.
3. Marpole, R.; Blackmore, A.M.; Gibson, N.; Cooper, M.S.; Langdon, K.; Wilson, A.C. Evaluation and Management of Respiratory Illness in Children With Cerebral Palsy. *Front. Pediatr.* **2020**, *8*, 333. [CrossRef] [PubMed]
4. Ryan, J.M.; Peterson, M.D.; Matthews, A.; Ryan, N.; Smith, K.J.; O'Connell, N.E.; Liverani, S.; Anokye, N.; Victor, C.; Allen, E. Noncommunicable disease among adults with cerebral palsy: A matched cohort study. *Neurology* **2019**, *93*, e1385–e1396. [CrossRef] [PubMed]
5. Blair, E.; Langdon, K.; McIntyre, S.; Lawrence, D.; Watson, L. Survival and mortality in cerebral palsy: Observations to the sixth decade from a data linkage study of a total population register and National Death Index. *BMC Neurol.* **2019**, *19*, 111. [CrossRef]
6. Blackmore, A.M.; Bear, N.; Blair, E.; Gibson, N.; Jalla, C.; Langdon, K.; Moshovis, L.; Steer, K.; Wilson, A.C. Prevalence of symptoms associated with respiratory illness in children and young people with cerebral palsy. *Dev. Med. Child Neurol.* **2016**, *58*, 780–781. [CrossRef]
7. Telfar Barnard, L.; Zhang, J. *The Impact of Respiratory Disease in New Zealand: 2018 Update*; University of Otago, Asthma and Respiratory Foundation NZ: Dunedin, New Zealand, 2019.
8. Byrnes, C.; Asher, I. *Trying to Catch Our Breath: The Burden of Preventable Breathing Diseases in Children and Young People: Summary*; Asthma and Respiratory Foundation of New Zealand: Wellington, New Zealand, 2006.
9. Twiss, J.; Metcalfe, R.; Edwards, E.; Byrnes, C. New Zealand national incidence of bronchiectasis "too high" for a developed country. *Arch. Dis. Child.* **2005**, *90*, 737–740. [CrossRef]
10. Simpson, J.D.M.; Oben, G.; Adams, J.; Wicken, A.; Pierson, M.; Lilley, R.; Gallagher, S. *Te Ohonga Ake: The Health of Māori Children and Young People in New Zealand Series Two*; New Zealand Child and Youth Epidemiology Service, University of Otago: Dunedin, New Zealand, 2017.
11. Robson, B.; Harris, R. *Hauora: Māori Standards of Health IV. A Study of the Years 2000–2005*; Te Rōpū Rangahau Hauora a Eru Pōmare: Wellington, New Zealand, 2007.
12. Becares, L.; Cormack, D.; Harris, R. Ethnic density and area deprivation: Neighbourhood effects on Maori health and racial discrimination in Aotearoa/New Zealand. *Soc. Sci. Med.* **2013**, *88*, 76–82. [CrossRef]
13. Mackey, A.; Williams, S.; Alzaher, W.; Sorhage, A.; Wilson, N.; Battin, M.; Stott, S. An evaluation of equity in the cerebral palsy diagnostic process in the New Zealand setting between Māori and non- Māori children. *Dev. Med. Child Neurol.* **2022**, *64*, 18. [CrossRef]
14. Blackmore, A.M.; Bear, N.; Blair, E.; Langdon, K.; Moshovis, L.; Steer, K.; Wilson, A.C. Predicting respiratory hospital admissions in young people with cerebral palsy. *Arch. Dis. Child.* **2018**, *103*, 1119–1124. [CrossRef]
15. Simpson, J.; Duncanson, M.; Oben, G.; Adams, J.; Wicken, A.; Morris, S.; Gallagher, S. *The Health of Children and Young People with Chronic Conditions and Disabilities in the Northern District Health Boards 2016*; New Zealand Child and Youth Epidemiology Service, University of Otago: Dunedin, New Zealand, 2016.

16. Simpson, J.D.M.; Oben, G.; Adams, J.; Wicken, A.; Morris, S.; Gallagher, S. *The Health of Children and Young People with Chronic Conditions and Disabilities in New Zealand 2016 (National)*; University of Otago: Wellington, New Zealand, 2016.
17. NZ Ministry of Health. National Health Index: Manatū Hauora Ministry of Health. 2022. Available online: https://www.health.govt.nz/our-work/health-identity/national-health-index (accessed on 21 September 2022).
18. NZ Ministry of Health. *National Minimum Dataset (Hospital Events)*; Manatū Hauora Ministry of Health: Wellington, New Zealand, 2021. Available online: https://www.health.govt.nz/nz-health-statistics/national-collections-and-surveys/collections/national-minimum-dataset-hospital-events (accessed on 7 August 2022).
19. NZ Ministry of Health. *Pharmaceutical Collection*; Manatū Hauora Ministry of Health: Wellington, New Zealand, 2022. Available online: https://www.health.govt.nz/nz-health-statistics/national-collections-and-surveys/collections/pharmaceutical-collection (accessed on 21 September 2022).
20. Cormack, D.; Robson, C. *Classification and Output of Multiple Ethnicities: Considerations for Monitoring Māori Health*; Te Rōpū Rangahau Hauora a Eru Pōmare, University of Otago: Wellington, New Zealand, 2011.
21. Statistics NZ Tatauranga Aotearoa. *Ethnicity Standard Classification: Findings from Public Consultation November*; Statistics New Zealand: Wellington, New Zealand, 2019.
22. Atkinson, J.; Salmond, C.; Crampton, P. *Socioeconomic Deprivation Indexes*; University of Otago: Wellington, New Zealand, 2014.
23. The R Foundation. The R Project for Statistical Computing 2022. Available online: https://www.r-project.org/ (accessed on 19 November 2022).
24. Blackmore, A.M.; Bear, N.; Langdon, K.; Moshovis, L.; Gibson, N.; Wilson, A. Respiratory hospital admissions and emergency department visits in young people with cerebral palsy: 5-year follow-up. *Arch. Dis. Child.* **2020**, *105*, 1126–1127. [CrossRef]
25. Johannesen, C.K.; van Wijhe, M.; Tong, S.; Fernandez, L.V.; Heikkinen, T.; van Boven, M.; Wang, X.; Boas, H.; Li, Y.; Campbell, H.; et al. Age-Specific Estimates of Respiratory Syncytial Virus-Associated Hospitalizations in 6 European Countries: A Time Series Analysis. *J. Infect. Dis.* **2022**, *226*, S29–S37. [CrossRef] [PubMed]
26. Speyer, R.; Cordier, R.; Kim, J.H.; Cocks, N.; Michou, E.; Wilkes-Gillan, S. Prevalence of drooling, swallowing, and feeding problems in cerebral palsy across the lifespan: A systematic review and meta-analyses. *Dev. Med. Child Neurol.* **2019**, *61*, 1249–1258. [CrossRef] [PubMed]
27. Pavone, P.; Gulizia, C.; Le Pira, A.; Greco, F.; Parisi, P.; Di Cara, G.; Falsaperla, R.; Lubrano, R.; Minardi, C.; Spalice, A.; et al. Cerebral Palsy and Epilepsy in Children: Clinical Perspectives on a Common Comorbidity. *Children* **2020**, *8*, 16. [CrossRef] [PubMed]
28. Boel, L.; Pernet, K.; Toussaint, M.; Ides, K.; Leemans, G.; Haan, J.; Van Hoorenbeeck, K.; Verhulst, S. Respiratory morbidity in children with cerebral palsy: An overview. *Dev. Med. Child Neurol.* **2019**, *61*, 646–653. [CrossRef] [PubMed]
29. Statistics New Zealand. Stats NZ Infoshare: Population Estimates Wellington. 2022. Available online: https://infoshare.stats.govt.nz/ (accessed on 5 August 2022).
30. MBIE; Whakatutuki, H. *Three Year Refugee Quota Programme 2019/20–2021/22*; Office of the Ministry of Immigration, New Zealand Government: Wellington, New Zealand, 2019.
31. Hobbs, M.R.; Grant, C.C.; Ritchie, S.R.; Chelimo, C.; Morton, S.M.B.; Berry, S.; Thomas, M.G. Antibiotic consumption by New Zealand children: Exposure is near universal by the age of 5 years. *J. Antimicrob. Chemother.* **2017**, *72*, 1832–1840. [CrossRef]
32. Burns, E.M.; Rigby, E.; Mamidanna, R.; Bottle, A.; Aylin, P.; Ziprin, P.; Faiz, O.D. Systematic review of discharge coding accuracy. *J. Public Health* **2012**, *34*, 138–148. [CrossRef]
33. Craig, E.; Dell, R.; Reddington, A.; Adams, J.; Oben, G.; Wicken, A. *Te Ohonga Ake, The Determinants of Health for Māori Children and Young People in New Zealand*; University of Otago's Dunedin School of Medicine, NZ Child and Youth Epidemiology Service: Dunedin, New Zealand, 2013.
34. Gerdung, C.A.; Tsang, A.; Yasseen, A.S., 3rd; Armstrong, K.; McMillan, H.J.; Kovesi, T. Association Between Chronic Aspiration and Chronic Airway Infection with Pseudomonas aeruginosa and Other Gram-Negative Bacteria in Children with Cerebral Palsy. *Lung* **2016**, *194*, 307–314. [CrossRef]
35. Owayed, A.F.; Campbell, D.M.; Wang, E.E. Underlying causes of recurrent pneumonia in children. *Arch. Pediatr. Adolesc. Med.* **2000**, *154*, 190–194. [CrossRef]
36. Young, N.; McCormick, A.; Gilbert, T.; Ayling-Campos, A.; Burke, T.; Fehlings, D.; Wedge, J. Reasons for Hospital Admissions Among Youth and Young Adults With Cerebral Palsy. *Arch. Phys. Med. Rehabil.* **2011**, *92*, 46–50. [CrossRef]
37. Langdon, K.; Cooper, M.S. Early identification of respiratory disease in children with neurological diseases: Improving quality of life? *Dev. Med. Child Neurol.* **2021**, *63*, 494–495. [CrossRef]
38. Blackmore, M.; Bear, N.; Langdon, K.; Moshovis, L.; Gibson, N.; Wilson, A. Risk Factors for Respiratory Hospital Admissions for Young People (1–26 Years) with Cerebral Palsy. *Arch. Dis. Child.* **2019**. [CrossRef]
39. Europe WHO. *Reducing Inequities in Health across the Life-Course: Early Years, Childhood and Adolescence*; Europe WHO: Copenhagen, Denmark, 2020.
40. Hobbs, M.; Ahuriri-Driscoll, A.; Marek, L.; Campbell, M.; Tomintz, M.; Kingham, S. Reducing health inequity for Maori people in New Zealand. *Lancet* **2019**, *394*, 1613–1614. [CrossRef] [PubMed]

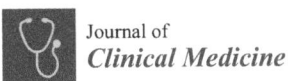

Article

Implementation of an Early Communication Intervention for Young Children with Cerebral Palsy Using Single-Subject Research Design

Roslyn Ward [1,2,*], Elizabeth Barty [3], Neville Hennessey [1], Catherine Elliott [1,4] and Jane Valentine [3,4]

1. School of Allied Health, Curtin University, Perth 6102, Australia
2. Institute of Health Research, University of Notre Dame Australia, Fremantle 6160, Australia
3. Department of Paediatric Rehabilitation, Perth Children's Hospital, Perth 6009, Australia
4. Telethon Kids Institute, Perth 6009, Australia
* Correspondence: r.ward@curtin.edu.au

Abstract: The implementation of an intervention protocol aimed at increasing vocal complexity in three pre-linguistic children with cerebral palsy (two males, starting age 15 months, and one female, starting age 16 months) was evaluated utilising a repeated ABA case series design. The study progressed until the children were 36 months of age. Weekly probes with trained and untrained items were administered across each of three intervention blocks. Successive blocks targeted more advanced protophone production and speech movement patterns, individualised for each participant. Positive treatment effects were seen for all participants in terms of a greater rate of achievement of target protophone categories and speech movement patterns. Tau coefficients for trained items demonstrated overall moderate to large AB phase contrast effect sizes, with limited evidence of generalisation to untrained items. Control items featuring protophones and speech movements not targeted for intervention showed no change across phases for any participant. Our data suggest that emerging speech-production skills in prelinguistic infants with CP can be positively influenced through a multimodal intervention focused on capitalising on early periods of plasticity when language learning is most sensitive.

Keywords: cerebral palsy; early intervention; infant vocalisations; infants; single-subject research design

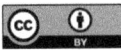

1. Introduction

Research shows as many as 85% of two-year-old children with cerebral palsy (CP) present with communication impairment, with only 10% expected to outgrow their delay by 4 years of age [1]. Early communication difficulties in young children with CP may be associated with sensory, motor and/or cognitive impairment [2] and are predictive of later language difficulties [3,4] that place children at risk of educational and social disadvantage and long-term activity and participation limitations [5].

Recent advances in the early identification of CP have seen the development of specific motor interventions for children less than two years of age [6,7]. These interventions were designed to mitigate the cascading consequences of impairment by capitalising on sensitive periods of neuroplasticity in early development [8,9]. In contrast, no such evidence-base of interventions exist for early communication impairment for children at-risk of CP [10]. This is despite the recognition that children who cross performance thresholds "earlier in life have better outcomes later" [11], p. 1609 and research demonstrating the impact of multi-modal experiences during sensitive periods of early development on later language learning [12].

For example, Kuhl and colleagues [9,12] identify the period between 6 months and 12 months of age as a sensitive period for phonetic learning, representing the earliest milestone in language acquisition [13]. The shaping or attunement of early speech perception and production to a child's native language is highly dependent on the multi-modal and bidirectional communicative exchanges that take place between a parent and infant [14]. Research has shown that infants of caregivers who engage in a high proportion of contingent communicative interactions show greater attunement and produce more mature vocalisations [15], with a direct positive influence on vocabulary development [16,17].

Moreover, there is good evidence to show that infant vocalisations provide a significant foundation for speech and language learning, as well as social, emotional, and cognitive abilities [18–20]. Infant vocalisations considered precursors to speech are termed protophones [21]. They follow a developmental trajectory of increasing vocal control and complexity [17]. For example, infants progress from pre-canonical vocalisations such as marginal babbling, containing consonant-like (closant) and vowel-like (vocant) elements with slow movement transitions, through to the canonical babble stage that features speech-like consonant–vowel (CV) syllables with quick transitions [22]. Whilst the age of emergence varies, it is typically reported infants gain control of basic canonical syllables between 5 and 10 months of age [21]. The canonical babbling stage progresses to more advanced or motorically complex forms and provides a foundation for the child to produce their first words with communicative intent. From this perspective, delays or restrictions in the development of infant vocalizations due to an underlying deficit should be predictive of ongoing constraints on the expansion of these vocal production skills into intelligible language, hence, contributing to communication impairment. Consistent with this expectation, research has shown that delayed emergence of canonical syllables predicts poor expressive language, particularly, vocabulary development, in children [18,20]. Furthermore, recent research focusing on identifying biomarkers in infant vocalisations [23,24] has been undertaken in children with neurodevelopmental conditions, such as autism [25] and Down Syndrome [26], contributing to the development of targeted early interventions designed to ameliorate the impact of communication impairment. The development of infant vocalisations in children with CP with the potential to identify communication impairment and intervene early has received limited attention.

In 1999, Levin [27] reported on the vocalisations of eight, 12-month-old infants with CP. The babbling of all eight participants was limited to monosyllables with the phonetic repertoire comprised largely of back vowels, plosives and velars. These vocal behaviors were associated with limited oral motor control that included the speech subsystems of respiration, phonation and articulation. Nyman and Lohmander [28] also reported on the canonical babble in three children with CP, representing a subset of 18 children with neurodevelopmental disability. They identified children with CP presented with significantly lower levels of canonical babble and limited phonetic repertoire. More recently, Ward et al. [29] reported longitudinal data of 18 infants with CP, as compared to TD infants, utilising the Infant Monitor of vocal Production (IMP). They identified divergence from typical development in the vocalisations of infants with CP at 9 and 12 months of age suggesting delays in the transition from the pre-canonical to canonical babble stage. Collectively, these findings provide evidence of impaired emergence of speech motor control in very young children with CP, and represent an opportunity for the development of CP specific early interventions to benefit their early speech production skills and subsequent communication development.

Currently, a multi-modal approach to very early intervention is recommended [30]. This includes supporting the social foundations of communication (i.e., joint attention for engagement, and play); building comprehension to facilitate the transition to spoken language [31]; and providing access to expressive communication including building speech production, all embedded in the child's routine to increase opportunities of practice of targeted skills [32]. These principles are consistent with research showing interventions that target parent–child interactions benefit the development of expressive language skills in children at risk of language impairment [33]. However, few interventions to date have been directed at the development of early vocalisations in infants at risk of motor-speech impairments including infants at risk of CP [34–36].

In light of the above, this paper reports on a multi-modal case-series intervention for children under 24 months with communication impairment associated with CP. Consideration was given to recommendations for principles of early communication intervention [33], including CP specific early intervention [10], and theoretical constructs that consider a child's development to arise from bi-directional interactions within the physical, social, cognitive and environmental domains.

The PROMPT approach we adopted in the present study encompasses each of the aforementioned elements [37]. PROMPT has previously been used in children with CP [38] and found to be effective in improving speech motor control and intelligibility in children aged 3 years to 14 years. It is an empirically supported and manualised approach guided by key tenets of Dynamic Systems Theory, as illustrated within the PROMPT conceptual framework [37]. Clinicians undertake a dynamic assessment of the physical–sensory, cognitive linguistic and social emotional domains utilising the Global Domain Evaluation to determine intervention goals and priorities for functional communication. This is based on the presumption that "all domains interact during communication and that audition and somatosensory information are equally important in the development and organisation of motor-speech behaviour" [37], p. 477. PROMPT trained clinicians will "alternate" their treatment priorities between the communication domains, with the first intervention priority chosen to achieve the greatest shift. For example, intervention with a child who is pre-linguistic and not engaging in reciprocity, will focus on the social–emotional domain, as their priority. All intervention goals and objectives are functionally motivated and developed with consideration given to the child's and family's environment, and sufficient opportunity for repetition and practice within the daily routine.

Within the physical–sensory domain, three intervention priorities are determined using the Systems Analysis Observation and Motor Speech Hierarchy (MSH) [37]. The MSH represents seven stages of motor-speech subsystem control and based upon the inter-hierarchical sequence of motor-speech development [39].

A PROMPT session must include tactile input that is used to (a) create an interactive awareness for communication with intention; (b) provide associative mapping for cognitive-linguistic input; and/or (c) develop speech subsystems at the sound, word, or phrase level. In addition to behavioural based studies that have demonstrated modifications to the speech system brought about through tactile input [40], more recent exploratory work by Fiori et al. [41] has identified neural changes in participants subsequent to intervention.

In summary, this study tests the hypothesis that intervention started before 2 years of age, framed within the PROMPT approach and utilising tactile input, will improve the vocal complexity of children with communication impairment secondary to CP. The single-subject experimental methodology was selected to (a) demonstrate proof-of-concept for a multi-modal intervention, focused on speech sound practice for young children at risk of communication impairment secondary to CP; (b) inform a larger scale research design; and (c) accommodate the heterogeneity of the participants.

Three intervention blocks, each using an ABA sequence, were designed to build successive complexity as follows. Block one focused primarily on preparing the child for learning by building social interaction and reciprocity, teaching targeted words within home-based daily routines and play activities. The tactile input was timed to precede or follow the turn-taking routine, avoiding disruption to the reciprocity of the interaction. It was hypothesised the tactile input during block one intervention would contribute to achieving the vocal production priorities developed for each child, our primary outcome of interest, although these changes may be minimal or not consistently sustained.

In contrast, block two and three focused more directly on building the complexity and diversity of vocalisations/speech produced with communicative intent and increasing motor control, in accordance with the developed motor-speech priorities for each child in each block. The tactile input was provided to shape articulator (i.e., motor) movements during speech production. It was hypothesised that intervention blocks two and three would be associated with an increase in the use of target vocal patterns or protophones (e.g., CV syllable production) and associated speech movements (e.g., closed to open and open to closed jaw transitions with phonation control) during vocal elicitation tasks.

Each intervention block included three word sets that targeted increasing motor control, as based on the MSH. Word set 1 contained words with the lowest level of complexity, targeted intervention priority one and were trained throughout the whole intervention phase. As Word set 2 contained a higher level of complexity, these were introduced half-way through the intervention phase to allow initial focus on the priority one word set. Word set 3 represented intervention priority three. These words acted as a control and were not actively trained but were embedded within meaningful daily interactions.

It was hypothesised a treatment effect would be observed for trained items that were part of the intervention. Untrained items, that is, different words containing the same target protophones and requiring the same speech movement pattern, were included in the elicitation tasks to test for generalisation effects to other items. The third word set represents the control goal and as such no treatment effect was expected.

2. Method

2.1. Research Design

A single-subject multiple-probe research design with three participants was conducted in compliance with the Single-Case Reporting Guideline in Behavioural Interventions (SCRIBE) Statement [42], and design standards described by Kratochwill et al. [43]. This involved (a) systematic manipulation of the independent variable; (b) systematic measurement of dependent variables by more than one blinded assessor; (c) replication of the study design across phases and participants to demonstrate an intervention effect and experimental control; and (d) a minimum of three data points during each pre-intervention baseline phase.

The study design involved repeated ABA phase sequences with the start of each subsequent intervention (B) phase targeting more complex vocalisations (i.e., AB_1A, AB_2A, AB_3A). The length of the first baseline (A) phase in each ABA sequence ranged from 3 to 4 weeks. This was followed by a 10-week intervention phase and then a 3 to 4 week post intervention baseline phase, also involving no treatment being delivered (A). There were three ABA phase sequences for two participants (P1 and P2) and two sequences for one participant (P3). The third intervention ABA block was not offered to P3 due to the COVID-19 pandemic [44].

2.2. Participants

Three infants (P1, P2, and P3) with CP were recruited through the 'at-risk' early intervention service at Perth Children's Hospital. The tertiary service adheres to recommendations for early diagnosis [45] and evidence-based practice principles.

Inclusion criteria were: identified as at high-risk of CP at less than 6 months of age, and enrolment in the It Takes Two to Talk (ITTT)—The Hanen Program® (Toronto, ON, Canada) [46] administered through the early intervention service at PCH at or by 12 months of age. The Hanen ITTT Program® is based on best practice principles of building parent–child interactions, utilising daily routines, and establishing a shared expectation of parent implemented intervention through joint planning and coaching [47].

Exclusion criteria were: English not spoken in the home, medically unstable, cortical visual impairment and uncorrected hearing impairment with thresholds greater than 25 dB.

Two participants (P1 and P2) formed a subset of data collected within a larger study, focused on profiling the longitudinal development of communication in young children at-risk of CP [29]. Both P1 and P2 were male and aged 15 months at the start of the present study. P3, a female, was referred into the study at 16 months by their managing speech pathologist, following completion of the Hanen ITTT Program® and a multi-site clinical trial for infants with hemiparesis. All parents completed all sessions of the Hanen ITTT Program®.

Table 1 shows the participant characteristics at baseline. All three were at the prelinguistic stage of language development at the onset of this study. Table 2 shows communication status, as measured at baseline across each of the study phases.

Table 1. Participant Characteristics at Study Onset.

Participant	P1	P2	P3
Age at Intervention Block One	15 months	15 months	16 months
Sex	M	M	F
Diagnosis	Spastic Quadraparesis	Dyskinetic	Spastic Hemiplegia
Gestational Age	Term	35 weeks	Term
Age of diagnosis	<6 months	<6 months	<6 months
GMFCS at 2 years	III	III	I
Hearing Status	WNL	Aided	WNL
Oral Pharyngeal Dysphagia	Oral	PEG	Oral
Epilepsy	No	No	Stable

Table 2. Communication Status as Measured Across the Study Phases.

	Age of Assessment							
	Participant 1			Participant 2			Participant 3	
	15	24	36	15	24	36	15	24
CSBS DP	SS (PR)	SS (PR)	[RS]	SS (PR) [RS]	SS (PR)	[RS]	SS (PR)	SS (PR)
Communication Composite	120 (91)	107 (68)	NA	82 (12)	79 (8)	NA	102 (55)	96 (39)
Cluster Scores				SS (PR) [RS]	SS (PR)	[RS]	SS (PR)	SS (PR)
Function	14 (91)	5 (5)	NA	9 (37)	7 (16)	NA	10 (50)	10 (50)
Gestural	10 (50)	5 (5)	NA	3 (1)	8 (25)	NA	10 (50)	8 (25)
Vocal	15 (98)	6 (9)	NA	8 (25)	3 (1)	NA	12 (75)	7 (16)
Consonants used [#different]	[8] (3)	[9] (4)	[12]	[2] (2)	[5] (3)	[5]	[4] (3)	[7] (3)
	/m/, /n/, /b/, /d/, /g/, /w/, /j/, /dz/	/m/, /n/, /ŋ/, /b/, /d/, /t/, /g/, /w/, /dz/	/m/, /n/, /ŋ/, /b/, /p/, /d/, /g/, /w/, /v/, /s/, /dz/, /ʃ/	/n/, /g/	/m/, /n/, /d/, /g/, /w/	/m/, /n/, /b/, /d/, /w/	/m/, /n/, /d/, /j/	/m/, /n/, /b/, /p/, /d/, /g/, /j/
Verbal	* 11 (63)	7 (16)	NA	7 (15)	6 (9)	NA	* 11 (63)	6 (9)
DW	[8]	[11]	[45]	[0]	[5]	[10]	[2]	[8]
DWC	[3]	[3]	[3]	[0]	[0]	[2]	[0]	[0]
Reciprocity	10 (50)	12 (63)	NA	8 (25)	8 (25)	NA	10 (50)	11 (63)
Social-affective signalling	14 (91)	13 (84)	NA	13 (84)	14 (91)	NA	10 (50)	13 (84)
REEL-3	SS (PR)	SS (PR)	SS (PR)	SS (PR)	SS (PR)	SS (PR)	SS (PR)	SS (PR)
Expressive	73 (3)	87 (19)	72 (3)	<55 (<1)	70 (2)	<55 (<1)	98 (45)	105 (63)
Receptive	81 (10)	82 (12)	108 (70)	<55 (<1)	<55 (<1)	85 (16)	72 (3)	78 (7)
Language Ability Score	109 (73)	81 (10)	88 (21)	<46 (<1)	54 (1)	64 (<1)	82 (12)	90 (25)

Note. CSBS DP = The Communication and Symbolic Behaviour Scales Developmental Profile; REEL-3 = Receptive-Expressive Emergent Language Test-3; SS = Standard Score; PR = percentile rank; RS = raw score; Function = Communication Function from CSBS; Gestural = Communication Means Gestural from CSBS; Vocal = Communication Means Vocal from CSBS; DW = Inventory of different words; DWC = Different word combination; NA = Not Applicable; * This standard score is reflective of a raw score of one word approximation.

2.3. Setting

This research study was conducted through the state-wide tertiary rehabilitation service at Perth Children's Hospital [29,48]. The study was framed within the integrated knowledge-to-action framework [49] and designed to transfer knowledge gained through the study directly into the clinical service.

The study phases were conducted within the family home. Home visits were conducted on a weekly basis and administered in collaboration with a primary caregiver, primarily the mother. Inclusion of fathers and grandparents took place on an ad hoc basis, around availability for P2 and P3.

2.4. Measures

2.4.1. Baseline Assessments

The following measures were used to assess each child prior to each pre-intervention baseline period.

The Receptive-Expressive Emergent Language Test-3 (REEL-3). The REEL-3 is a standardised assessment of emerging language in children from birth to 3 years of age. Information is obtained through parent interview. Raw scores from the receptive and expressive language scales were converted to standard ability scores ($M = 100$, $SD = 15$) with percentile ranks, and a combined language ability standard score was also obtained. The REEL-3 has been identified as a reference standard for early language assessment [50], with established psychometric properties [51]. In addition, Rome-Flanders and Cronk [52] report longitudinal stability, with predictive validity of later testing results at 15 months and 18 months.

The Communication and Symbolic Behaviour Scales Developmental Profile (CSBS DP). The Communication and Symbolic Play Scales (CSBS) DP Behaviour Sample [53] is a standardised measure of early communication and symbolic skills for children 6 months to 2 years of age. Information is obtained through the administration of standardised behavioural sampling that includes communicative temptations, books, construction, and symbolic play. The behaviour sample derives a composite score ($M = 100$, $SD = 15$) from six cluster scores ($M = 10$, $SD = 3$): Communication Function, Communication Means Gestural, Communication Means Vocal, Communication Means Verbal, Reciprocity, and Social-Affective Signalling. Reliability and validity are reported to be high, with the three composite scores a significant predictor of receptive and receptive language outcomes [54].

2.4.2. Dependent Variables

The two primary outcome measures reported in this study are the number of probe items (i.e., words within each word set) produced with communicative intent [55] showing (a) achievement of the targeted protophone category [21], and (b) achievement of the targeted *motor-speech movement pattern* (e.g., bilabial closing and opening gesture) reflecting emergence of speech motor control. These measures were extracted via weekly probes administered in the day of each session in each study phase.

Speech Probes. A wordbook containing personalised pictures/photos representing the individual target words for each intervention priority, was developed for each child. For example, the probe word "bye" requires production of the target CV protophone, as well as a bilabial closing and opening speech movement pattern. Expressive speech probes were selected based on the intervention priorities and the MSH, daily routines and play interests, family relevance and communicative functions, including social words, requesting, nouns, action words, and pronouns [35].

The Appendix A provides the word sets for each participant across the intervention blocks. Target words for each participant were selected prior to the commencement of each intervention block and divided into three groups based on motor-speech control as described in the systems analysis observation and the MSH. Word set 1 and 2 both contained trained and untrained words based on the increasing complexity of the MSH represented in priorities one and two, respectively. An equal number of trained to untrained words were allocated a priori to each word set. However, a small number of words (no greater than 3 per participant), were re-allocated during the intervention phase in response to participant interest and motivation (see Appendix A).

Word set 3 contained control words based on intervention priority three. These words were not targeted and acted as a control probe condition throughout the study.

2.5. Procedure

Approval for this study was obtained from the Child and Adolescent Health Services Ethics Committee (study number 2015221). In addition to the intervention being conducted within the family home, parents agreed to an all-day recording of their infant's vocalisations up to two times a week, as captured through the Language Environmental Analysis (LENA) Digital Language Processor (DLP).

All participants completed standardised assessments of communication within a 2 week period prior to the commencement of each intervention block. Standards assessments took place within the family home, administered by the first author. Following completion and scoring of the standardised assessments, a second home visit was conducted within 7 days to discuss the assessment results and in collaboration with the family determined the intervention goals, priorities and vocabulary (trained, untrained and control) for each intervention block. Figure 1 illustrates the study phases and timepoints. The speech sample obtained during administration of the CSBS was used to inform the three motor-speech priorities targeted in each intervention block. All sessions in each phase of the study were video recorded (Sony Handycam HDR-CX405).

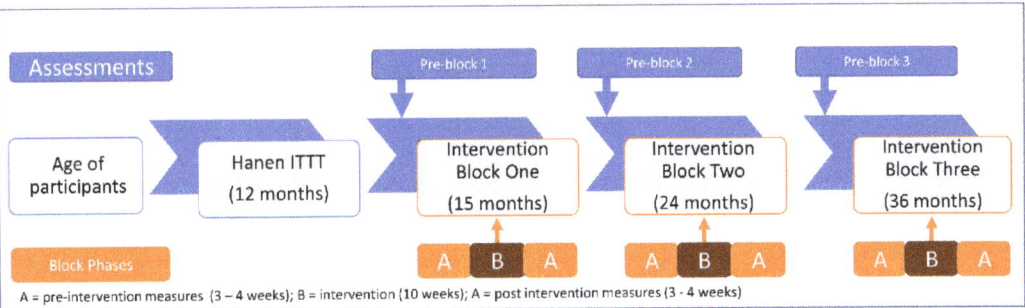

Figure 1. Study phases and timeline.

Administration of Speech Probes

Baseline phase. Weekly home visits were conducted to administer the expressive speech probes. Participants were offered a maximum of five opportunities to elicit the targeted verbal response. The planned elicitation strategy was a mand-model (e.g., say X), or open ended prompt (e.g., holding the picture or object represented in the picture book and asking "this is a ?"). However, upon commencement of baseline for intervention block one, it became clear not all participants could respond to these elicitation strategies. As a result, a hierarchy of elicitation procedures was developed and included: cloze with time delay when the word was elicited through a familiar nursery rhyme (e.g., row, row, row your …) and information (e.g., use your lips, /b/). When participants attempted multiple repetitions and self-correction, the best of the first two trials was scored. The elicitation task took between 10 and 20 min to complete for each child, with the order of presentation varied.

Intervention phase. Following completion of each home-based therapy session across all intervention blocks, participants were presented with their books to elicit the target word, using the same procedure as the baseline sessions. The exception to this was the speech probes for P2 in block one. P2 was unable to complete the speech probes at the end of the intervention sessions in block one, therefore, the parent was asked to elicit the probes on a selected day at the same time during the week whilst wearing the LENA device. With the investigator given permission to extract the audio file, the parents were asked to identify a period in the day where the speech probes were elicited. The extracted wav files were then used for analysis. The speech movement targets that rely on visual as well as audio information could not be scored during that intervention block.

2.6. Scoring of Speech Probes

Video recordings of the speech probes were converted to wav files, exported to Praat software [56] and visually inspected using the time-amplitude waveform and wide-band spectrograms. Onsets and offsets for each of the target words were annotated in a Praat textgrid and coded using broad phonetic transcription ready for scoring. Three independent PROMPT trained speech-language pathologists (referred to as raters), blinded to the ages of the child, phases of the study, intervention blocks and intervention objectives, completed the scoring of the dependent variables. The individual sessions and target words were randomised during scoring, using the Excel random function.

Protophone coding. Rater 1, who coded the elicited vocal productions, has a master's degree in linguistics and more than 30 years paediatric clinical experience working with neurodevelopmental disorders, including CP; as well as research experience in the coding of protophones according to Stark protocol [21].

The operational definitions used to code the protophones of the vocalisations/word approximations elicited were based on the Stark Assessment of Early Vocal Development-Revised (SAEDV-R) [21]. A binary scoring (1 or 0) was used where the vocalisation was scored for the presence (i.e., achievement) (1) or absence (score = 0) of the targeted protophone for each target word for each participant, with a maximum score of 1 allocated to each word.

Speech movement patterns (speech motor control). Raters 2 and 3 coded the speech movement patterns of elicited vocal productions of the participants. Rater 2 has worked clinically as a PROMPT trained clinician for 20+ years, with a clinical caseload that includes children with motor-speech disorders, including CP. In addition, rater 2 has experience coding speech movement patterns as a research assistant. Rater 3 is a speech-language pathologist with 8 years clinical experience in the assessment and management of speech sound disorders, including CP. She has been trained in the scoring the Motor Speech Hierarchy Probe Words [57]. Similar to protophone scoring the targeted movement pattern was then scored from the digital video recordings for the presence (1) or absence (0) of the identified speech movement pattern for each word, with a maximum score of 1 allocated, with the most accurate production of the first two vocal attempts selected.

Reliability. Inter-rater agreement for protophone coding was assessed by the first author and rater 1 both scoring a separate data set, with the amount equivalent to 10% of the coding of the present study, to ensure independence from the data analysis. Good levels of agreement in both percentage (89%) and correlation for agreement using Cohen's kappa (0.864, $p < 0.001$) was obtained (Hartman et al., 2004).

Good level of inter-rater agreement using Cohen's kappa of speech movement coding between rater 2 and rater 3, calculated on 10% of the data, was achieved, K = 0.681 (95% CI, 0.600 to 0.748), $p < 0.001$.

Intervention Protocol

Intervention priorities were selected to address the social–emotional, cognitive-linguistic and physical–sensory domains, for each child, as represented within the PROMPT conceptual framework [37]. The intervention routines were developed in consultation with the family and targeted the following three activities: daily routine/play activity, social routine (songs and nursery rhymes), and interactive book-share. Therapy routines were established to allow children to anticipate the targeted vocabulary. For example, cloze techniques during song routines (e.g., "row, row, row your ... [boat])" and activities (e.g., stacking cups "up" when placing cups on top of each other).

Block one prioritised turn-taking within parent–child interactions. Activities at the cognitive-linguistic level included building spatial concepts and following single stage instructions. Linguistic input was supported by key word signs and picture supports, as required by the child. The aim was to increase comprehension of salient and meaningful vocabulary for active participation in daily routines and activities. Additionally, the physical–sensory domain of block one informed the three articulatory subsystem priorities that were identified using the MSH and systems analysis observation, as based on the CSBS DP speech sample administered during the pre-baseline assessments.

In blocks two and three, the social routines established in block one were extended or modified in keeping with the child's interests. Linguistic input continued to be supported by key word signs and picture supports, as required by the child. Within the physical–sensory domain, three articulatory subsystem priorities were identified using the MSH and systems analysis observation, as based on the CSBS DP speech sample administered in the pre-baseline assessments, as well as the level of success achieved in the preceding block. The emphasis on speech subsystem organisation was increased with the introduction of the motor phoneme warm-up at the commencement of each therapy session. Tactile input was used to facilitate the formation of sensory-motor pathways for speech production.

Table 3 details the intervention goals for each participant across the study phases. For P1 and P3, intervention blocks one and two focused on refining objectives within the same levels of the MSH. Intervention block three also targeted increased motor complexity at a higher level of the MSH. For P2, the treatment priorities established in intervention block one were further refined in treatment blocks two and three with a focused on increasing the accuracy and variability in syllable structure.

Table 3. Intervention Priorities for each Participant across the Three Intervention Blocks.

Priority	Participant One	Participant Two	Participant Three
		Block One	
1	Production of /m/, /b/ and /a/ with jaw transitions moving from closed to open (closant–vocant) and open to closed (vocant–closant) in target words, with controlled phonation.	Produce vocalisations with communicate intent, within a turn-taking routine (Decrease vocalisations without communicative intent)	Controlled phonation of the sounds /m/, /b/ and /a/ with communicate intent, in target words
2	Lip-to-lip contact producing bilabials in words that contain movements with broad lip rounding (e.g., moo, push, boo) or retraction (e.g., me, bee) in CV syllables	Increase complexity of vocalisations in target words as coded on SAEDV-R. Responsive vocalisations to include isolated continuant closant (m, b, a) or closant–vocants	Jaw transitions moving from closed to open and open to closed, producing consonant–vowel and vowel–consonant combinations
3	Achieve tongue separation from jaw in production of the phonemes /n/, d/, /t/ in target words	Jaw transitions moving from closed to open and open to closed, with phonation	Broad lip rounding (e.g., moo, push, boo) or retraction (e.g., me, bee) in CV syllable structures
		Block Two	
1	Jaw transitions moving from closed to open and open to closed, in syllables containing CV, CVCV, VC and CVC structures	Increase complexity of vocalisations in target words as coded on SAEDV-R with communicate intent (b, m, a) closant–vocant or vocant–closant (marginal babble)	Jaw transitions moving from closed to open and open to closed, producing consonant–vowel and vowel–consonant combinations

Table 3. Cont.

Priority	Participant One	Participant Two	Participant Three
2	Broad lip rounding or retraction in CV syllable structures	Jaw transitions moving from closed to open and open to closed, producing targeted closant–vocant and vocant–closant combinations	Broad lip rounding (e.g., moo, push, boo) or retraction (e.g., me, bee) in CV syllable structures
3	Tongue separation from jaw in production of the phonemes /n/, d/, /t/ in CVC, VCV and VC words	Produce anterior lingual sounds /d/, /n/ in target words	Separation of tongue from jaw in CV, VC and CVC syllable structures
Block Three			
1	Engage lower lip for production of fricatives /f/ and /v/	Increase complexity of vocalisations in target words as coded on SAEDV-R with communicate intent, CV, VC or VCV	
2	Tongue separation of jaw in production of the phonemes /n/, /d/, /s/	Jaw transitions moving from closed to open and open to closed, producing targeted consonant–vowel and vowel–consonant combinations	
3	Sequenced movements over two syllables	Produce the anterior lingual sounds /d/, /n/ in target words	

Note. Bold font = targeted priorities 1 and 2. Priority 3 is a control goal and not targeted.

Participants received therapy once a week for a duration of approximately 45 min. The first 5–10 min were spent in parent discussion reviewing intervention goals and home practice during the week, followed by 30 min active therapy with parent coaching, and the last 10 min were spent planning implementation within the daily routine. The speech probe elicitations for that session were then carried out. The therapy format was individualised to each participant, with the same format followed throughout the intervention block.

Intervention fidelity. Intervention fidelity was secured for all participants through the delivery of the intervention protocols by a certified to fidelity PROMPT Instructor (RW), who also has 30+ years' clinical experience. The instructor has collaborated with Ms Deborah Hayden (PROMPT founder and research director) in previous research protocols [38,58], as well as validation of the PROMPT fidelity checklist [59] and Motor-Speech Hierarchy-Probe Words scoring system [60], and ongoing development of the PROMPT approach to intervention [37]. RW prepared the data for analysis but did not contribute to the scoring of the data.

Procedural fidelity: dosage. Fidelity to intervention intensity, as described by Warren, Fey and Yoder [61], was recorded and extracted for 50% of the intervention sessions. Table 4 illustrates the total number of intervention sessions attended, with the average therapy duration and dosage of the active ingredient based on the analysed sessions. Dosage of the active ingredient includes a count of the teaching episodes with tactile input, per minute, where the child was actively engaged in a play routine. Furthermore, the proportion of word set 1 and word set 2 words trained, was calculated. Our data show the active treatment ingredient was administered at more than 1 teaching episode per minute for all participants, except for P3 block one.

Table 4. Fidelity to Intervention Dosage.

	Block One			Block Two			Block Three	
	P1	P2	P3	P1	P2	P3	P1	P2
Teaching Episodes Per Minute	1.56	1.03	0.95	1.40	1.24	1.11	1.5	1.29
No of sessions attended	10	10	10	10	10	10	10	10
Active Therapy Duration	35.80	35.00	26.80	35.25	31.13	37.00	34	22.8
Proportion Word set 1/Word set 2	3.60	1.04	3.40	2.90	1.20	2.40	4.80	1.60

2.7. Analyses

Visual inspection was undertaken to determine evidence of a relationship between the independent variable (intervention) and the dependent variable (outcome measures). Within and between-phase data patterns were evaluated for change in magnitude (level), trend (direction of performance), variability (degree of overall scatter) between the study phases and consistency of data patterns across the study phases.

Visual analysis was supplemented with the nonparametric Tau-U analysis to determine statistically significant change. Tau-U measures nonoverlap between pre-intervention baseline and intervention phases, and provides a non-parametric Tau coefficient (varies between −1 and 1) to yield effect size estimates [62]. The following Tau benchmarks were applied to document treatment effects: <0.20 small, 0.20 to <0.60 moderate, 0.60 to <0.80 large, and >0.80 very large [63]. A Tau-U phase contrast p value < 0.1, where Tau was positive (i.e., 0.05 one-tailed probability test equivalent), was considered statistically significant.

Finally, the numerical difference between the mean of the post-intervention baseline values, expressed as a percentage of items within the corresponding word set, and pre-intervention baseline percentage values for each ABA time series was calculated to capture the increase in level of performance (i.e., percentage increase in the number of achievements of the target vocalisation pattern) after the intervention stopped relative to the pre-intervention baseline.

3. Results

The speech probe data plotted across the study phases for each intervention block are shown in Figures 2–4 for P1, Figures 5–7 for P2, and Figures 8 and 9 for P3. Each data point represents the number of elicited vocal productions coded as achieved within each word set for protophone targets (in panel A) and speech movement targets (in panel B). The number achieved for trained items is given on the left vertical axis, and the number of achieved untrained items is given on the right, with the maximum value of each scale adjusted according to the total number of items for that word set condition. Visual analysis indicates the initial baselines for each intervention block were relatively stable with low or no variability for all participants. A positive treatment effect, that is, an increase in the number of trained items from word sets 1 and 2 achieving the target priorities compared to pre-intervention baseline counts, was seen for all participants for some intervention blocks. The magnitude of treatment effect is reported in Table 5 for protophone targets and Table 6 for speech movement targets. As an overall summary across participants and outcome measures, the mean Tau coefficient effect size for trained items in word set 1 (i.e., items trained throughout the intervention block) was 0.61 ($SD = 0.27$, range 0.22–1.0), a large effect size. Of those 15 Tau coefficients, five were statistically significant with large or very large effect size. The mean difference in percent for the word set 1 trained items between the post-intervention and pre-intervention baselines was positive and averaged 37% ($SD = 24.9$, range 6.7–75.0). The Tau coefficient also correlated strongly with the mean difference scores ($r = 0.86$, $p < 0.001$, $n = 15$), confirming larger effects during the intervention phase for trained word set 1 items tended to be associated with a higher post-intervention mean (see also Figures 2–9).

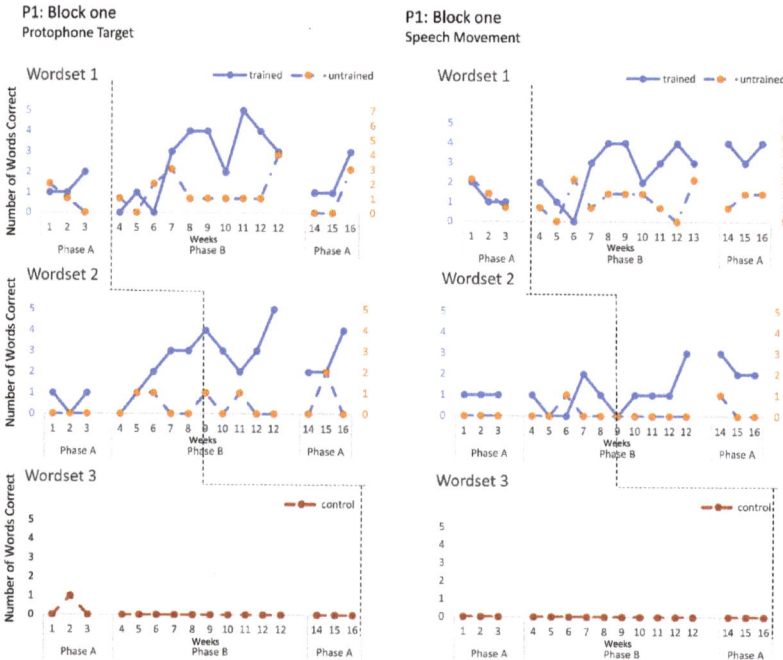

Figure 2. Accuracy of performance on the speech probes as scored for protophone target (**left**) and motor-speech movements (**right**) block one, participant 1.

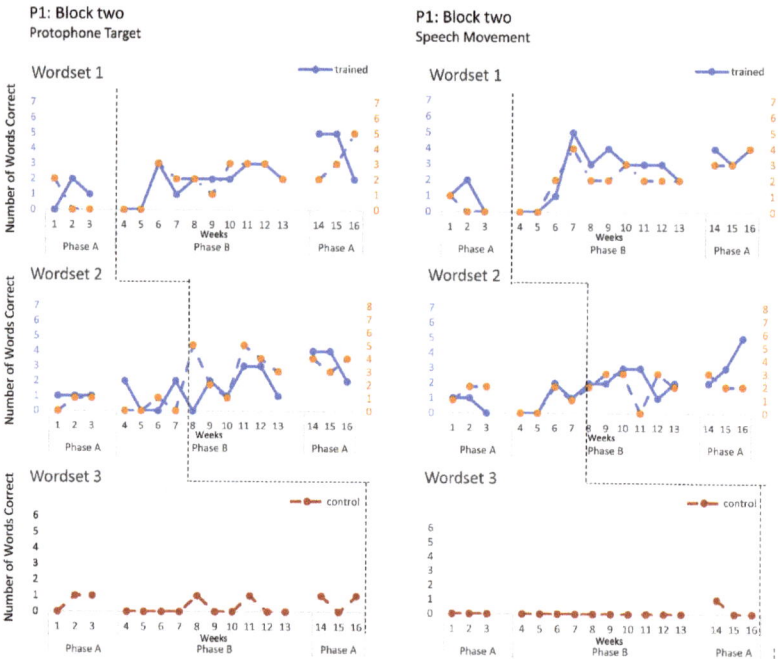

Figure 3. Accuracy of performance on the speech probes as scored for protophone target (**left**) and motor-speech movements (**right**) block two, participant 1.

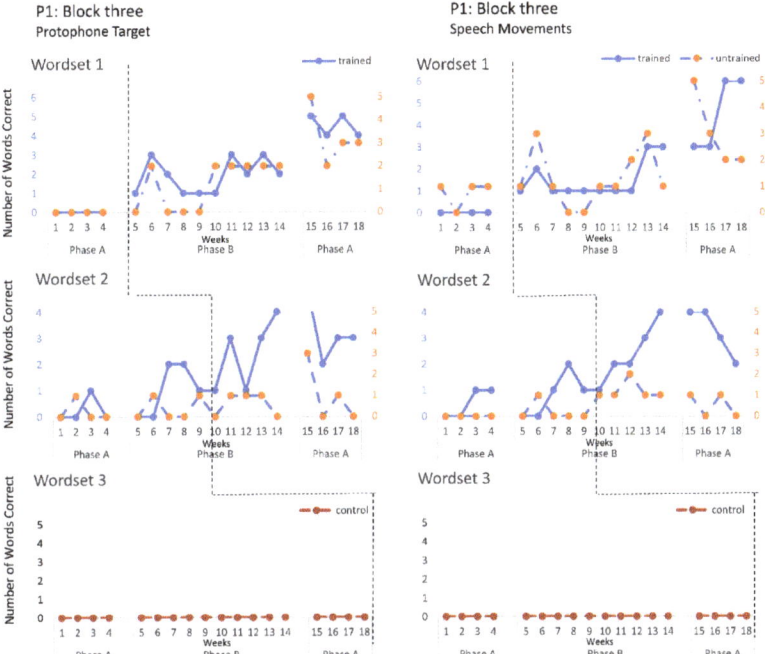

Figure 4. Accuracy of performance on the speech probes as scored for protophone target (**left**) and motor-speech movements (**right**) block three, participant 1.

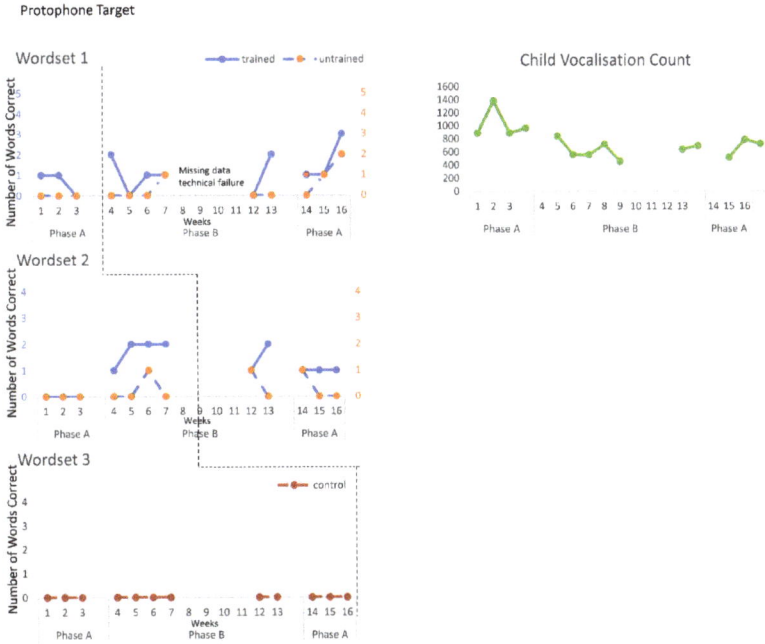

Figure 5. Accuracy of performance on the speech probes as scored for protophone target block one, participant 2 (vocalisation counts obtained from LENA device over same periods as block one).

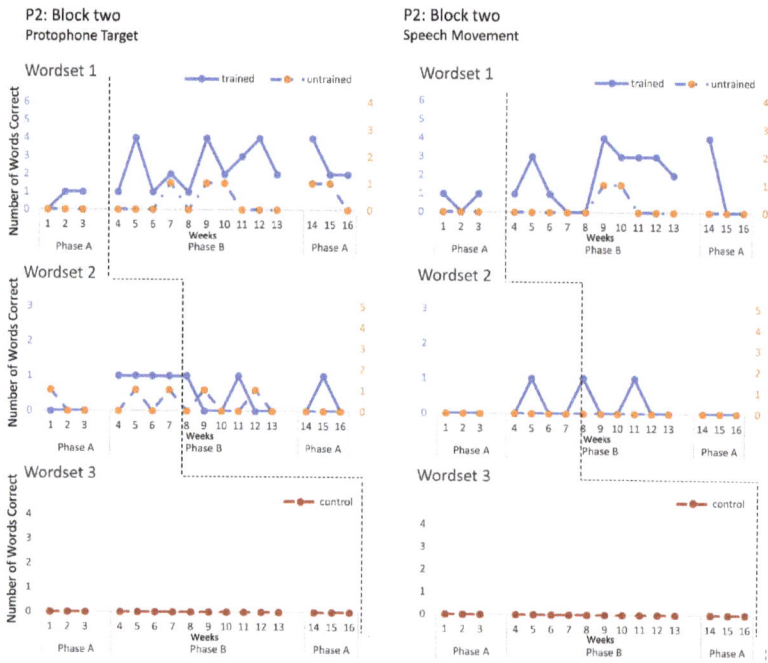

Figure 6. Accuracy of performance on the speech probes as scored for protophone target (**left**) and motor-speech movements (**right**) block two, participant 2.

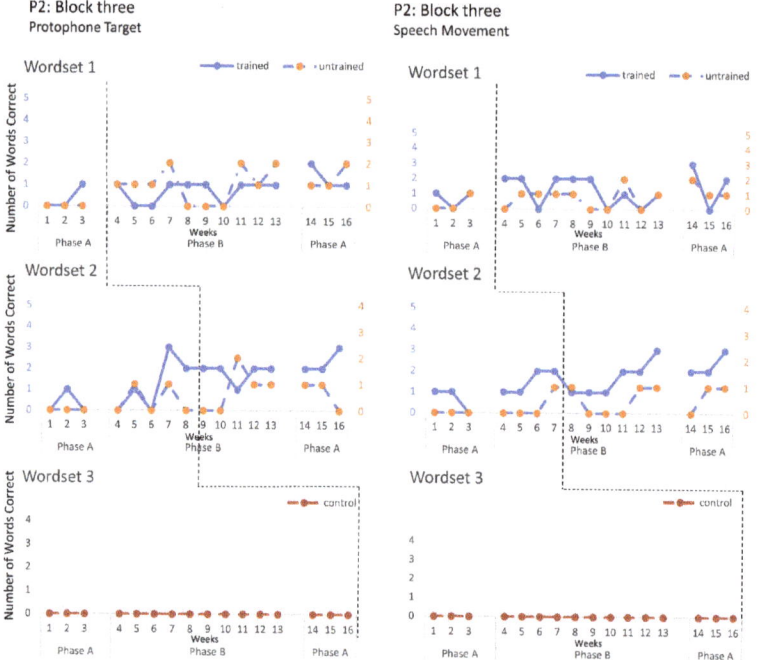

Figure 7. Accuracy of performance on the speech probes as scored for protophone target (**left**) and motor-speech movements (**right**) block three, participant 2.

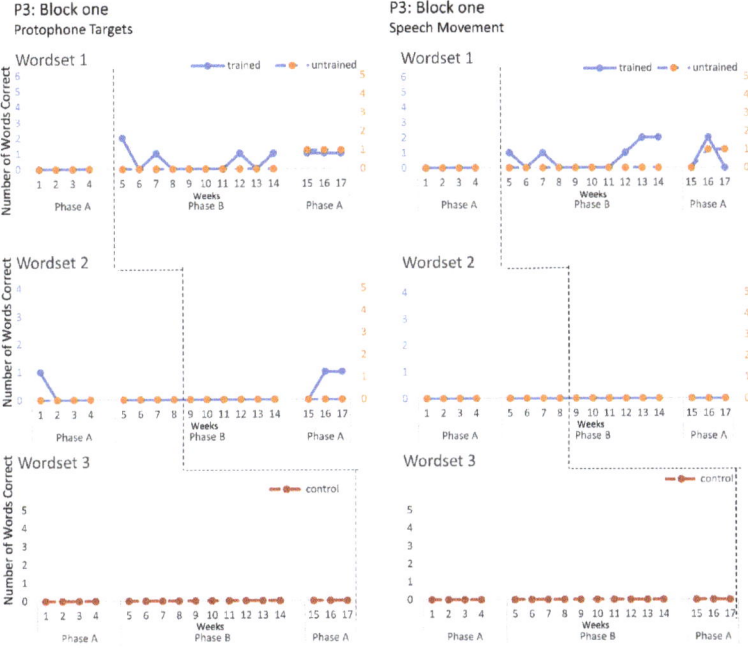

Figure 8. Accuracy of performance on the speech probes as scored for protophone target (**left**) and motor-speech movements (**right**) block one, participant 3.

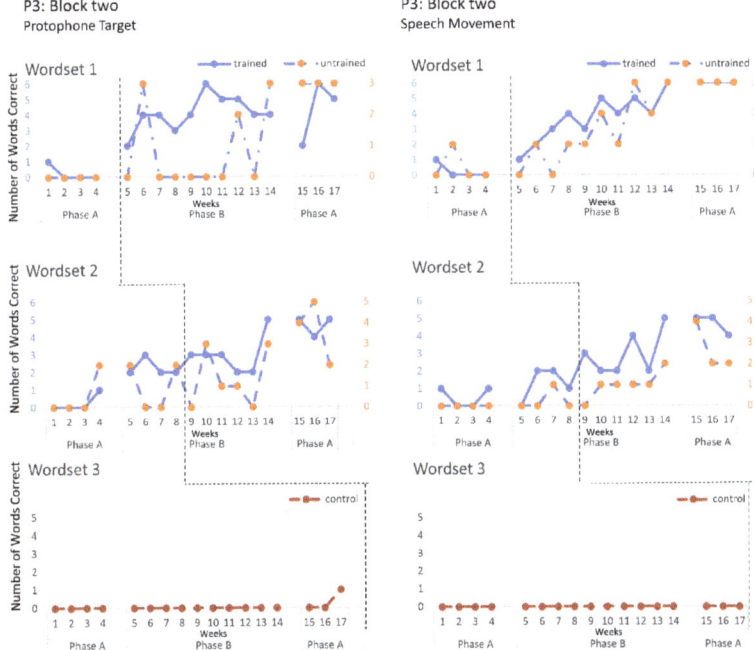

Figure 9. Accuracy of performance on the speech probes as scored for protophone target (**left**) and motor-speech movements (**right**) block two, participant 3.

Table 5. Tau coefficient, z, p values and pre to post mean differences in percent for each word set for protophone scoring across Intervention Blocks.

	Participant 1				Participant 2				Participant 3			
	Tau	z	p	%M_{diff}	Tau	z	p	%M_{diff}	Tau	z	p	%M_{diff}
Word set					Block One							
Word set 1 TR	0.43	1.10	0.272	6.67	0.22	0.52	0.606	20.00	0.40	1.13	0.26	16.67
Word set 1 UT	0.20	0.51	0.612	0.00	0.17	0.39	0.699	20.00	0.00	0.00	1.00	20.00
Word set 2 TR	**0.77**	**1.94**	**0.052**	40.00	**1.00**	**2.32**	**0.020**	25.00	0.00	0.00	1.00	10.42
Word set 2 UT	0.40	1.01	0.311	13.33	0.33	0.77	0.439	8.33	0.10	0.28	0.78	0.00
Word set 3 control	−0.33	−0.85	0.398	−6.67	0.00	0.00	1.000	0.00	0.00	0.00	1.00	0.00
					Block Two							
Word set 1 TR	0.43	1.10	0.272	42.86	**0.80**	**2.03**	**0.043**	33.33	**1.00**	**2.83**	**0.005**	68.06
Word set 1 UT	0.57	1.44	0.151	38.10	0.30	0.76	0.447	16.7	0.30	0.85	0.396	100.0
Word set 2 TR	0.20	0.51	0.612	33.33	0.60	1.52	0.128	11.11	**1.00**	**2.83**	**0.005**	73.61
Word set 2 UT	0.37	0.93	0.353	37.50	0.07	0.17	0.866	−6.67	0.35	0.99	0.322	63.33
Word set 3 control	−0.47	−1.18	0.237	0.00	0.00	0.00	1.000	0.00	0.00	0.00	1.000	6.67
					Block Three							
Word set 1 TR	**1**	**2.83**	**0.016**	75.00	0.37	0.93	0.353	20.00				
Word set 1 UT	**0.60**	**1.70**	**0.090**	65.00	**0.70**	**1.77**	**0.076**	26.67				
Word set 2 TR	**0.68**	**1.91**	**0.056**	75.00	**0.67**	**1.69**	**0.091**	40.00				
Word set 2 UT	0.25	0.71	0.480	15.00	0.50	1.27	0.205	16.67				
Word set 3 control	0.00	0.00	1.000	0.00	0.00	0.00	1.000	0.00				

Note. TR = trained, UT = Untrained. Bold font = statistically significant, p value < 0.1, where Tau was positive.

Table 6. Tau coefficient, z, p values, and pre to post mean difference in percent for each word sets for motor-speech movement patterns, scored across the Intervention Blocks.

	Participant 1				* Participant 2				Participant 3			
	Tau	z	p	%M_{diff}	Tau	z	p	%M_{diff}	Tau	z	p	%M_{diff}
Word set					Block One							
Word set 1 TR	0.60	1.52	0.128	46.67					0.50	1.41	0.157	11.11
Word set 1 UT	−0.17	−0.42	0.673	−4.76					0.00	0.00	1.000	13.33
Word set 2 TR	−0.10	−0.25	0.800	26.67					0.00	0.00	1.000	0.00
Word set 2 UT	0.10	0.25	0.800	6.667					0.00	0.00	1.000	0.00
Word set 3 control	0.00	0.00	1.000	0.00					0.00	0.00	1.000	0.00
					Block Two							
Word set 1 TR	0.60	1.52	0.128	38.1	0.53	1.35	0.176	11.11	**0.98**	**2.76**	**0.006**	70.83
Word set 1 UT	**0.73**	**1.86**	**0.063**	42.86	0.20	0.51	0.612	0.00	**0.65**	**1.84**	**0.066**	66.67
Word set 2 TR	0.53	1.35	0.176	38.1	0.30	0.76	0.447	0.00	**0.80**	**2.26**	**0.024**	50.00
Word set 2 UT	0.03	0.08	0.933	8.333	0.00	0.00	1.000	0.00	**0.60**	**1.70**	**0.090**	40.00
Word set 3 control	0.00	0.00	1.000	5.556	0.00	0.00	1.000	0.00	0.00	0.00	1.000	0.00
					Block Three							
Word set 1 TR	**1**	**2.83**	**0.005**	75.00	0.30	0.76	0.447	20.00				
Word set 1 UT	0.28	0.78	0.437	45.00	0.23	0.59	0.554	20.00				
Word set 2 TR	0.55	1.55	0.120	68.75	**0.73**	**1.86**	**0.063**	33.33				
Word set 2 UT	**0.60**	**1.70**	**0.090**	10.00	0.40	1.01	0.311	16.67				
Word set 3 control	0.00	0.00	1.000	0.00	0.00	0.00	1.000	0.00				

Note. TR = trained, UT = Untrained. Bold font = statistically significant, p value < 0.1, where Tau was positive.
* = Participant 2 block one motor-speech movements were not targeted.

The mean Tau coefficient effect size for trained word set 2 items, also calculated across participants and outcome measures, was 0.51 (SD = 0.36, range −0.1–1.0), a moderate to large effect size, with seven out of 15 coefficients being statistically significant with a large or very large effect size. The pre to post-intervention mean differences in percent averaged 35% (SD = 24.4, range 0.0 to 75) for trained word set 2 items. The correlation between the Tau coefficient and the mean difference for the same items was positive and statistically significant (r = 0.57, p = 0.026, n = 15).

There was some limited evidence of generalisation to untrained items with five out of 30 Tau coefficients, all from either block two or three, being statistically significant with a large or very large effect size. The average mean difference across word set 1 and 2 untrained items was 23% (SD = 25.2, range −6.67–100). No changes were recorded in the control goal for any participant.

P1. In block one, intervention targeted controlled phonation, whilst moving the jaw from closed to open (closant–vocant) and open to closed (vocant–closant) syllable shapes, with target words containing predominantly bilabials. A moderate treatment effect was recorded for the protophone targets and speech movements on trained word set 1. In addition, a large and significant treatment effect was also observed in protophone targets for trained words containing bilabials in word set 2. Block two recorded a moderate treatment effect on trained word set 1 with generalisation to the untrained word set (moderate effect), where intervention targeted the production of protophones requiring open–close (vowel–consonant), close–open (consonant–vowel). Furthermore, a moderate treatment effect was observed on speech movements for the word set 2 trained items, and a significant effect for the untrained word set 2 items, showing the targeted vowels contained rounded and retracted lip movements. Block three recorded the largest treatment effects for protophone targets in word sets 1 and 2 and for speech movement targets in trained word sets 1 for items containing labial-fricatives (e.g., /f/, /v/) and lingual sounds (e.g., /d/, /g/), with large or very large effect sizes. Overall, there was a trend for larger and more consistent effects in block three for P1 compared to block one and two, which indicates a possible cumulative response to intervention.

P2. Treatment effects were observed in the intentional use of vocalisations and target protophones and speech movements across all three intervention blocks. Block one targeted the production of protophone vocalisations with communicative intent, thereby decreasing non-communicative vocalisations. The data for four intervention sessions are missing due to technical failure. Nonetheless, the data show a large treatment effect on word set 2. Furthermore, the child vocalisation count, automatically generated from the LENA DLP, revealed a significant treatment effect, with decreasing vocalisations recorded within the home environment (Tau = −1, z = −2.393, p = 0.017). Block two recorded a moderate treatment effect on speech movement in trained word sets 1 and 2, where the intervention targeted jaw transitions from open-to-closed and closed-to-open; however, performance was variable. These changes in motor-speech control coincided with a large treatment effect in the number of target protophones for word set 1 trained items, with evidence of closant–vocant and vocant–closant productions, not previously sampled with communicative intent. Block three recorded treatment effects consistent with block two (e.g., significant effect for trained items from word set 2 for both protophone and speech movement targets), and showed evidence of generalisation of target protophone production in untrained words (word set 1). Treatment effects were greater for word set 2 than word set 1 for protophone production and speech movement targets, with evidence of CV (i.e., consonant–vowel), VC and CVCV productions, the phonemes /m/, /b/, /d/, /h/ and low vowels (e.g., /a/), for words such as bubble, bye and more.

P3. P3 participated in two intervention blocks. During block one, there was a moderate increase in the production of controlled phonation on single protophones in word set 1, with no controlled phonation evident during baseline. Jaw transitions from closed-to-open and closed-to-open were not produced with communicative intent. These treatment effects were not maintained during post-intervention baseline. In contrast to block one, block two reveals a very large and significant treatment effect on trained word sets 1 and 2, for both protophone and speech movement targets, and large significant effects on word sets

1 and 2 untrained items for speech movement target for CV, VC and CVC words containing bi-labials (/b/, /p/, /m/), alveolars (t/d/ and the velar (/g/). Post intervention data show the treatment effects were maintained for word sets 1 and 2.

4. Discussion

The purpose of this study was to investigate the implementation of an early intervention protocol specifically designed for very young children with communication impairment secondary to CP. Our primary outcome measures focused specifically on (a) increasing the complexity of infant vocalisations produced with communicative intent, and (b) the establishment of motor-speech movements that would support the development of a core oral vocabulary.

Intervention blocks were multi-modal and framed within a Dynamic Systems Theory perspective, that posits increasing complexity arises from the bi-directional interaction of the components of a complex system [37]. Consequently, intervention block one was designed to build social interaction, with tactile input used to build the associate map between perception and speech production for the target vocabulary. Blocks two and three targeted motor-speech control more directly, with intervention priorities based on building subsystem control, as assessed using the MSH. Tactile input was used to shape key speech movement patterns required for the production of the target vocabulary. Our findings are presented with consideration given to the intervention priorities across the intervention blocks.

4.1. Block One: Building the Social Routine and Enriching the Environment

Intervention block one focused on building the social routine and creating activity dependent sensorimotor experiences for the shaping of motor-speech control. Our data show moderate treatment effects were observed in block one for participants 1 and 3 on the trained word set, with limited generalisation to the untrained word set. Treatment effects were not observed for the control word set. These results are consistent with our hypothesis of minimal change during this block, but are encouraging given all participants were pre-linguistic and had yet to establish communicative intent in their vocalisations.

Previous studies show that language learning is dependent on building social routines and parent responsiveness to interactions [36]; with the reciprocity of the interactions contributing to increased vocal complexity [33]. Numerous studies have further demonstrated the effectiveness of training parent–child interactions in children with language impairment [32]. In addition, Pennington et al. [64] have also reported improved parent–child interactions in children with motor impairment following participation in the ITTT Hanen Program®. Accordingly, the increasing complexity of protophone production observed in this intervention block, could be considered a result of the increased responsiveness to the facilitated social feedback loop [65].

However, the fact that parents of participants in this study had all completed the ITTT Hanen Program® as an entry requirement would suggest that the parents already were responsive to their child's communication signals. As such, the therapeutic effect cannot be solely attributed to ongoing parent–child interaction. We postulate the tactile input that was mapped to the target words during the social routines and activities, provided a scaffold on which to build a template for word learning, and primed the child for word production [66]. Whilst the role of tactile input in building an associative map to enhance receptiveness to building oral vocabulary has not been fully explored in very young children, there is increasing evidence to support the role of auditory–tactile input connected with speech articulation [66]. Vihman et al. [67] suggest infants acquire language by the "implicit tallying of repeatedly experienced regularities in sensory input" [67], p. 129, with sound-meaning links more likely to be established when the input is highly familiar.

Furthermore, the literature has also identified that tactile input may reduce cognitive load [68] with haptic guidance enhancing motor learning by developing anticipatory activities and enhancing the "user's presence and cooperation" [69], p. 37. Neurophysiological studies in adults suggest that congruent multi-sensory tactile input reduces ambiguity through cross-modal congruency [70]. It is therefore possible that the auditory–tactile input focused the child's attention to the motor-speech action, making them more meaningful [66]. This warrants further investigation, particularly given the well documented risk of attention and memory deficits in children with CP [71].

We further postulate the experience of input from treatment block one positively influenced what Saffran and Kirkham [72] refer to as "downstream learning". That is, the pre-existing vocal routines established in block one may have provided a "low-cost" communicative environment on which to build more complex vocal productions [72]. Therefore, the multi-dimensional focus of the first intervention block that focused on building routines that promoted turn-taking and the anticipation of the targeted vocabulary, along with the tactile input that linked the cognitive–linguistic input with the targeted output, may have been foundational to building motor-speech control in the subsequent intervention blocks.

4.2. Block Two and Three: Facilitating Motor-Speech Control

All participants continued to demonstrate increased production of target protophones and change in speech movement patterns that reflect increasing protophone complexity, in treatment blocks two and three. There was a trend for larger effect sizes during subsequent intervention blocks compared to treatment block one. This suggests a greater magnitude of treatment effect was observed in the intervention blocks where tactile input was used to shape motor-speech production.

Neurophysiological studies have shown difficulty planning and executing motor end goals experienced by children with CP may arise from impaired neural oscillatory activity in the sensorimotor cortices [73] and altered somatosensory organisation [74]. Speech production and ultimately language learning is a perceptuo-motor experience [75] with the role of the somatosensory input in building complexity through the proprioceptive consequences of the child's own production, gaining increasing attention. For example, Choi et al. [14] identified when the proprioceptive-kinaesthetic information of an infant's vocal tract is constrained, speech perception is disrupted. Conversely, when supplemental multimodal information is provided during active vocal play (e.g., contact of the fingers or an object on the lips), vocal complexity is increased [76]. We, therefore, hypothesise the tactile input assisted participants in acquiring the speech movement representation [40] and this is consistent with the literature supporting the role of augmentative feedback in improving motor learning in children with CP [77].

The contribution of tactile input in inducing therapeutic neuroplasticity has been demonstrated by Fiori et al. [41] in older children presenting with a motor-speech disorder. Whilst based on a small sample size, Fiori et al. [41] provide preliminary data that suggest the coupling of specific sensory information with specific movements can lead to treatment induced neuroplasticity. They identified not only changes in motor-speech control in children with the motor-speech disorder, childhood apraxia of speech, but also identified changes in white matter microstructural properties. The role of tactile input in children, in improving motor-speech control for infants with CP, therefore, warrants further attention.

It is noted that participants responded differently across the study phases, with change in level of performance greater on word set 1 than word set 2 for most participants, thus reflecting the first intervention priority as based on the MSH, in this intervention phase. This may be related to treatment dosage, with the rate of training in word set 1 at times three times more than word set 2. However, this finding is also consistent with the previous findings reported by Ward et al. [38,58] in older children with CP. Their research tested and supported the hypothesis that changes in motor-speech control at one level of the MSH would facilitate changes at the subsequent level of the motor-speech hierarchy as a result of inter-articulator coupling.

Participant data also showed variability within the intervention phases, across the intervention blocks. This is expected and consistent with the literature reporting younger children experience more variability than older children [78]. This is observed not only in the development of language in typically developing infants, with the order and emergence of milestones variable [79,80], but also considered a hallmark of motor development [81], with variability considered the ongoing search for a solution to the motor strategy required.

Our focus on infant vocalisations challenges what Brady et al. [82] has reported to be the prevailing clinical practice of abandoning efforts to increase speech production in children who are at risk of severe communication impairment and likely to be users of augmentative and alternative communication. Increasingly, emphasis is being placed on the potential therapeutic role of targeting infant vocalisations in infants at predicted risk of communication impairment to mitigate the severity of impairment.

It is argued that by supporting oral communication, the very act of practice and effort builds a more robust memory of representation that shapes phonological memory for later language learning [75]. A clear demonstration of the mediating effect of early intervention is evident in the research directed at children born deaf but provided with early access to hearing through cochlear implants. Infants who receive implants at less than 12 months typically progress to first words without delay and continue to perform well on language measures at a later age [83]. In contrast, children who receive implants later than 12 months can show deficits in the acquisition of first words and continue to perform more poorly on language measures.

Similar access to early intervention in the emergence of canonical vocalisations in infants at-risk of CP may mitigate the cascading consequences of underlying impairment to speech motor control. Notably, we found the participants in this study continued to demonstrate improvements in their expressive language skills, as measured on the REEL-3. This contrasts with the findings of Ward et al. [29] who reported a worsening developmental trajectory at 24 months of age. This finding lends further support to our conclusion that the intervention was responsible for bringing about therapeutic change. The findings of this study could therefore be used to inform a larger longitudinal study.

The focus on oral vocalisations for this study was based on a strong research foundation that has identified the critical importance of vocal play in developing later language skills, with the expectation that " ... intervening at the prelinguistic stage may alter a child's trajectory for producing spoken words" [84], p. 203, as well as semantic processing [67]. Oral motor dysfunction affecting speech related movements of the jaw, lips and tongue is high in children with CP [85]. These impairments can have significant functional consequences on speech intelligibility and communication. Thus, if infants at risk of communication impairment associated with CP are afforded the opportunity to experience more complex vocal play, we may ameliorate secondary impairments.

5. Limitations

There are a number of limitations to consider with this study. The highest level of single-subject research design (SSRD) is a randomised n-of-1 design, which may include random assignment of participant to treatment or order of treatment administration, as well as extended baselines when responses are more variable. This standard, whilst desirable, was not able to be met. At the time of this study, two additional multisite research trials were in process within this clinical population and age group. However, we mitigated risks to internal validity through the minimum of three data points per phase, systematic manipulation and assessment of the dependent variables by more than one assessor, and replication with at least three demonstrations of the experimental effect [42,43].

SSRD research requires repeated measures that are standardised, sensitive to change, reliable and valid. Given SSRD has been heralded as a methodology with clinical relevance, outcome measures should also be feasible to administer. The coding of speech probes for this study, however, required phonetic transcription, manual coding of the protophones, and visual-perceptual analysis of speech movements. The analysis was therefore labor intensive, and this potentially limits the clinically feasibility of the intervention.

Furthermore, the outcome measures of this study required the a priori compilation of trained and untrained word sets with equal numbers of items in each word set. However, in response to participant interest and motivation, or the fact that some items did not get trained as intended, some words moved from their assigned word set resulting in a different number of items in the trained and untrained conditions (see Appendix A). A greater number of items within a condition may result in more opportunities to show improvement. This potential bias in effect size from differences in item numbers when comparing the trained and untrained data should be taken into account. However, we do note that the imbalance in item numbers does not systematically favour either the trained or untrained item conditions across participants.

Finally, whilst parents were provided with a LENA device to record the elicitation of the speech probes once per week during intervention block one, and two times per week during intervention blocks two and three, home practice was not monitored to track cumulative treatment intensity.

6. Conclusions

Children with CP are at predictable risk of communication impairment with impaired speech production being the most common form [1–3]. Yet, to date the earliest reported interventions for children with CP is greater than 2 years of age, well after the critical period where infants are primed for learning the basic building blocks required for later language and speech development and perceptual narrowing has already taken place [9,86]. The lack of evidence-based interventions for young infants with communication impairment and neurodevelopmental disability is well recognised [10]. The dearth of research in this space, therefore, places young infants with CP at increased risk of communication impairment. Our data suggest the speech skills of young children with CP can be positively influenced through a multimodal intervention thus capitalising on early periods of plasticity, when language learning is most sensitive.

Author Contributions: R.W. conceptualised the research design; secured financial support for the project; participated in data collection and preparation of the data for analysis as well as interpretation of the data; writing the original manuscript preparation, editing and reviewing subsequent drafts and final revision of the manuscript. E.B. contributed to the data preparation; contributed to scoring the data as a blinded assessor; participated in the preparation and revision of the manuscript. N.H. contributed to the data preparation, analysis and interpretation, contributed to writing the draft manuscript and final review and editing. C.E. contributed to the research design, acquisition of financial support for the project, and final writing review and editing. J.V. contributed to the research design; acquisition of financial support for the project; provided resources including the clinical management of research participants, and final writing review and editing. All authors have read and agreed to the published version of the manuscript.

Funding: This research was funded by the Health Translation Network Early Career Fellowship and the Australian Government's Medical Research Future Fund (MRFF) as part of the Rapid Applied Research Translation program (2019); and Telethon Child and Adolescent Health Allied Health Fellowship (2015).

Institutional Review Board Statement: Approval for this study was obtained from the Child and Adolescent Health Services Ethics Committee (study number 2015221).

Informed Consent Statement: Informed consent was obtained from all participants involved in the study.

Data Availability Statement: The data are not publicly available in accordance with consent provided by participants on the use of confidential data.

Acknowledgments: This research was embedded within the Early Intervention (EI) at-risk of CP Service PCH. Our thanks go to the EI service staff and families. Without their dedication and support this research would not have been possible. Our thanks also go to the speech pathologists who completed the blinded assessments and rating of the speech probes—Taryn Bond and Linda Orton; and Eve Blair for her contribution to the research design.

Conflicts of Interest: The authors declare no conflict of interest.

Appendix A

The word-lists for each participant across the intervention blocks.

P1

Word set 1		Word set 2		Word set 3
Trained	Untrained	Trained	Untrained	Control
Block One				
mama	mine	ball	boom	go
bu(bble)	bang	(peeka)boo	knee	dator (grandpa)
up	arm	more	bow	kaka (brother)
down	done	moo	pooh	push
out	oh oh	bee	pea	eat
	ta			
	Bye [a]			
Block Two				
mine	pan	up	pull	go
yum	bag	pour	bow	dator (grandpa)
hot	hat	me	knee	kaka (brother)
out	arm	do	pooh	push
more	bang	bye	boom	eat
(bar)bie (BBQ)	one	here	pea	door
bubble	nigh nigh	done	two	
Block Three				
four	feet	dinner	allah	icecream
give	phone	mine	amen	marshmallow
sun	horse	dog	soup	hungry
have	knife	off	and	spaghetti
need	bought		sand	yoghurt
done				

[a] A trained item that did not get trained, added to untrained data.

P2

Word set 1		Word set 2		Word set 3
Trained	Untrained	Trained	Untrained	Control
Block One				
up	bu(bble)	more	oh oh	here
ou(t)	mama	moo	poo-ie	down
ah	oh	ball	wee	dada
arm	boat	baa	boo	bang
done	bye			
Block Two				
ou(t)	done	baa	poo (i)	here
ah	oh	mama	oh oh	down
more	bye	moo	boo	dada
bu(bble)	boat		wee (i)	bang
up			Me [a]	
arm [b]				
Block Three				
ball	bowl	out	bird	boat
mama	hat	up	bee	down
open	bye	boo(k)	baby	put
mine	done	more	pull	shoe
dada	apple	bubble		

[a] A trained item that did not get trained, added to untrained data. [b] An untrained item that did get trained, added to trained data.

	P3				
	Word set 1		Word set 2		Word set 3
	Trained	Untrained	Trained	Untrained	Control
Block One	baa	bag	ball	pooh	out
	bubble	paper	go	boo	cat
	under	bye	arm	do	eat
	up	hat	push	bee	dirty
	more	done		me	nose
	moo [c]				
Block Two	more	paper	bubble	pooh	push
	up	bye	out	boo	cat
	arm	baa	bag	do	nose
	ball		me	bee	dirty
	hat [b]		go	moo	eat
	done [b]		under		

[b] An untrained item that did get trained, added to trained data. [c] Moved from word set 2 trained to word set 1 trained.

References

1. Hustad, K.C.; Allison, K.; McFadd, E.; Riehle, K. Speech and language development in 2-year-old children with cerebral palsy. *Dev. Neurorehabilit.* **2013**, *17*, 167–175. [CrossRef]
2. Pennington, L.; Dave, M.; Rudd, J.; Hidecker, M.J.C.; Caynes, K.; Pearce, M.S. Communication disorders in young children with cerebral palsy. *Dev. Med. Child Neurol.* **2020**, *62*, 1161–1169. [CrossRef] [PubMed]
3. Hustad, K.C.; Gorton, K.; Lee, J. Classification of Speech and Language Profiles in 4-Year-Old Children with Cerebral Palsy: A Prospective Preliminary Study. *J. Speech Lang. Heart Res.* **2010**, *53*, 1496–1513. [CrossRef] [PubMed]
4. Hidecker, M.J.C.; Slaughter-Acey, J.; Abeysekara, P.; Ho, N.T.; Dodge, N.; Hurvitz, E.A.; Workinger, M.S.; Kent, R.D.; Rosenbaum, P.; Lenski, M.; et al. Early Predictors and Correlates of Communication Function in Children with Cerebral Palsy. *J. Child Neurol.* **2018**, *33*, 275–285. [CrossRef]
5. Langbecker, D.; Snoswell, C.; Smith, A.; Verboom, J.; Caffery, L. Long-term effects of childhood speech and language disorders: A scoping review. *South Afr. J. Child. Educ.* **2020**, *10*, 13. [CrossRef]
6. Novak, I.; Morgan, C.; Adde, L.; Blackman, J.; Boyd, R.N.; Brunstrom-Hernandez, J.; Cioni, G.; Damiano, D.; Darrah, J.; Eliasson, A.C.; et al. Early, accurate diagnosis and early intervention in cerebral palsy: Advances in diagnosis and treatment. *JAMA Pediatr.* **2017**, *171*, 897–907. [CrossRef] [PubMed]
7. te Velde, A.; Morgan, C.; Novak, I.; Tantsis, E.; Badawi, N. Early Diagnosis and Classification of Cerebral Palsy: An Historical Perspective and Barriers to an Early Diagnosis. *J. Clin. Med.* **2019**, *8*, 1599. [CrossRef] [PubMed]
8. Choi, D.; Black, A.K.; Werker, J.F. Cascading and multisensory influences on speech perception development. *Mind Brain Educ.* **2018**, *12*, 212–223. [CrossRef]
9. Kuhl, P.K. Brain Mechanisms in Early Language Acquisition. *Neuron* **2010**, *67*, 713–727. [CrossRef]
10. Morgan, C.; Fetters, L.; Adde, L.; Badawi, N.; Bancale, A.; Boyd, R.N.; Chorna, O.; Cioni, G.; Damiano, D.L.; Darrah, J.; et al. Early intervention for children aged 0 to 2 years with or at high risk of cerebral palsy: International clinical practice guideline based on systematic reviews. *JAMA Pediatr.* **2021**, *175*, 846–858. [CrossRef]
11. Hustad, K.C.; Sakash, A.; Natzke, P.E.M.; Broman, A.T.; Rathouz, P.J. Longitudinal Growth in Single Word Intelligibility Among Children with Cerebral Palsy From 24 to 96 Months of Age: Predicting Later Outcomes from Early Speech Production. *J. Speech. Lang. Heart Res.* **2019**, *62*, 1599–1613. [CrossRef] [PubMed]
12. Kuhl, P.K. Infant Speech Perception: Integration of Multimodal Data Leads to a New Hypothesis—Sensorimotor Mechanisms Underlie Learning. In *Minnesota Symposia on Child Psychology: Human Communication: Origins, Mechanisms, and Functions*; Wiley Online Library: Hoboken, NJ, USA, 2021; pp. 113–158.
13. Zhao, T.C.; Boorom, O.; Kuhl, P.K.; Gordon, R. Infants' neural speech discrimination predicts individual differences in grammar ability at 6 years of age and their risk of developing speech-language disorders. *Dev. Cogn. Neurosci.* **2021**, *48*, 100949. [CrossRef]
14. Choi, D.; Bruderer, A.G.; Werker, J.F. Sensorimotor influences on speech perception in pre-babbling infants: Replication and extension of Bruderer et al. (2015). *Psychon. Bull. Rev.* **2019**, *26*, 1388–1399. [CrossRef] [PubMed]
15. Marklund, E.; Marklund, U.; Gustavsson, L. An Association Between Phonetic Complexity of Infant Vocalizations and Parent Vowel Hyperarticulation. *Front. Psychol.* **2021**, *12*, 2873. [CrossRef] [PubMed]
16. Best, C.T.; Goldstein, L.M.; Nam, H.; Tyler, M.D. Articulating What Infants Attune to in Native Speech. *Ecol. Psychol.* **2016**, *28*, 216–261. [CrossRef] [PubMed]

17. Goldstein, M.H.; Schwade, J.A.; Bornstein, M.H. The Value of Vocalizing: Five-Month-Old Infants Associate Their Own Noncry Vocalizations with Responses from Caregivers. *Child Dev.* **2009**, *80*, 636–644. [CrossRef]
18. Morgan, L.; Wren, Y.E. A Systematic Review of the Literature on Early Vocalizations and Babbling Patterns in Young Children. *Commun. Disord. Q.* **2018**, *40*, 3–14. [CrossRef]
19. Abney, D.H.; Warlaumont, A.S.; Oller, D.K.; Wallot, S.; Kello, C.T. Multiple Coordination Patterns in Infant and Adult Vocalizations. *Infancy* **2016**, *22*, 514–539. [CrossRef]
20. Oller, D.K.; Ramsay, G.; Bene, E.; Long, H.L.; Griebel, U. Protophones, the precursors to speech, dominate the human infant vocal landscape. *Philos. Trans. R. Soc. B* **2021**, *376*, 20200255. [CrossRef]
21. Nathani, S.; Ertmer, D.J.; Stark, R.E. Assessing vocal development in infants and toddlers. *Clin. Linguist. Phon.* **2006**, *20*, 351–369. [CrossRef]
22. Ramsdell-Hudock, H.L.; Warlaumont, A.S.; Foss, L.E.; Perry, C. Classification of Infant Vocalizations by Untrained Listeners. *J. Speech Lang. Heart Res.* **2019**, *62*, 3265–3275. [CrossRef] [PubMed]
23. Einspieler, C.; Freilinger, M.; Marschik, P.B. Behavioural biomarkers of typical Rett syndrome: Moving towards early identification. *Wien. Med. Wochenschr.* **2016**, *166*, 333–337. [CrossRef] [PubMed]
24. Yankowitz, L.D.; Schultz, R.T.; Parish-Morris, J. Pre- and Paralinguistic Vocal Production in ASD: Birth Through School Age. *Curr. Psychiatry Rep.* **2019**, *21*, 126. [CrossRef]
25. Trembath, D.; Westerveld, M.F.; Teppala, S.; Thirumanickam, A.; Sulek, R.; Rose, V.; Tucker, M.; Paynter, J.; Hetzroni, O.; Keen, D.; et al. Profiles of vocalization change in children with autism receiving early intervention. *Autism Res.* **2019**, *12*, 830–842. [CrossRef] [PubMed]
26. LeJeune, L.M.; Lemons, C.J.; Hokstad, S.; Aldama, R.; Næss, K.-A.B. Parent-Implemented Oral Vocabulary Intervention for Children with Down Syndrome. *Top. Early Child. Spéc. Educ.* **2021**, *42*, 175–188. [CrossRef]
27. Levin, K. Babbling in infants with cerebral palsy. *Clin. Linguist. Phon.* **1999**, *13*, 249–267. [CrossRef]
28. Nyman, A.; Lohmander, A. Babbling in children with neurodevelopmental disability and validity of a simplified way of measuring canonical babbling ratio. *Clin. Linguist. Phon.* **2017**, *32*, 114–127. [CrossRef]
29. Ward, R.; Hennessey, N.; Barty, E.; Elliott, C.; Valentine, J.; Moore, R.C. Clinical utilisation of the Infant Monitor of vocal Production (IMP) for early identification of communication impairment in young infants at-risk of cerebral palsy: A prospective cohort study. *Dev. Neurorehabilit.* **2021**, *25*, 101–114. [CrossRef]
30. Snell, M.E.; Brady, N.; McLean, L.; Ogletree, B.T.; Siegel, E.; Sylvester, L.; Mineo, B.; Paul, D.; Romski, M.A.; Sevcik, R. Twenty Years of Communication Intervention Research with Individuals Who Have Severe Intellectual and Developmental Disabilities. *Am. J. Intellect. Dev. Disabil.* **2010**, *115*, 364–380. [CrossRef]
31. Kaiser, A.P.; Roberts, M. Advances in Early Communication and Language Intervention. *J. Early Interv.* **2011**, *33*, 298–309. [CrossRef]
32. Windsor, K.S.; Woods, J.; Kaiser, A.P.; Snyder, P.; Salisbury, C. Caregiver-Implemented Intervention for Communication and Motor Outcomes for Infants and Toddlers. *Top. Early Child. Spéc. Educ.* **2018**, *39*, 73–87. [CrossRef]
33. Heidlage, J.K.; Cunningham, J.E.; Kaiser, A.P.; Trivette, C.M.; Barton, E.E.; Frey, J.R.; Roberts, M.Y. The effects of parent-implemented language interventions on child linguistic outcomes: A meta-analysis. *Early Child. Res. Q.* **2019**, *50*, 6–23. [CrossRef]
34. Peter, B.; Davis, J.; Finestack, L.; Stoel-Gammon, C.; VanDam, M.; Bruce, L.; Kim, Y.; Eng, L.; Cotter, S.; Landis, E.; et al. Translating principles of precision medicine into speech-language pathology: Clinical trial of a proactive speech and language intervention for infants with classic galactosemia. *Hum. Genet. Genom. Adv.* **2022**, *3*, 100119. [CrossRef] [PubMed]
35. Kaiser, A.P.; Scherer, N.J.; Frey, J.R.; Roberts, M.Y. The Effects of Enhanced Milieu Teaching with Phonological Emphasis on the Speech and Language Skills of Young Children with Cleft Palate: A Pilot Study. *Am. J. Speech-Lang. Pathol.* **2017**, *26*, 806–818. [CrossRef] [PubMed]
36. Ferjan Ramírez, N.; Lytle, S.R.; Kuhl, P.K. Parent coaching increases conversational turns and advances infant language development. *Proc. Natl. Acad. Sci. USA* **2020**, *117*, 3484–3491. [CrossRef]
37. Hayden, D.; Namasivayam, A.K.; Ward, R.; Clark, A.; Eigen, J. The PROMPT Approach. In *Interventions for Speech Sound Disorders in Children*, 2nd ed.; William, A.L., McLeod, S., McCauley, R.J., Eds.; Brookes Publishing: Baltimore, MD, USA, 2020.
38. Ward, R.; Leitão, S.; Strauss, G. An evaluation of the effectiveness of PROMPT therapy in improving speech production accuracy in six children with cerebral palsy. *Int. J. Speech-Lang. Pathol.* **2014**, *16*, 355–371. [CrossRef]
39. Namasivayam, A.K.; Huynh, A.; Bali, R.; Granata, F.; Law, V.; Rampersaud, D.; Hard, J.; Ward, R.; Helms-Park, R.; van Lieshout, P.; et al. Development and Validation of a Probe Word List to Assess Speech Motor Skills in Children. *Am. J. Speech Lang. Pathol.* **2021**, *30*, 622–648. [CrossRef]
40. Dale, P.S.; Hayden, D.A. Treating Speech Subsystems in Childhood Apraxia of Speech with Tactual Input: The PROMPT Approach. *Am. J. Speech Lang. Pathol.* **2013**, *22*, 644–661. [CrossRef]
41. Fiori, S.; Pannek, K.; Podda, I.; Cipriani, P.; Lorenzoni, V.; Franchi, B.; Pasquariello, R.; Guzzetta, A.; Cioni, G.; Chilosi, A. Neural Changes Induced by a Speech Motor Treatment in Childhood Apraxia of Speech: A Case Series. *J. Child Neurol.* **2021**, *36*, 958–967. [CrossRef]
42. Tate, R.L.; Perdices, M.; Rosenkoetter, U.; Shadish, W.; Vohra, S.; Barlow, D.H.; Horner, R.; Kazdin, A.; Kratochwill, T.; McDonald, S.; et al. The Single-Case Reporting Guideline in Behavioural Interventions (SCRIBE) 2016 Statement. *Phys. Ther.* **2016**, *96*, e1–e10. [CrossRef]

43. Kratochwill, T.R.; Hitchcock, J.H.; Horner, R.H.; Levin, J.R.; Odom, S.L.; Rindskopf, D.; Shadish, W.R. Single-Case Intervention Research Design Standards. *Remedial Spéc. Educ.* **2012**, *34*, 26–38. [CrossRef]
44. Romeiser-Logan, L.; Slaughter, R.; Hickman, R. Single-subject research designs in pediatric rehabilitation: A valuable step towards knowledge translation. *Dev. Med. Child Neurol.* **2017**, *59*, 574–580. [CrossRef] [PubMed]
45. Novak, I.; Morgan, C.; McNamara, L.; Velde, A.T. Best practice guidelines for communicating to parents the diagnosis of disability. *Early Hum. Dev.* **2019**, *139*, 104841. [CrossRef] [PubMed]
46. Manolson, A. *It Takes Two to Talk. A parent's Guide to Helping Children Communicate*; Hanen Centre: Toronto, ON, Canada, 1992.
47. Ward, R.; Reynolds, J.E.; Pieterse, B.; Elliott, C.; Boyd, R.; Miller, L. Utilisation of coaching practices in early interventions in children at risk of developmental disability/delay: A systematic review. *Disabil. Rehabil.* **2019**, *42*, 2846–2867. [CrossRef] [PubMed]
48. Davidson, S.-A.; Ward, R.; Elliott, C.; Harris, C.; Bear, N.; Thornton, A.; Salt, A.; Valentine, J. From guidelines to practice: A retrospective clinical cohort study investigating implementation of the early detection guidelines for cerebral palsy in a state-wide early intervention service. *BMJ Open* **2022**, *12*, e063296. [CrossRef]
49. Graham, I.D.; McCutcheon, C.; Kothari, A. Exploring the frontiers of research co-production: The Integrated Knowledge Translation Research Network concept papers. *Health Res. Policy Syst.* **2019**, *17*, 88. [CrossRef]
50. Gilkerson, J.; Richards, J.A.; Greenwood, C.R.; Montgomery, J.K. Language assessment in a snap: Monitoring progress up to 36 months. *Child Lang. Teach. Ther.* **2016**, *33*, 99–115. [CrossRef]
51. Hurford, D.P.; Stutman, G. *The 16th Mental Measurements Yearbook*; The Buros Institute of Mental Measurements: Lincoln, NE, USA, 2004.
52. Rome-Flanders, T. Stability and usefulness of language test results under two years of age Stabilite et fiabilite des resultats de tests linguistiques chez les moins de deux ans. *J. Speech Lang. Pathol. Audiol.* **1998**, *22*, 2.
53. Wetherby, A.M.; Prizant, B.M.; Barry, M. *Communication and Symbolic Behavior Scales*; APA PsycTests: Washington, DC, USA, 2003.
54. Wetherby, A.M.; Goldstein, H.; Cleary, J.; Allen, L.; Kublin, K. Early identification of children with communication disorders: Concurrent and predictive validity of the CSBS Developmental Profile. *Infants Young Child.* **2003**, *16*, 161–174. [CrossRef]
55. McDaniel, J.; Yoder, P.; Estes, A.; Rogers, S.J. Validity of Vocal Communication and Vocal Complexity in Young Children with Autism Spectrum Disorder. *J. Autism Dev. Disord.* **2019**, *50*, 224–237. [CrossRef]
56. Boersma, P.; Weenink, D. Praat: Doing Phonetics by Computer (Version 5.2.34) [Computer software]. 2007. Available online: https://www.fon.hum.uva.nl/praat/ (accessed on 17 November 2022).
57. Namasivayam, A.K.; Huynh, A.; Granata, F.; Law, V.; van Lieshout, P. PROMPT intervention for children with severe speech motor delay: A randomized control trial. *Pediatr. Res.* **2020**, *89*, 613–621. [CrossRef] [PubMed]
58. Ward, R.; Strauss, G.; Leitão, S. Kinematic changes in jaw and lip control of children with cerebral palsy following participation in a motor-speech (PROMPT) intervention. *Int. J. Speech-Lang. Pathol.* **2012**, *15*, 136–155. [CrossRef] [PubMed]
59. Hayden, D.; Namasivayam, A.K.; Ward, R. The assessment of fidelity in a motor speech-treatment approach. *Speech Lang. Heart* **2014**, *18*, 30–38. [CrossRef] [PubMed]
60. Choi, D.; Dehaene-Lambertz, G.; Peña, M.; Werker, J.F. Neural indicators of articulator-specific sensorimotor influences on infant speech perception. *Proc. Natl. Acad. Sci. USA* **2021**, *118*, e2025043118. [CrossRef]
61. Warren, S.F.; Fey, M.E.; Yoder, P.J. Differential treatment intensity research: A missing link to creating optimally effective communication interventions. *Ment. Retard. Dev. Disabil. Res. Rev.* **2007**, *13*, 70–77. [CrossRef]
62. Parker, R.I.; Vannest, K.J.; Davis, J.L.; Sauber, S.B. Combining Nonoverlap and Trend for Single-Case Research: Tau-U. *Behav. Ther.* **2011**, *42*, 284–299. [CrossRef]
63. Vannest, K.J.; Ninci, J. Evaluating Intervention Effects in Single-Case Research Designs. *J. Couns. Dev.* **2015**, *93*, 403–411. [CrossRef]
64. Pennington, L.; Thomson, K.; James, P.; Martin, L.; McNally, R. Effects of It Takes Two to Talk—The Hanen Program for Parents of Preschool Children with Cerebral Palsy: Findings from an Exploratory Study. *J. Speech Lang. Heart Res.* **2009**, *52*, 1121–1138. [CrossRef]
65. Tenenbaum, E.J.; Carpenter, K.L.; Sabatos-DeVito, M.; Hashemi, J.; Vermeer, S.; Sapiro, G.; Dawson, G. A six-minute measure of vocalizations in toddlers with autism spectrum disorder. *Autism Res.* **2020**, *13*, 1373–1382. [CrossRef]
66. Shen, G.; Meltzoff, A.N.; Marshall, P.J. Touching lips and hearing fingers: Effector-specific congruency between tactile and auditory stimulation modulates N1 amplitude and alpha desynchronization. *Exp. Brain Res.* **2017**, *236*, 13–29. [CrossRef]
67. Vihman, M.M.; DePaolis, R.A.; Keren-Portnoy, T. The Role of Production in Infant Word Learning. *Lang. Learn.* **2014**, *64*, 121–140. [CrossRef]
68. Shams, L.; Seitz, A.R. Benefits of multisensory learning. *Trends Cogn. Sci.* **2008**, *12*, 411–417. [CrossRef] [PubMed]
69. Sigrist, R.; Rauter, G.; Riener, R.; Wolf, P. Augmented visual, auditory, haptic, and multimodal feedback in motor learning: A review. *Psychon. Bull. Rev.* **2012**, *20*, 21–53. [CrossRef] [PubMed]
70. Riecke, L.; Snipes, S.; van Bree, S.; Kaas, A.; Hausfeld, L. Audio-tactile enhancement of cortical speech-envelope tracking. *Neuroimage* **2019**, *202*, 116134. [CrossRef]
71. Stadskleiv, K.; Jahnsen, R.; Andersen, G.L.; von Tetzchner, S. Neuropsychological profiles of children with cerebral palsy. *Dev. Neurorehabilit.* **2017**, *21*, 108–120. [CrossRef]
72. Saffran, J.R.; Kirkham, N.Z. Infant statistical learning. *Annu. Rev. Psychol.* **2018**, *69*, 181. [CrossRef]

73. Kurz, M.J.; Becker, K.M.; Heinrichs-Graham, E.; Wilson, T.W. Neurophysiological abnormalities in the sensorimotor cortices during the motor planning and movement execution stages of children with cerebral palsy. *Dev. Med. Child Neurol.* **2014**, *56*, 1072–1077. [CrossRef]
74. Papadelis, C.; Butler, E.E.; Rubenstein, M.; Sun, L.; Zollei, L.; Nimec, D.; Snyder, B.; Grant, P.E. Reorganization of the somatosensory cortex in hemiplegic cerebral palsy associated with impaired sensory tracts. *NeuroImage Clin.* **2017**, *17*, 198–212. [CrossRef]
75. Vihman, M.M.; DePaolis, R.A.; Keren-Portnoy, T.; Allen, S.; Bryant, J.B.; Behrens, H.; Berman, R.A.; Clark, E.V.; Crain, S.; Curtin, S.; et al. *A Dynamic Systems Approach to Babbling and Words*; Cambridge University Press: Cambridge, UK, 2012; pp. 163–182. [CrossRef]
76. Zuccarini, M.; Guarini, A.; Savini, S.; Iverson, J.M.; Aureli, T.; Alessandroni, R.; Faldella, G.; Sansavini, A. Object exploration in extremely preterm infants between 6 and 9 months and relation to cognitive and language development at 24 months. *Res. Dev. Disabil.* **2017**, *68*, 140–152. [CrossRef]
77. Schoenmaker, J.; Houdijk, H.; Steenbergen, B.; Reinders-Messelink, H.A.; Schoemaker, M.M. Effectiveness of different extrinsic feedback forms on motor learning in children with cerebral palsy: A systematic review. *Disabil. Rehabil.* **2022**, 1–14. [CrossRef]
78. Cheng, M.; Anderson, M.; Levac, D.E. Performance Variability During Motor Learning of a New Balance Task in a Non-immersive Virtual Environment in Children with Hemiplegic Cerebral Palsy and Typically Developing Peers. *Front. Neurol.* **2021**, *279*, 12. [CrossRef] [PubMed]
79. To, C.K.S.; McLeod, S.; Sam, K.L.; Law, T. Predicting Which Children Will Normalize Without Intervention for Speech Sound Disorders. *J. Speech Lang. Heart Res.* **2022**, *65*, 1724–1741. [CrossRef] [PubMed]
80. Fernald, A.E.; Marchman, V.A. Causes and Consequences of Variability in Early Language Learning. In *Experience, Variation and Generalization: Learning a First Language.*; John Benjamins Publishing Company: Amsterdam, The Netherlands, 2011; pp. 181–202. [CrossRef]
81. Adolph, K.E.; Cole, W.G.; Vereijken, B. Intraindividual Variability in the Development of Motor Skills in Childhood. In *Handbook of Intraindividual Variability Across the Life Span*; Routledge: London, UK, 2014; pp. 79–103.
82. Brady, N.C.; Storkel, H.L.; Bushnell, P.; Barker, R.M.; Saunders, K.; Daniels, D.; Fleming, K. Investigating a Multimodal Intervention for Children with Limited Expressive Vocabularies Associated with Autism. *Am. J. Speech-Lang. Pathol.* **2015**, *24*, 438–459. [CrossRef] [PubMed]
83. Nicholas, J.G.; Geers, A.E. Spoken Language Benefits of Extending Cochlear Implant Candidacy Below 12 Months of Age. *Otol. Neurotol.* **2013**, *34*, 532–538. [CrossRef] [PubMed]
84. McDaniel, J.; Slaboch, K.D.; Yoder, P. A meta-analysis of the association between vocalizations and expressive language in children with autism spectrum disorder. *Res. Dev. Disabil.* **2017**, *72*, 202–213. [CrossRef] [PubMed]
85. Mei, C.; Fern, B.; Reilly, S.; Hodgson, M.; Reddihough, D.; Mensah, F.; Morgan, A. Communication behaviours of children with cerebral palsy who are minimally verbal. *Child Care Health Dev.* **2020**, *46*, 617–626. [CrossRef]
86. Werker, J.; Hensch, T. Critical periods in speech perception: New directions. *Annu. Rev. Psychol.* **2015**, *66*, 173–196. [CrossRef]

Disclaimer/Publisher's Note: The statements, opinions and data contained in all publications are solely those of the individual author(s) and contributor(s) and not of MDPI and/or the editor(s). MDPI and/or the editor(s) disclaim responsibility for any injury to people or property resulting from any ideas, methods, instructions or products referred to in the content.

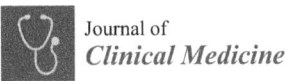

Article

Parental Coping, Representations, and Interactions with Their Infants at High Risk of Cerebral Palsy

Silja Berg Kårstad [1,2,*], Åse Bjørseth [1], Johanna Lindstedt [3], Anne Synnøve Brenne [1], Helene Steihaug [2] and Ann-Kristin Gunnes Elvrum [4,5,6]

1. Regional Centre for Child and Youth Mental Health and Child Welfare (RKBU Central Norway), Department of Mental Health, Faculty of Medicine and Health Sciences, Norwegian University of Science and Technology, 7130 Trondheim, Norway
2. Child and Adolescent Mental Health Services, St. Olav's Hospital, Trondheim University Hospital, 7130 Trondheim, Norway
3. Department of Psychology and Speech-Language Pathology, University of Turku, 20500 Turku, Finland
4. Department of Neuromedicine and Movement Science, Faculty of Medicine and Health Sciences, Norwegian University of Science and Technology, 7130 Trondheim, Norway
5. Department of Clinical and Molecular Medicine, Faculty of Medicine and Health Sciences, Norwegian University of Science and Technology, 7130 Trondheim, Norway
6. Clinical Services, St. Olav's Hospital, Trondheim University Hospital, 7130 Trondheim, Norway
* Correspondence: silja.b.karstad@ntnu.no; Tel.: +47-9775-2958

Abstract: The aim of this study is to describe parental coping, representations, and interactions during the time of inclusion in the Small Step early intervention program for infants at high risk of cerebral palsy (CP) in Norway (ClinicalTrials.gov: NCT03264339). Altogether, 11 infants (mean age 4.8 months, SD: 1.5) and their parents (mothers: n = 10, fathers: n = 9) were included. Parental coping was assessed using the Parenting Stress Index-Short Form (PSI-SF) and the Hospital Anxiety and Depression Scale (HADS). Parental representations and parent–infant interactions were assessed using the Working Model of the Child Interview (WMCI) and the Parent–Child Early Relational Assessment (PCERA). Parents' PSI-SF and HADS scores were within normal range; however, 26.7% showed symptoms of stress, 52.6% showed symptoms of anxiety, and 31.6% showed symptoms of depression above the cut-off. WMCI results indicate that 73.7% of the parents had balanced representations. For PCERA, the subscale Dyadic Mutuality and Reciprocity was of concern, while two other subscales were in areas of strength and three subscales in some concern areas. There were no differences between mothers and fathers. Most of the parents had balanced representations, some had mental or stress symptoms and many were struggling with aspects of the parent–infant interaction. This knowledge could be useful when developing more family-centered interventions.

Keywords: CP; infant; stress; anxiety; depression; parents; fathers; parent–infant interaction; representations

Citation: Kårstad, S.B.; Bjørseth, Å.; Lindstedt, J.; Brenne, A.S.; Steihaug, H.; Elvrum, A.-K.G. Parental Coping, Representations, and Interactions with Their Infants at High Risk of Cerebral Palsy. *J. Clin. Med.* **2023**, *12*, 277. https://doi.org/10.3390/jcm12010277

Academic Editor: Umberto Aguglia

Received: 18 November 2022
Revised: 16 December 2022
Accepted: 27 December 2022
Published: 29 December 2022

Copyright: © 2023 by the authors. Licensee MDPI, Basel, Switzerland. This article is an open access article distributed under the terms and conditions of the Creative Commons Attribution (CC BY) license (https://creativecommons.org/licenses/by/4.0/).

1. Introduction

Cerebral palsy (CP) results from a lesion or maldevelopment in the immature brain and is the most common severe motor disability in childhood [1]. The motor disorder is frequently accompanied by disturbances of cognition, communication, and epilepsy [2]. The birth prevalence varies from 1.4 to 2.5 per 1000 live births in high-income countries and is even higher in low- to middle-income countries [3–7]. About half of all infants with CP have identifiable risk factors in the newborn period, such as prematurity, low birthweight for gestational age, genetic abnormalities, or encephalopathy [8]. New guidelines recommend diagnosing high risk of CP at 4 to 6 months so that interventions can start as early as possible [8,9]. Recent research is focusing on habilitation services that provide more accurate knowledge about the psychological needs of parents and their infants at high risk of CP in order to develop more family-centered habilitative interventions [10,11].

Becoming a parent can be a stressful experience that demands great responsibility for the newborn child and can cause concerns about their development and health [12–17]. However, when risk of brain damage occurs during pregnancy, labor, or shortly after birth, parents are substantially more prone to experiencing high levels of stress [18–20], which might lead to the development of mental health problems such as depression and anxiety [21–23]. Parents of infants at high risk of disease are often hospitalized with their newborn, and it may be traumatic to witness their infant experience various medical procedures and assessments [24]. Worries for potential sequala or diagnosis may put an additional strain on parents [25]. Studies of older children with CP have found that mothers experience more stress than fathers [26], while the experience of stress among mothers and father of infants diagnosed with a high risk of CP is largely unknown.

Parents of children and adolescents with CP are found to have an increased risk for mental health problems. This has been proposed in a systematic review [23], which indicates that symptoms of depression and anxiety are more prevalent in parents of children with CP compared to healthy controls. The results from this review suggest that the severity of a child's condition and the time required to care for the child are risk factors for developing mental health problems. Another review reveals that parental coping ranges from parents who do not perceive their child's disabilities as stressful, to parents who report negative stress and describe their lives as challenging [26]. Thus far, few studies have described parental coping at the time when their infant is diagnosed with a high risk of CP, yet most of these studies include mothers. One recent study from Sweden describes that almost one-third of mothers with an infant at high risk of CP scored above the cut-off value for symptoms of anxiety and depression [27]. This percentage exceeds what has been reported in population-based studies without any known risk factors, showing a prevalence of 15% for postnatal anxiety symptoms for mothers [13] and 7% for fathers [28], as well as 11.9% for depression during the perinatal period for mothers [29] and 3–5% for fathers [30,31]. There is a need to investigate further the anxiety and depression rates in mothers and fathers of infants with a high risk of CP to gain knowledge regarding potential risks for mental health problems.

Parents' relationship with their infants may also be at risk when parents experience stress and worries concerning their infants' health [32–35]. Typically, the development of a parent–infant relationship begins before the infant is born through the parents' mental representations of themselves, combined with their thoughts and feelings about the unborn child [36–38]. Parental representations assessed with the Working Model of the Child Interview (WMCI) are classified into the global categories: balanced, disengaged, or distorted [39]. It has been found that in clinical populations of infants and toddlers at risk, or with a diagnosis, most parents' representations were disengaged (34.2%) and distorted (43.6%) [32]. To our knowledge, no studies have assessed parents' mental representations at the time their infant was given the diagnosis at high risk of CP. Some studies have found more balanced representations in mothers of full-term infants compared to mothers of pre-term infants using the WMCI [35,40], while other studies indicated no differences [33,41]. Furthermore, a few studies have found a relationship between non-balanced representations in mothers and higher levels of depression both in clinical and non-clinical samples [33,34]. Getting to know more about parents' representations of their infant at high risk of CP may help professionals set up suitable support and interventions adjusted to the needs of the families [42].

Despite the knowledge that fathers spend much time with their infants, few studies have focused on the father–infant relationship. A recent longitudinal study of fathers with typical developing infants showed that higher levels of sensitivity, and lower levels of withdrawal behaviors were more often observed in fathers with balanced compared to unbalanced prenatal representations [38]. In another longitudinal study of fathers of typical developing infants, they found that early attachment representations of the infant predicted the quality of future father–infant interaction [43]. Similar findings have been found with mothers showing positive relationship between balanced representations and better quality of infant-mother interaction [44,45]. Since there are few studies including both genders, the present study will describe the representations of both mothers and fathers of infants at high risk of CP and investigate if there are any differences.

The quality of parent–infant interactions contribute to an infant's cognitive, emotional, and social development [46,47]. Previous studies have investigated parent–infant interactions when the infant is at risk of different conditions [45,48–53], and for parents with, or at risk of, mental health problems [54–57]. In a recent review of the parent–infant interaction of infants at risk of CP compared to healthy populations, it was found that infants at risk were generally less active and showed fewer facial expressions. Furthermore, mothers were more intrusive, and parent–infant dyads were described as less synchronized, with fewer sensitive responses [48]. However, the studies included in that systematic review did not use the new, recommended guidelines for setting a diagnosis with a high risk of CP [8]. Rather, prematurity was used as the main inclusion criteria to indicate high risk in several studies; only one study included fathers, and they found no differences between the interaction qualities of mothers and fathers [58]. Thus, there is an urgent need for studies that investigate the early dyadic interaction between parents and their infant who is diagnosed with a high risk of CP. The present study aims to (1) describe parental coping, parental representations, and parent–infant interaction during inclusion in the Small Step early intervention program for infants at high risk of CP (i.e., when the infant is between 4 and 6 months old), and (2) assess if there are differences between mothers and fathers in coping, representations, and the quality of parent-infant interaction.

2. Materials and Methods

2.1. Design

This study is part of the Small Step early intervention study performed at St. Olavs hospital, Trondheim, Norway from September 2017 to July 2020 (ClinicalTrials.gov: NCT03264339). The study was performed in collaboration with the researchers who developed the Small Step early intervention program at the Karolinska Institute, Sweden [27,59]. In the Small Step study, a single subject research design was used, with each participant serving as his/her own control through multiple testing at baseline and during intervention and withdrawal periods [60]. In the current study, data collected through the baseline period were applied. The Small Step study was approved by the Regional Ethical Committee (REC) for Medical Research in Mid-Norway (2016/1366).

2.2. Participants

Eligible participants were families with an infant diagnosed with CP, or at high risk of CP, at the regular clinical follow-up at three months corrected age for infants with known complications before, during or shortly after birth. The guidelines for setting the diagnosis with a high risk of CP were used, i.e., assessment of general movements (GMs), neonatal magnetic resonance imaging (MRI), and neurological assessment with Hammersmith Infant Neurological Examination (HINE) [8]. In addition, motor development was assessed using the Alberta Infant Motor Scale (AIMS) [61].

2.3. Procedurals

During the baseline period, parental coping, parental representations, and parent-infant interactions were assessed once for each parent. In addition, the infants were tested at three time-points with various motor tests that are outside the scope of the current study. The testing took place either in the family's home or at the hospital.

Parental coping was measured with the Parenting Stress Index-Short Form third edition (PSI-SF) [62]. The PSI-SF is a 36-item, self-report measure of parenting stress where parents rate items on a 5-point scale. The PSI-SF includes a Total Stress scale and three subscales: Parental Distress, Parent–Child Dysfunctional Interaction and Difficult Child. In the present study, we used the Total Stress scale. The Total Stress scale ranges from 36 to 180 and is seen as an indicator of a parent's overall experience of parenting stress. The 90th percentile of the PSI-SF score represents a "clinically significant" level of parenting stress and can be used as an indicator that counseling or other support is required. The PSI-SF demonstrates high internal consistency, test–retest reliability, and validity [63–65].

In addition, we used the Hospital Anxiety and Depression Scale (HADS) to investigate parental coping [66]. The HADS consists of 14 questions, seven measure symptoms of anxiety and seven measure symptoms of depression. Each question has four answer categories ranging from zero to three, where category three indicates the highest level of the symptom. The HADS is divided into a scale for anxiety (HADS-A) and a scale for depression (HADS-D), with scores ranging from 0 to 21. Scores between 0 and 7 are within the normal range, while scores between 8 and 10 indicate mild symptoms, scores between 11 and 14 indicate moderate symptoms, and scores between 15 and 21 indicate severe symptoms. The HADS has been shown to have a good factor structure, discriminant validity and internal consistency [67,68].

Parental representations of their infant were assessed with the Working Model of the Child Interview (WMCI) [39]. The WMCI is a semi-structured interview where caregivers are asked about their subjective experiences and perceptions of their child, parenting and their relationship with the child. The caregiver's narratives are classified into six qualitative scales (i.e., Richness of Perceptions, Openness to Change, Intensity of Involvement, Coherence, Caregiving Sensitivity, and Acceptance). High scores in the qualitative scales indicate positive parental narrative qualities, except for the scale of Intensity of Involvement, where a score of 3 is the most optimal. The WMCI also includes two content scales (i.e., Infant Difficulty and Fear for Safety), where high scores represent negative parental narrative content. In addition, the caregiver's affective tone of the representations is coded, identifying how much joy, pride, anger, disappointment, anxiety, guilt, indifference, or other emotions were expressed throughout the interview. Parents' representations were classified into three main categories (balanced, disengaged or distorted). The two latter categories can be classified as non-balanced representations. The WMCI has good psychometric properties, and the reliability of the clinical scales is found to be satisfactory in a Norwegian sample of infants [32,69]. The WMCI interviews lasted approximately 30–90 min and were videotaped and scored by certified coders not involved in the intervention study. The main coder (A.S.B) scored all the 19 interviews using a 5-point Likert scale and another certified coder (Å.B) scored six interviews (30%). They agreed upon the main categories in 4 of the 6 interviews corresponding to an interrater agreement of 0.67. The two interviews that were coded differently were discussed and consensus was made by the two coders on both categorical and scale levels. Thus, the main coder's scorings were used for 17 of the interviews and the consensus scores for two interviews.

Parent–infant interactions were assessed during five minutes of videotaped free play using the Parent–Child Early Relational Assessment (PCERA) [70]. The PCERA is widely used in the Nordic countries as an observation method that measures the quality of affect and behavior in parent–infant interactions and it is shown to have acceptable psychometric properties [38,50,51,54,71]. The videos were recorded either in the family's home or at the hospital. The parents were filmed with their infants on separate occasions. The parents received the following instruction: "Play with your infant as you normally do. You can use the toys if you like or play without the toys". The PCERA free play situations were rated according to the manual [70] by two trained coders. The complete PCERA consists of 65 independent items. In the present study, 60 PC-ERA items were rated since some of the items are not ratable for infants under 6–9 months. The main coder (A.-K.G.E.) rated all video recordings, and 20% of the videos were double rated by another certified coder (J.L.). To retain interrater agreement, drift sessions between coders were held throughout the assessment process. All PCERA items were rated on a five-point Likert scale. The coders considered the frequency, duration, and intensity of the behaviors when rating each item. After rating all the videos, the coders decided that the item "mirroring" had to be removed, since five parents used their native language in the play situation. Thus, it was difficult to score "mirroring", i.e., parent's attunements with their child's emotional state, including consideration of parents labeling of their infants' internal feeling state. Before the interrater agreement calculation, all items were recoded into a three-point scale describing areas of concern (scores 1 and 2), areas of some concern (score 3) and areas of strength (scores 4 and 5), as conducted in previous studies [38,50,54]. The interrater agreement was calculated by the mean percentile of the raters' overall agreement. The interrater agreement between the two coders was 0.80, which is considered acceptable [72]. Before analyzing the data, 52 items were combined into 6 subscales using the five-point scale according to the "4 Month feeding factors" described in the PCERA manual [70]: (1) Parent Positive Affective Involvement, Sensitivity, and Responsiveness; (2) Parent Negative Affect and Behavior; (3) Infant Positive Affect, Communicative and Social Skills; (4) Infant Dysregulation and Irritability; (5) Dyadic Mutuality and Reciprocity; and (6) Dyadic Tension. High PCERA scores indicate positive affect or/and behavior; therefore, high scores on subscales 2, 4, and 6 indicate a lack of negative affect and/or behavior. In this study, Cronbach's α coefficients for calculating the internal consistency of the six PCERA subscales ranged between excellent and acceptable [73]: 0.95 (subscale 1), 0.89 (subscale 2), 0.85 (subscale 3), 0.90 (subscale 4), 0.83 (subscale 5), and 0.78 (subscale 6).

2.4. Statistical Analysis

We used the IBM SPSS statistics 27 program to analyze the data [74]. Descriptive statistics with means, standard deviations, confidence intervals and percentages were used to present the data. The variables were normally distributed according to Q–Q plots and we used a paired-sample t test to compare means between mothers' and fathers' coping scores, qualitative and content WMCI scores, and the PCERA subscales. An alpha level of 0.05 was used to determine statistical significance.

3. Results

3.1. Sample Characteristics

Altogether, 19 parents (10 mothers and 9 fathers) of 11 infants from ten families consented to participate in the Small Step early intervention study. Two more families were invited, however one family declined due to long travels, and the other family could not be included because of the involvement from the child protective service. All 11 infants had a clinical history indicating a risk for CP. Four of the infants were born premature. Among these, three were twins and one was born extremely premature because of placental abruption. One of the infants born at term had microcephaly, two had difficult births causing asphyxia, and four had various complications within the first ten days after birth. At the regular clinical hospital follow-up at three months corrected age, the infants had the following high-risk factors for CP: absent ($n = 6$) or sporadic ($n = 5$) fidgety GMs, suboptimal HINE scores < 57 ($n = 10$), abnormal MRI ($n = 11$), and delayed motor gross motor skills, as indicated by AIMS scores at or below the fifth percentile ($n = 6$) or between the fifth and tenth percentile ($n = 5$).

The baseline testing was performed during three timepoints between two and six weeks after the time of diagnosis, except for one infant where summer holidays delayed the baseline testing (age at first baseline: 5.7 months) and another infant where hospital stays prolonged the baseline period till 10 weeks. See Table 1 describing parent and infant characteristics. About 2/3 of the parents had university degrees, equally distributed between mothers ($n = 6$) and fathers ($n = 6$). Five of the parents were not native Norwegians; therefore, three of the WMCI interviews were conducted in English, and two with an interpreter.

Table 1. Sample characteristics parents ($n = 19$) and infants ($n = 11$).

Characteristics Parents	Total $n = 19$	Mothers $n = 10$	Fathers $n = 9$
Language (*n*)			
Norwegian	10	7	7
Other *	5	3	2
Mean age in years (min-max)	34 (25–57) [2]	32 (25–42) [1]	36 (28–57) [1]
Highest degree (*n*)			
Upper secondary school	3	3	0
Vocational training	4	2	2
Bachelor's degree	7	4	3
Master's or doctoral degree	5	2	3
Characteristics infants	**Total $n = 11$**		
Gender: Female/Male (*n*)	4/7		
Gestational age			
Mean gestational age: weeks (range; ± SD)	35.6 (24.6–41.4; ± 5.3)		
Term/preterm (*n*)	7/4		
Risk factors for cerebral palsy (*n*)			
GMs: absent/sporadic fidgety movements	6/5		
HINE scores: suboptimal < 57/normal	10/1		
MRI: abnormal	11		
AIMS: ≤ 5th percentile/5th - 10th percentile	6/5		
Additional impairments (*n*)			
Epilepsy	2		
Cortical visual impairment	2		
Hearing impairment	2		
Hydrocephalus, shunt	2		
Nasogastric intubation	2		
Bronchopulmonary dysplasia	1		
Corrected age at baseline			
Mean age baseline 1: months (range; ± SD)	4.2 (3.5–6.7; ± 0.9)		
Mean age baseline 2: months (range; ± SD)	4.8 (4.0–7.2; ± 0.8)		
Mean age baseline 3: months (range; ± SD)	5.3 (4.5–7.7; ± 0.9)		
Family (*n*)			
Living with both parents: Yes/No	9/2		
Number of siblings: 0/1/2/3	1/8/1/1		

Note: *n* = number, * = English as second language, min = minimum, max = maximum, [2] = age missing for $n = 2$; [1] = age missing for $n = 1$; SD = Standard Deviation, GMs = General Movements, HINE = Hammersmith Infant Neurological Examination, MRI = Magnetic Resonance Imaging, AIMS = Alberta Infant Motor Scale.

3.2. Parental Coping

The PSI-SF was completed by 17 of the 19 parents, and two forms were excluded because of missing scores. For four forms the score for one item was missing and imputation was done according to the manual [62]. For two forms there were missing scores for three and five items, respectively, and we decided to exclude these forms. The results for the remaining 15 parents indicate that the parents' mean stress scores were within normal range; however, $\frac{1}{4}$ showed stress above normal range in the clinically area. There was no significant difference between mothers' and fathers' mean stress scores. Parents' mean anxiety and depression scores measured with the HADS were within normal range, although as shown in Table 2, almost half of the parents (52.6%) scored above cut-off for anxiety (from score 8) and 31.6% showed depression symptoms. Mothers' mean scores for anxiety and depression were higher than fathers' mean scores, but these differences were not significant.

Table 2. Percent and mean scores of the Parenting Stress Index-Short Form third edition (PSI-SF) and the Hospital Anxiety and Depression Scale (HADS) for the group and for the mothers and fathers.

Variable	Percentages (n)	Mean (SD)	95% CI
Parenting stress			
PSI-SF total [1]	100 (15)	77.4 (26.5)	61.7–93.5
Fathers		78.0 (27.6)	56.9–99.1
Mothers		76.5 (27.5)	47.5–105.5
Low level [2]	26.7 (4)		
Normal level [2]	46.6 (7)		
High level [2]	0		
Clinically [2]	26.7 (4)		
Anxiety (HADS-A) [3]			
Total	100 (19)	7.5 (4.9)	4.0–9.7
Fathers		6.2 (4.6)	2.7–9.8
Mothers		8.6 (5.1)	4.9–12.3
Normal	47.4 (9)		
Borderline	15.8 (3)		
Abnormal	36.8 (7)		
Depression (HADS-D) [3]			
Total	100 (19)	5.3 (4.2)	2.4–7.5
Fathers		3.8 (3.3)	1.3–6.3
Mothers		6.7 (4.5)	3.5–9.9
Normal	68.4 (13)		
Borderline	15.8 (3)		
Abnormal	15.8 (3)		

Note: SD = Standard deviation. CI = Confidence interval. n = number. [1] PSI-SF = Parenting Stress Index-Short Form. [2] PSI-SF Total scores: 36–55 = low stress, 56–85 normal stress, 86–90 = high stress and above 90 = clinically significant stress level. [3] Anxiety and Depression total scores: 0–7 = Normal, 8–10 = Borderline, and 11–21 = Abnormal. HADS = Hospital Anxiety and Depression Scale, D = depression and A = anxiety.

3.3. Parental Representations

The results from the WMCI interviews indicate that, at the categorical level, 73.7% (n = 14) of parents' representations were balanced, 21.1% (n = 4) were disengaged, and 5.2% (n = 1) were distorted. The mean scores for the eight WMCI scales are shown in Table 3.

As a group, all means for the qualitative and content scales shown in Table 3 are within the non-concerned range. Counting the frequency of the individual parents' mean scores on the eight scales reveals that 0–15.8% were in the concerned range on the qualitative scales and 5.3–10.6% on the content scales. Furthermore, the following affective contents of the representations during the interview were most common: joy (*mean* = 3.0, SD = 1.1), pride (*mean* = 3.3, SD = 1.3) and sadness/sorrow (*mean* = 4.1, SD = 2.2). We found no significant differences between mothers' and fathers' mean scores on the qualitative or content scales with independent *t*-tests.

Table 3. Mean scores of the Qualitative and Content Scales of the Working Model of the Child Interview (WMCI) measuring parents' representations of their infants for the group and for the mothers and fathers.

WMCI	n	Mean (SD)	95% CI
Qualitative Scales			
Richness of Perceptions	19	3.7 (1.0)	3.2–4.1
Fathers	8	3.9 (0.4)	2.9–4.8
Mothers	11	3.6 (0.3)	2.9–4.2
Openness to Change	19	3.7 (1.0)	3.3–4.2
Fathers	8	4.0 (0.3)	3.2–4.8
Mothers	11	3.6 (0.3)	2.9–4.2
Intensity of Involvement	19	3.6 (1.1)	3.1–4.1
Fathers	8	3.9 (0.4)	2.9–4.8
Mothers	11	3.5 (0.3)	2.8–4.1
Coherence	19	4.0 (0.9)	3.5–4.4
Fathers	8	4.1 (0.3)	3.4–4.8
Mothers	11	3.8 (0.3)	3.2–4.4
Caregiving Sensitivity	19	3.9 (0.9)	3.5–4.3
Fathers	8	4.1 (0.2)	3.6–4.7
Mothers	11	3.7 (0.3)	3.1–4.4
Acceptance	19	3.8 (1.0)	3.4–4.3
Fathers	8	3.9 (0.4)	3.1–4.7
Mothers	11	3.8 (0.3)	3.1–4.5
Content Scales			
Infant Difficulty	19	2.4 (1.1)	1.8–2.9
Father	8	2.5 (0.3)	1.7–3.3
Mother	11	2.3 (0.4)	1.4–3.1
Fear for the Infant's Safety	19	2.7 (0.9)	2.3–3.1
Father	8	2.5 (0.3)	1.9–3.1
Mother	11	2.8 (0.3)	2.2–3.5

Note: SD = Standard deviation. CI = Confidence interval. n = number. High scores in the qualitative scales indicate positive parental narrative qualities, except for the scale of Intensity of Involvement, where a score of 3 is the most optimal. The two content scales (i.e., Infant Difficulty and Fear for Safety) high scores represent negative parental narrative content.

3.4. Parent–Infant Interaction

The mean scores for the PCERA subscales are presented in Table 4. The high mean scores on parental subscales 2 (Negative Affect and Behavior) and infant subscale 4 (Dysregulation and Irritability) indicate strength areas in parent–infant interactions, suggesting low levels of negative affect both in parents and infants. For the parent subscale 1 (Positive Affective Involvement, Sensitivity and Responsiveness), infant subscale 3 (Positive Affect, Communicative and Social Skills) and parent–infant subscale 6 (Dyadic Tension), mean scores indicate areas of some concern, while the mean score for parent–infant subscale 5 (Dyadic Mutuality and Reciprocity) indicates an area of concern.

Figure 1 shows the six subscales with a percentage distribution for the three PCERA categories. As seen in the figure, most of the parents were in the "some concern" area on subscales 1, 3, 5 and 6, and the concern area was highest in subscales 1 and 5.

To describe the parent–infant interactions in more detail, we report in Table 5 the items that showed mean scores above four in the strengths area (16 of 52 items) and items that had mean scores below three (6 of 52 items), indicating items of concern. High item scores indicate positive affect or/and behavior or a lack of negative affect and/or behavior.

Table 4. The Parent–Child Early Relational Assessment subscales mean scores measuring the parent–infant interactions for the group and for mothers and fathers.

Subscales	n	Mean (SD)	95% CI
Parental Positive Affective Involvement, Sensitivity and Responsiveness	19	3.5 (0.5)	3.2–3.7
Fathers	8	3.3 (0.2)	2.9–3.8
Mothers	11	3.6 (0.1)	3.3–3.9
Parental Negative Affect and Behavior	19	4.0 (0.4)	3.7–4.1
Fathers	8	3.8 (0.2)	3.5–4.2
Mothers	11	4.1 (0.1)	3.8–4.3
Infant Positive Affect, Communicative and Social Skills	19	3.3 (0.5)	2.9–3.5
Fathers	8	3.4 (0.2)	3.0–3.8
Mothers	11	3.2 (0.1)	2.9–3.5
Infant Dysregulation and Irritability	19	4.1 (0.4)	3.8–4.2
Fathers	8	4.1 (0.1)	3.9–4.3
Mothers	11	4.0 (0.1)	3.7–4.3
Dyadic Mutuality and Reciprocity	19	2.9 (0.6)	2.5–3.2
Fathers	8	3.0 (0.3)	2.4–3.6
Mothers	11	2.9 (0.1)	2.5–3.2
Dyadic Tension	19	3.5 (0.5)	3.2–3.7
Fathers	8	3.5 (0.2)	3.1–4.0
Mothers	11	3.5 (0.2)	3.2–3.9

Note: SD = Standard deviation. CI = Confidence interval. n = number. Scores 1 and 2 describes areas of concern, score 3 means areas of some concern and scores 4 and 5 are areas of strength.

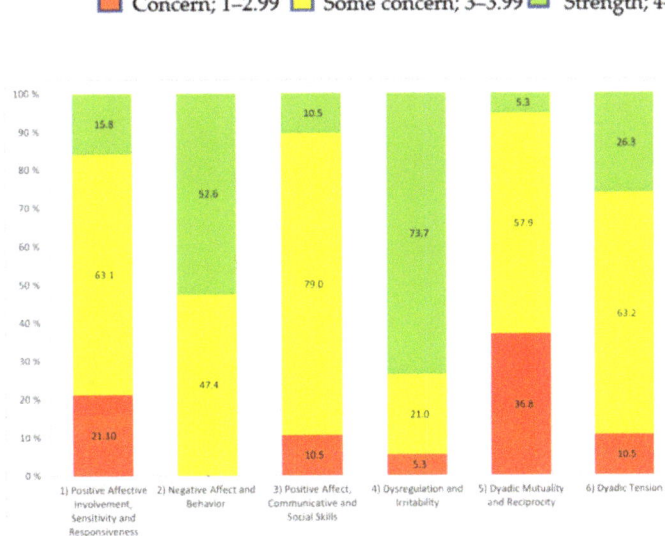

Figure 1. The six subscales with percentages in the three Parent–Child Early Relational Assessment categories: concern, some concern, and strengths.

Table 5. The Parent–Child Early Relational Assessment items mean scores in the strength and concern area.

Items	n	Mean (SD)	95% CI
Parental items strength area			
Annoyed, Angry, Hostile Tone of Voice	19	4.9 (0.3)	4.7–5.1
Warm, Kind Tone of Voice	19	4.2 (0.7)	3.8–4.5
Expressed Negative Affect	19	4.4 (0.6)	4.1–4.7
Irritable/Frustrated/Angry Mood	19	4.9 (0.2)	4.8–5.1
Depressed Mood	19	4.2 (0.8)	3.8–4.6
Displeasure, Disapproval, Criticism	19	4.6 (0.5)	4.3–4.8
Negative Physical Contact	19	4.4 (0.7)	4.0–4.7
Amount of Visual Contact with Child	19	4.4 (0.5)	4.1–4.6
Responsivity to Child's Negative or Unresponsive behavior	19	4.3 (0.6)	4.0–4.6
Infant items strength area			
Apathetic, Withdrawn, Depressed Mood	19	4.0 (0.7)	3.7–4.3
Irritable/Frustrated/Angry Mood	19	4.2 (0.5)	4.0–4.5
Emotion Lability	19	4.9 (0.2)	4.8–5.1
Robustness	19	4.3 (0.6)	4.0–4.6
Consolability/Soothability	19	4.6 (0.7)	4.1–5.1
Dyad items strength area			
Frustrated, Angry, Hostile	19	4.5 (0.5)	4.2–4.7
Tension, Anxiety	19	4.0 (0.7)	3.6–4.4
Parent items concern area			
Amount of Verbalization	19	2.8 (0.8)	2.4–3.6
Infant items concern area			
Social Behavior of Infant-Initiates	19	2.9 (0.9)	2.5–3.4
Quality of Exploratory Play	19	2.8 (1.0)	2.3–3.3
Communicative Competence	19	2.7 (0.6)	2.4–3.0
Dyadic items concern area			
Mutual Enthusiasm, Joyfulness, Enjoyment, Dyadic "Joie de Vivre"	19	2.8 (0.7)	2.5–3.1
Reciprocity	19	2.7 (0.7)	2.4–3.0

Note: SD = Standard deviation. CI = Confidence interval. n = number.

We found no significant differences between mothers' and fathers' mean parent–infant interaction subscale scores.

4. Discussion

Our results indicate that parents' mean stress, anxiety and depression symptoms were within normal range. However, some parents reported symptoms of stress (26.7%), anxiety (52.6%, including both borderline and abnormal scores) and depression (31.6%, including both borderline and abnormal scores) above normal level. Parents' representations of their infant were primarily balanced (73.7%), and there were low levels of negative affect in both parents and infants. However, there were some concerns regarding parents' affective involvement, sensitivity, and responsiveness towards their infants, as well as the infants' communicative and social competence. This may have affected the parent–infant dyad, causing some tension between the infant and the parent, and decreasing dyadic mutuality and reciprocity. We found no significant differences between mothers and fathers in coping, representations, and the quality of parent-infant interaction.

There was a large variation in reported stress levels and symptoms of anxiety and depression among the parents in our study. For most of the parents, feelings of stress, anxiety, or depression were within normal levels. Additionally, we found no differences between mothers' and fathers' levels of stress, anxiety, and depression symptoms. Knowing that all the included infants had a history of complications before, during, or shortly after birth, and that they had recently received the diagnosis at high risk of CP, may indicate that there are factors beyond birth-related trauma and receiving a diagnosis that affected coping in this group of parents. This is in accordance with a review that demonstrated great differences in how parents deal with having a child with CP [26]. Some parents may have protective factors such as being in a stable relationship and having a supportive family that makes them more resilient to traumatic experiences and more able to cope with stress and trauma [26,75]. Furthermore, the relatively high educational level among the parents in the current study might be a protective factor [26]. Nonetheless, about one quarter of the included parents had stress symptoms in clinical areas, and symptoms of anxiety and depression were similar or higher than in comparable populations [27] and much higher than reported in populations without any known risk factors [13,28–31]. This indicates that it is important to assess the levels of stress, anxiety, and depression in parents of infants at risk of CP and to promote potential protective factors to increase parental coping [75].

According to parental representations, assessed with the WMCI, the percentage of balanced representations (73.7%) in this study was higher than for parents of prematurely born infants (20–55%) [35,40,50] and for parents of low- to moderate-risk infants in Norway (58.3%) [69]. One possible explanation for these differences may be a lower number of parents in the present study compared to previous studies [33,35,40]. Another explanation might be that nearly half of the infants in the current study ($n = 4$) were born at full term after non-complicated pregnancies. It is possible that the parents of these infants had already developed balanced representations during pregnancy, and research has shown that these representations are often quite stable [37]. Additionally, there were no differences between the mothers' and fathers' representations. This may indicate that mothers and fathers develop similar patterns of thoughts and feelings towards their relationship with their infant at high risk of CP, however this finding needs to be replicated with studies with larger number of participants.

In this study, the parents displayed little, or no displeasure, annoyance, frustration, or anger towards their infant, and the infants were easily soothed by their parents. This is considered an interactive strength and may suggest that having an infant at high risk of CP does not increase the risk of physical abuse [76]. Nonetheless, the decreased mutuality and reciprocity of the interaction was of concern, with low mean scores for turn taking, mutual enthusiasm, joyfulness, and enjoyment. This could be due to several infants having decreased communicative skills, with reduced or delayed responses to social initiatives made by the parents. Similar results have been found in other studies, indicating that reduced communicative abilities affect the parent–infant dyad [34,48]. Motor impairments and the reduced quality of the exploratory play could place additional limitations on playfulness and enjoyment in the interaction. Our results also indicate some concerns when it comes to the parents' sensitivity and responsiveness towards their infant. Previous studies reported that mothers of infants at risk of CP were less sensitive and demonstrated less smiling compared to mothers of healthy controls [48,49,77]. Few studies have investigated the dyad between fathers and infants, but one study from Finland investigated this for fathers of typically developing infants during their first months of life [38]. In this Finnish study, similar patterns to those in our study for areas of strengths and concerns were identified, except with less dyadic tension in the parent–infant dyad for fathers of typically developing infants. In our study, we did not find any differences between the scores for mothers and fathers. Thus, it seems that the concerns identified in our study may be related to having an infant at high risk of CP and not related to the fact that we included both mothers and fathers.

Overall, our results indicate that there may be both protective and risk factors in our sample of parents of infants at high risk of CP. Most of the parents had balanced representations, and stress, anxiety, and depression symptoms were within normal range. However, some parents experienced mental health problems or stress above normal level, and many struggled with aspects of parent–infant interactions. Thus, our results underscore the need for assessments, preventive strategies, and interventions, not only focusing on the infants, but also targeting parents' stress levels, mental health, and interactions with their infant.

One of the strengths of this study was the use of diverse assessments, such as self-report questionaries, interviews, and observations, to illuminate parental coping, representations, and interactions with their infants at high risk of CP. This provides a broader understanding of the psychological challenges parents may encounter when having an infant at high risk of CP and how this may affect parent–infant relationships. Secondly, our sample included fathers, which are seldom studied in research on postnatal mental health, and even more lacking in studies of infants at risk [26,31]. Recent research shows that some fathers have mental health problems regarding the parenting of healthy babies [28,31,78]; therefore, it is important to understand more about fathers of infants at high risk of CP. The health system in Norway continues to mainly assess mothers' mental health on a regular basis, so we need increased attention to the fact that fathers also may struggle. Finally, our study included infants at very high risk of CP according to recent diagnostic guidelines [8]. Most previous studies included premature infants, with unknown additional risks for CP.

Our study also has some limitations. We only recorded parent–infant interactions during play activities using the PCERA. It would have been preferrable to include recordings of an additional situation, for example feeding or diaper changing. However, it was necessary to reduce the number of assessments to avoid fatigue for both the infants and the parents. Furthermore, in some of the parent-infant situations the other parent was present, in addition to the one who was filming. It is possible that this affected the behavior of the parent being filmed, however there was no interaction between the parents, and the other parent was in another section of the room. Additionally, we did not double code all the WMCI videotapes because double coding all instruments was time-consuming and expensive. This could possibly have strengthened the presentation of the level of interrater reliability. Finally, the cross-sectional design used in this study precludes any causal implications, and because of the low number of participants, we cannot generalize our findings. Thus, our findings need to be further investigated in a larger sample, including both mothers and fathers of infants at high risk of CP. In addition, we need more longitudinal studies following infants and parents over an extended period to describe the trajectories of their mental health and quality of interactions.

Author Contributions: Conceptualization, S.B.K., Å.B., J.L., A.S.B., H.S. and A.-K.G.E.; methodology, S.B.K., J.L. and A.-K.G.E.; formal analysis, S.B.K. and A.-K.G.E.; investigation, S.B.K., Å.B., J.L., A.S.B., H.S. and A.-K.G.E. resources, S.B.K. and A.-K.G.E.; data curation, S.B.K. and A.-K.G.E.; writing—original draft preparation, S.B.K., Å.B., J.L., A.S.B. and A.-K.G.E.; writing—review and editing, S.B.K., Å.B., J.L., A.S.B., H.S. and A.-K.G.E.; visualization, S.B.K. and A.-K.G.E.; project administration, A.-K.G.E.; funding acquisition, A.-K.G.E. All authors have read and agreed to the published version of the manuscript.

Funding: This research was funded by "Samarbeidsorganet" between the Central Norway Regional Health Authority and the Norwegian University of Science and Technology (NTNU) in Trondheim, Norway, grant number 90056100 and 46055600-102/153.

Institutional Review Board Statement: The study was conducted in accordance with the Declaration of Helsinki and approved by the Regional Ethical Committee (REC) for Medical Research in Mid-Norway (2016/1366) for studies involving humans.

Informed Consent Statement: Informed consent was obtained from all parents involved in the study.

Data Availability Statement: The data presented in this study are available on request from the corresponding author. The data are not publicly available due to ethical restrictions.

Acknowledgments: We thank the children and their families who participated in this research. In addition, we want to acknowledge collaborators in the Small Step single subject research design study at the Karolinska Institute, Stockholm, Sweden, and at St. Olavs hospital, Trondheim, Norway.

Conflicts of Interest: The authors declare no conflict of interest. The funders had no role in the design of the study; in the collection, analyses, or interpretation of data; in the writing of the manuscript, or in the decision to publish the results.

References

1. Korzeniewski, S.J.; Slaughter, J.; Lenski, M.; Haak, P.; Paneth, N. The complex aetiology of cerebral palsy. *Nat. Rev. Neurol.* **2018**, *14*, 528–543. [CrossRef] [PubMed]
2. Rosenbaum, P.; Paneth, N.; Leviton, A.; Goldstein, M.; Bax, M. A report: The definition and classification of cerebral palsy-April 2006. *Dev. Med. Child Neurol.* **2007**, *49*, 8–14. [CrossRef]
3. Sellier, E.; Platt, M.J.; Andersen, G.L.; Krageloh-Mann, I.; De La Cruz, J.; Cans, C.; Networ, S.C.P. Decreasing prevalence in cerebral palsy: A multi-site European population-based study, 1980 to 2003. *Dev. Med. Child Neurol.* **2016**, *58*, 85–92. [CrossRef] [PubMed]
4. Galea, C.; McIntyre, S.; Smithers-Sheedy, H.; Reid, S.M.; Gibson, C.; Delacy, M.; Watson, L.; Goldsmith, S.; Badawi, N.; Blair, E.; et al. Cerebral palsy trends in Australia (1995–2009): A population-based observational study. *Dev. Med. Child Neurol.* **2019**, *61*, 186–193. [CrossRef] [PubMed]
5. Bufteac, E.G.; Andersen, G.L.; Torstein, V.; Jahnsen, R. Cerebral palsy in Moldova: Subtypes, severity and associated impairments. *BMC Pediatr.* **2018**, *18*, 332. [CrossRef]
6. Kakooza-Mwesige, A.; Andrews, C.; Peterson, S.; Mangen, F.W.; Eliasson, A.C.; Forssberg, H. Prevalence of cerebral palsy in Uganda: A population-based study. *Lancet Glob. Health* **2017**, *5*, E1275–E1282. [CrossRef] [PubMed]
7. McIntyre, S.; Goldsmith, S.; Webb, A.; Ehlinger, V.; Hollung, S.J.; McConnell, K.; Arnaud, C.; Smithers-Sheedy, H.; Oskoui, M.; Khandaker, G.; et al. Global prevalence of cerebral palsy: A systematic analysis. *Dev. Med. Child Neurol.* **2022**, *64*, 1494–1506. [CrossRef]
8. Novak, I.; Morgan, C.; Adde, L. Early, accurate diagnosis and early intervention in cerebral palsy: Advances in diagnosis and treatment. *JAMA Pediatr* **2017**, *171*, 897–907. [CrossRef]
9. Morgan, C.; Fetters, L.; Adde, L.; Badawi, N.; Bancale, A.; Boyd, R.N.; Chorna, O.; Cioni, G.; Damiano, D.L.; Darrah, J.; et al. Early Intervention for Children Aged 0 to 2 Years With or at High Risk of Cerebral Palsy International Clinical Practice Guideline Based on Systematic Reviews. *JAMA Pediatr* **2021**, *175*, 846–858. [CrossRef]
10. Aydin, R.; Nur, H. Family-centered approach in the management of children with cerebral palsy. *Turkiye Fiz. Tip Ve Rehabil. Derg.* **2012**, *58*, 229–235. [CrossRef]
11. King, S.; Teplicky, R.; King, G.; Rosenbaum, P. Family-Centered Service for Children With Cerebral Palsy and Their Families: A Review of the Literature. *Semin. Pediatr. Neurol.* **2004**, *11*, 78–86. [CrossRef] [PubMed]
12. Eberhard-Gran, M.; Engelsen, L.Y.; Al-Zirqi, I.; Vangen, S. Depressive symptoms and experiences of birthing mothers during COVID-19 pandemic. *Tidsskr. Nor. Laegeforen.* **2022**, *142*, 1–9. [CrossRef]
13. Dennis, C.-L.; Falah-Hassani, K.; Shiri, R. Prevalence of antenatal and postnatal anxiety: Systematic review and meta-analysis. *Br. J. Psychiatry* **2017**, *210*, 315–323. [CrossRef]
14. Sørbø, M.F.; Grimstad, H.; Bjørngaard, J.H.; Lukasse, M.; Schei, B. Adult physical, sexual, and emotional abuse and postpartum depression, a population based, prospective study of 53,065 women in the Norwegian Mother and Child Cohort Study. *BMC Pregnancy Childbirth* **2014**, *14*, 316. [CrossRef]
15. Condon, J.T.; Boyce, P.; Corkindale, C.J. The First-Time Fathers Study: A prospective study of the mental health and wellbeing of men during the transition to parenthood. *Aust. N. Z. J. Psychiatry* **2004**, *38*, 56–64. [CrossRef] [PubMed]
16. Skjothaug, T.; Smith, L.; Wentzel-Larsen, T.; Moe, V. Prospective fathers' adverse childhood experiences, pregnancy-related anxiety, and depression during pregnancy. *Infant Ment Health J.* **2015**, *36*, 104–113. [CrossRef] [PubMed]
17. Paulson, J.F.; Bazemore, S.D. Prenatal and postpartum depression in fathers and its association with maternal depression: A meta-analysis. *JAMA* **2010**, *303*, 1961–1969. [CrossRef]
18. Pinquart, M. Parenting stress in caregivers of children with chronic physical condition-A meta-analysis. *Stress Health* **2018**, *34*, 197–207. [CrossRef]
19. Wang, H.-Y.; Jong, Y.-J. Parental Stress and Related Factors in Parents of Children with Cerebral Palsy. *Kaohsiung J. Med. Sci.* **2004**, *20*, 334–340. [CrossRef]
20. Ketelaar, M.; Volman, M.J.M.; Gorter, J.W.; Vermeer, A. Stress in parents of children with cerebral palsy: What sources of stress are we talking about? *Child Care Hlth Dev* **2008**, *34*, 825–829. [CrossRef]
21. Gugala, B.; Penar-Zadarko, B.; Pieciak-Kotlarz, D.; Wardak, K.; Lewicka-Chomont, A.; Futyma-Ziaja, M.; Opara, J. Assessment of Anxiety and Depression in Polish Primary Parental Caregivers of Children with Cerebral Palsy Compared to a Control Group, as well as Identification of Selected Predictors. *Int. J. Environ. Res. Public Health* **2019**, *16*, 4173. [CrossRef] [PubMed]
22. Cheshire, A.; Barlow, J.H.; Powell, L.A. The psychosocial well-being of parents of children with cerebral palsy: A comparison study. *Disabil. Rehabil.* **2010**, *32*, 1673–1677. [CrossRef] [PubMed]
23. Barreto, T.M.; Bento, M.N.; Barreto, T.M.; Jagersbacher, J.G.; Jones, N.S.; Lucena, R.; Bandeira, I.D. Prevalence of depression, anxiety, and substance-related disorders in parents of children with cerebral palsy: A systematic review. *Dev. Med. Child Neurol.* **2020**, *62*, 163–168. [CrossRef] [PubMed]
24. Obeidat, H.M.; Bond, E.A.; Callister, L.C. The parental experience of having an infant in the newborn intensive care unit. *J. Perinat. Educ.* **2009**, *18*, 23–29. [CrossRef]

25. Cousino, M.K.; Hazen, R.A. Parenting Stress Among Caregivers of Children With Chronic Illness: A Systematic Review. *J. Pediatr. Psychol.* **2013**, *38*, 809–828. [CrossRef]
26. Rentinck, I.C.M.; Ketelaar, M.; Jongmans, M.J.; Gorter, J.W. Parents of children with cerebral palsy: A review of factors related to the process of adaptation. *Child Care Health Dev.* **2007**, *33*, 161–169. [CrossRef]
27. Holmstrom, L.; Eliasson, A.C.; Almeida, R.; Furmark, C.; Weiland, A.L.; Tedroff, K.; Lowing, K. Efficacy of the Small Step Program in a Randomized Controlled Trial for Infants under 12 Months Old at Risk of Cerebral Palsy (CP) and Other Neurological Disorders. *J. Clin. Med.* **2019**, *8*, 1016. [CrossRef]
28. Bradley, R.; Slade, P.; Leviston, A. Low rates of PTSD in men attending childbirth: A preliminary study. *Br. J. Clin. Psychol.* **2008**, *47*, 295–302. [CrossRef]
29. Woody, C.A.; Ferrari, A.J.; Siskind, D.J.; Whiteford, H.A.; Harris, M.G. A systematic review and meta-regression of the prevalence and incidence of perinatal depression. *J. Affect. Disord.* **2017**, *219*, 86–92. [CrossRef]
30. Bronte-Tinkew, J.; Moore, K.A.; Matthews, G.; Carrano, J. Symptoms of Major Depression in a Sample of Fathers of Infants: Sociodemographic Correlates and Links to Father Involvement. *J. Fam. Issues* **2007**, *28*, 61–99. [CrossRef]
31. Madsen, S.A.; Juhl, T. Paternal depression in the postnatal period assessed with traditional and male depression scales. *J. Men's Health Gend.* **2007**, *4*, 26–31. [CrossRef]
32. Vreeswijk, C.; Maas, A.; van Bakel, H.J.A. Parental representations: A systematic review of the working model of the child interview. *Infant Ment. Health J.* **2012**, *33*, 314–328. [CrossRef] [PubMed]
33. Korja, R.; Savonlahti, E.; Haataja, L.; Lapinleimu, H.; Manninen, H.; Piha, J.; Lehtonen, L. Attachment representations in mothers of preterm infants. *Infant Behav. Dev.* **2009**, *32*, 305–311. [CrossRef]
34. Minde, K.; Tidmarsh, L.; Hughes, S. Nurses' and physicians' assessment of mother-infant mental health at the first postnatal visits. *J. Am. Acad. Child Adolesc. Psychiatry* **2001**, *40*, 803–810. [CrossRef] [PubMed]
35. Borghini, A.; Pierrehumbert, B.; Miljkovitch, R.; Muller-Nix, C.; Forcada-Guex, M.; Ansermet, F. Mother's attachment representations of their premature infant at 6 and 18 months after birth. *Infant Ment. Health J.* **2006**, *27*, 494–508. [CrossRef] [PubMed]
36. Ahlqvist-Bjorkroth, S.; Korja, R.; Junttila, N.; Savonlahti, E.; Pajulo, M.; Raiha, H.; Aromaa, M.; Grp, S.S. Mothers' and Fathers' Prenatal Representations in Relation to Marital Distress and Depressive Symptoms. *Infant Ment. Health J.* **2016**, *37*, 388–400. [CrossRef]
37. Benoit, D.; Parker, K.C.H.; Zeanah, C.H. Mothers' Representations of Their Infants Assessed Prenatally: Stability and Association with Infants' Attachment Classifications. *J. Child Psychol. Psychiatry* **1997**, *38*, 307–313. [CrossRef]
38. Lindstedt, J.; Korja, R.; Vilja, S.; Ahlqvist-Bjorkroth, S. Fathers' prenatal attachment representations and the quality of father-child interaction in infancy and toddlerhood. *J. Fam. Psychol.* **2021**, *35*, 478–488. [CrossRef]
39. Zeanah, C.H.; Benoit, D.; Barton, M.; Hirshberg, L. Working model of the child interview coding manual. 1996; *unpublished manuscript*.
40. Forcada-Guex, M.; Borghini, A.; Pierrehumbert, B.; Ansermet, F.; Muller-Nix, C. Prematurity, maternal posttraumatic stress and consequences on the mother–infant relationship. *Early Hum. Dev.* **2011**, *87*, 21–26. [CrossRef]
41. Meijssen, D.; Wolf, M.-J.; van Bakel, H.; Koldewijn, K.; Kok, J.; van Baar, A. Maternal attachment representations after very preterm birth and the effect of early intervention. *Infant Behav. Dev.* **2011**, *34*, 72–80. [CrossRef]
42. Barfoot, J.; Meredith, P.; Ziviani, J.; Whittingham, K. Parent-child interactions and children with cerebral palsy: An exploratory study investigating emotional availability, functional ability, and parent distress. *Child Care Health Dev.* **2017**, *43*, 812–822. [CrossRef] [PubMed]
43. Hall, R.A.; De Waard, I.E.; Tooten, A.; Hoffenkamp, H.N.; Vingerhoets, A.J.; van Bakel, H.J. From the father's point of view: How father's representations of the infant impact on father-infant interaction and infant development. *Early Hum. Dev.* **2014**, *90*, 877–883. [CrossRef] [PubMed]
44. Sokolowski, M.S.; Hans, S.L.; Bernstein, V.J.; Cox, S.M. Mothers' representations of their infants and parenting behavior: Associations with personal and social-contextual variables in a high-risk sample. *Infant Ment. Health J.* **2007**, *28*, 344–365. [CrossRef] [PubMed]
45. Korja, R.; Ahlqvist-Björkroth, S.; Savonlahti, E.; Stolt, S.; Haataja, L.; Lapinleimu, H.; Piha, J.; Lehtonen, L. Relations between maternal attachment representations and the quality of mother-infant interaction in preterm and full-term infants. *Infant Behav. Dev.* **2010**, *33*, 330–336. [CrossRef]
46. Magill-Evans, J.; Harrison, M.J.; Burke, S.O. Parent-Child Interactions and Development of Toddlers Born Preterm. *West. J. Nurs. Res.* **1999**, *21*, 292–312. [CrossRef]
47. Feldman, R. Parent–infant synchrony and the construction of shared timing; physiological precursors, developmental outcomes, and risk conditions. *J. Child Psychol. Psychiatry* **2007**, *48*, 329–354. [CrossRef]
48. Festante, F.; Antonelli, C.; Chorna, O.; Corsi, G.; Guzzetta, A. Parent–infant Interaction during the First Year of Life in Infants at High Risk for Cerebral Palsy: A Systematic Review of the Literature. *Neural Plast.* **2019**, *2019*, 5759694. [CrossRef]
49. Minde, K.; Perrotta, M.; Marton, P. Maternal Caretaking and Play with Full-Term and Premature-Infants. *J. Child Psychol. Psychiatry* **1985**, *26*, 231–244. [CrossRef]
50. Korja, R.; Maunu, J.; Kirjavainen, J.; Savonlahti, E.; Haataja, L.; Lapinleimu, H.; Manninen, H.; Piha, J.; Lehtonen, L.; Grp, P.S. Mother-infant interaction is influenced by the amount of holding in preterm infants. *Early Hum. Dev.* **2008**, *84*, 257–267. [CrossRef]

51. Misund, A.R.; Braten, S.; Nerdrum, P.; Pripp, A.H.; Diseth, T.H. A Norwegian prospective study of preterm mother-infant interactions at 6 and 18months and the impact of maternal mental health problems, pregnancy and birth complications. *BMJ Open* **2016**, *6*, e009699. [CrossRef]
52. Steiner, A.M.; Gengoux, G.W.; Smith, A.; Chawarska, K. Parent–Child Interaction Synchrony for Infants At-Risk for Autism Spectrum Disorder. *J. Autism Dev. Disord.* **2018**, *48*, 3562–3572. [CrossRef] [PubMed]
53. Pijl, M.K.J.; Bontinck, C.; Rommelse, N.N.J.; Begum Ali, J.; Cauvet, E.; Niedzwiecka, A.; Falck-Ytter, T.; Jones, E.J.H.; Van den Boomen, C.; Bölte, S.; et al. Parent-child interaction during the first year of life in infants at elevated likelihood of autism spectrum disorder. *Infant Behav. Dev.* **2021**, *62*, 101521. [CrossRef] [PubMed]
54. Anke, T.M.S.; Slinning, K.; Moe, V.; Brunborg, C.; Siqveland, T.S.; Skjelstad, D.V. Mothers with and without bipolar disorder and their infants: Group differences in mother-infant interaction patterns at three months postpartum. *BMC Psychiatry* **2019**, *19*, 292. [CrossRef]
55. Riordan, D.; Appleby, L.; Faragher, B. Mother-infant interaction in post-partum women with schizophrenia and affective disorders. *Psychol. Med.* **1999**, *29*, 991–995. [CrossRef] [PubMed]
56. Hipwell, A.E.; Kumar, R. Maternal psychopathology and prediction of outcome based on mother-infant interaction ratings (BMIS). *Br. J. Psychiatry* **1996**, *169*, 655–661. [CrossRef]
57. Parfitt, Y.; Pike, A.; Ayers, S. The impact of parents' mental health on parent-baby interaction: A prospective study. *Infant Behav. Dev.* **2013**, *36*, 599–608. [CrossRef]
58. Feldman, R. Maternal versus child risk and the development of parent-child and family relationships in five high-risk populations. *Dev. Psychopathol.* **2007**, *19*, 293–312. [CrossRef]
59. Eliasson, A.C.; Holmstrom, L.; Aarne, P.; Nakeva von Mentzer, C.; Weiland, A.L.; Sjostrand, L.; Forssberg, H.; Tedroff, K.; Lowing, K. Efficacy of the small step program in a randomised controlled trial for infants below age 12 months with clinical signs of CP; a study protocol. *BMC Pediatr.* **2016**, *16*, 175. [CrossRef]
60. Romeiser-Logan, L.; Slaughter, R.; Hickman, R. Single-subject research designs in pediatric rehabilitation: A valuable step towards knowledge translation. *Dev. Med. Child Neurol.* **2017**, *59*, 574–580. [CrossRef]
61. Piper, M.C.; Pinnell, L.E.; Darrah, J.; Maguire, T.; Byrne, P.J. Construction and Validation of the Alberta Infant Motor Scale (Aims). *Can. J. Public Health-Rev. Can. Sante Publique* **1992**, *83*, S46–S50.
62. Abidin, R.R. *Parenting Stress Index*, 3rd ed.; Psychological Assessment Resource: Odessa, FL, USA, 1995.
63. Barroso, N.E.; Hungerford, G.M.; Garcia, D.; Graziano, P.A.; Bagner, D.M. Psychometric Properties of the Parenting Stress Index-Short Form (PSI-SF) in a High-Risk Sample of Mothers and Their Infants. *Psychol. Assess.* **2016**, *28*, 1331–1335. [CrossRef] [PubMed]
64. Whiteside-Mansell, L.; Ayoub, C.; McKelvey, L.; Faldowski, R.A.; Hart, A.; Shears, J. Parenting Stress of Low-Income Parents of Toddlers and Preschoolers: Psychometric Properties of a Short Form of the Parenting Stress Index. *Parenting* **2007**, *7*, 26–56. [CrossRef]
65. Haskett, M.E.; Ahern, L.S.; Ward, C.S.; Allaire, J.C. Factor structure and validity of the parenting stress index-short form. *J. Clin. Child Adolesc. Psychol.* **2006**, *35*, 302–312. [CrossRef] [PubMed]
66. Zigmond, A.S.; Snaith, R.P. The Hospital Anxiety and Depression Scale. *Acta Psychiatr. Scand.* **1983**, *67*, 361–370. [CrossRef] [PubMed]
67. Bjelland, I.; Dahl, A.A.; Haug, T.T.; Neckelmann, D. The validity of the Hospital Anxiety and Depression Scale-An updated literature review. *J. Psychosom. Res.* **2002**, *52*, 69–77. [CrossRef]
68. Kjaergaard, M.; Wang, C.E.A.; Waterloo, K.; Jorde, R. A study of the psychometric properties of the Beck Depression Inventory-II, the Montgomery and Asberg Depression Rating Scale, and the Hospital Anxiety and Depression Scale in a sample from a healthy population. *Scand. J. Psychol.* **2014**, *55*, 83–89. [CrossRef]
69. Sandnes, K.; Lydersen, S.; Karstad, S.B.; Berg-Nielsen, T.S. Measuring mothers' representations of their infants: Psychometric properties of the clinical scales of the working model of the child interview in a low- to moderate-risk sample. *Infant Ment. Health J.* **2021**, *42*, 690–704. [CrossRef]
70. Clark, R. *The Parent– Child Early Relational Assessment: Instrument and Manual*; University of Wisconsin: Madison, WI, USA, 1985.
71. Lotzin, A.; Lu, X.; Kriston, L.; Schiborr, J.; Musal, T.; Romer, G.; Ramsauer, B. Observational tools for measuring parent–infant interaction: A systematic review. *Clin. Child Fam. Psychol. Rev.* **2015**, *18*, 99–132. [CrossRef]
72. Gisev, N.; Bell, J.S.; Chen, T.F. Interrater agreement and interrater reliability: Key concepts, approaches, and applications. *Res. Soc. Adm. Pharm.* **2013**, *9*, 330–338. [CrossRef]
73. George, D.; Mallery, P. *SPSS for Windows Step by Step: A Simple Guide and Reference. 11.0 Update*, 4th ed.; Allyn & Bacon: Boston, MA, USA, 2003.
74. Corp, I. *IBM SPSS Statistics for Windows, Version 27.0.*; IBM Corp: Armonk, NY, USA, 2020.
75. Whittingham, K.; Wee, D.; Sanders, M.R.; Boyd, R. Sorrow, coping and resiliency: Parents of children with cerebral palsy share their experiences. *Disabil. Rehabil.* **2013**, *35*, 1447–1452. [CrossRef]
76. Austin, A.E.; Lesak, A.M.; Shanahan, M.E. Risk and protective factors for child maltreatment: A review. *Curr. Epidemiol. Rep.* **2020**, *7*, 334–342. [CrossRef] [PubMed]

77. Schmücker, G.; Brisch, K.H.; Köhntop, B.; Betzler, S.; Österle, M.; Pohlandt, F.; Pokorny, D.; Laucht, M.; Kächele, H.; Buchheim, A. The influence of prematurity, maternal anxiety, and infants' neurobiological risk on mother-infant interactions. *Infant Ment. Health J.* **2005**, *26*, 423–441. [CrossRef] [PubMed]
78. Bradley, R.; Slade, P. A review of mental health problems in fathers following the birth of a child. *J. Reprod. Infant Psychol.* **2011**, *29*, 19–42. [CrossRef]

Disclaimer/Publisher's Note: The statements, opinions and data contained in all publications are solely those of the individual author(s) and contributor(s) and not of MDPI and/or the editor(s). MDPI and/or the editor(s) disclaim responsibility for any injury to people or property resulting from any ideas, methods, instructions or products referred to in the content.

Article

Characteristics and Challenges of Epilepsy in Children with Cerebral Palsy—A Population-Based Study

Ana Dos Santos Rufino [1,2,3,*], Magnus Påhlman [1,4], Ingrid Olsson [1,5] and Kate Himmelmann [1,5]

1. Paediatric Neurology, Queen Silvia Children's Hospital, Sahlgrenska University Hospital, 41685 Gothenburg, Sweden
2. Epilepsy Center Frankfurt Rhine-Main, Center of Neurology and Neurosurgery, University Hospital, Goethe-University Frankfurt, 60590 Frankfurt am Main, Germany
3. LOEWE Center for Personalized Translational Epilepsy Research (CePTER), Goethe-University Frankfurt, 60590 Frankfurt am Main, Germany
4. Gillberg Neuropsychiatry Centre, Institute of Neuroscience and Physiology, Sahlgrenska Academy, University of Gothenburg, 41119 Gothenburg, Sweden
5. Department of Pediatrics, Institute of Clinical Sciences, Sahlgrenska Academy, University of Gothenburg, 41685 Gothenburg, Sweden
* Correspondence: ana.rufino@vgregion.se

Abstract: The aim of this population-based study was to describe the prevalence and characteristics of epilepsy in children with cerebral palsy (CP), focusing on antiseizure medication (ASM) and seizure outcome. Findings were related to CP type, gross motor function and associated impairments. Data on all 140 children with CP born in 2003–2006 were taken from the CP register of Western Sweden. Medical records were reviewed at ages 9–12 and 13–16 years. In total 43% had a diagnosis of epilepsy. Epilepsy was more common in children with dyskinetic CP, who more often had a history of infantile spasms, continuous spike-and-wave during sleep and status epilepticus. Neonatal seizures, severe intellectual disability, severe motor disability and autism were associated with a higher risk of epilepsy. Many children were on polytherapy, and valproate was frequently used, even in girls. At age 13–16 years, 45% of the children with epilepsy were seizure free for at least one year. Onset after 2 years of age, female sex and white matter injury were associated with good seizure outcome. Despite the risk of relapse, reduction or discontinuation of ASM could be an option in selected cases. It is important to optimize ASM and to consider the possibility of epilepsy surgery.

Keywords: epilepsy; cerebral palsy; children; neuroimaging; seizure outcome

1. Introduction

Children with cerebral palsy (CP) often have associated impairments and disorders. Epilepsy is a common comorbidity and occurs in 15–55% of children and adults with CP [1] while in the general childhood population, the prevalence of epilepsy is between 3.2 and 5.5 per 1000 in developed countries [2].

In a previous report from the CP register of western Sweden on children born in 1999–2002, 44% had epilepsy. This was a higher occurrence of epilepsy compared to previous birth-year cohorts, possibly due to an increase in cortical/subcortical lesions documented by neuroimaging [3].

Up to 50% of children with CP and epilepsy have been reported to have seizures despite antiseizure medication (ASM) [4,5]. A model has been described for predicting drug resistant epilepsy in children with CP, using four independent predictors: low Apgar score at 5 min, neonatal seizures, focal epilepsy clinically and on routine electroencephalogram (EEG) [6].

A recent study has shown that epilepsy in CP can remit with ASM in about 50% of all cases, and in up to 20% in spastic quadriplegia or hemiplegia even with previous status epilepticus or daily seizures, up to 10 years from epilepsy onset. ASM could be discontinued without relapse in 14%. In that study, older age, perinatal aetiology and improvement on EEG were favourable factors for terminating ASM [7].

The aims of the present study were to describe the prevalence of epilepsy in children with CP in a population-based cohort born in 2003–2006 from the CP register of western Sweden, to explore the epilepsy characteristics, EEG findings and treatment in relation to CP type, gross motor function and associated impairments, and explore seizure outcome at follow-up. Furthermore, we intended to compare characteristics of children with and without epilepsy and identify factors that may favour seizure remission.

2. Material and Methods

The medical records of all children with CP born from 2003 to 2006 in the CP register of western Sweden and currently living in the county of Västra Götaland, Sweden, were reviewed and data of the selected cohort were analyzed at two different timepoints: at ages 9–12 (data collected between July and October 2015) and 13–16 years (follow-up data collected in 2019). At the first timepoint the following data were analyzed: age of epilepsy onset, type of seizures, frequency of seizures, status epilepticus, EEG findings, use of ASM, and non-pharmacological treatment, cognitive level, and neuropsychiatric diagnosis. For the analyses at the second timepoint updated information about new cases of epilepsy, seizure freedom and type of ASM was collected. Information about cognitive function and neuropsychiatric diagnoses was obtained from another study from our centre [8].

The whole cohort comprised 140 children (61 girls and 79 boys) and was part of a larger cohort that has previously been reported [3]. Information about type and aetiology of CP, gestational age, Apgar score at 5 min, gross motor function, neuroimaging findings and history of neonatal seizures was taken from the CP register of western Sweden.

The aetiological period was defined as prenatal when the brain insult occurred during pregnancy until the onset of labour resulting in delivery, and as peri/neonatal from the onset of labour up to day 28. Data on aetiological period for this cohort have previously been published [3].

Neonatal seizures were defined as seizures occurring up to 72 h of age.

Magnetic resonance imaging (MRI) findings were classified according to the MRI classification system for children with cerebral palsy (MRICS) into five categories: maldevelopments, predominant white matter injury, predominant grey matter injury, miscellaneous and normal. The group with predominant grey matter injury was divided into: basal ganglia/thalamus lesions, cortical-subcortical lesions, and arterial infarctions [9]. Computer tomography (CT) findings were included in the absence of MRI and classified in a similar way [3,10].

The definition of CP was the one agreed upon at an international consensus meeting in Bethesda: Cerebral palsy (CP) describes a group of disorders of the development of movement and posture, causing activity limitation, that are attributed to non-progressive disturbances that occurred in the developing foetal or infant brain. The motor disorders of cerebral palsy are often accompanied by disturbance of sensation, cognition, communication, perception, and/or behaviour, and/or by a seizure disorder [11].

The CP types were classified into unilateral spastic (USCP), bilateral spastic (BSCP), dyskinetic or ataxic CP according to the Surveillance of Cerebral Palsy in Europe (SCPE 2000) [12], and according to Hagberg into hemiplegia, diplegia, tetraplegia, dyskinetic CP and ataxia [13]. To describe the gross motor function the Gross Motor Function Classification System (GMFCS) was used [14].

The 2014 definition of epilepsy according to the International League Against Epilepsy (ILAE) was used [15]. The types of epileptic seizures during the last two years were documented. Information about previous seizure types, including infantile spasms, was also registered. Seizures were classified according to the ILAE classification of seizure types in which the mode of seizure onset is subdivided into generalized, focal, and unknown [16]. The term 'multiple seizure types' was used when children had a combination of both focal and generalized seizures.

Seizure freedom was defined as absence of seizures (with or without ASM) for at least one year preceding data collection [17,18].

Seizure frequency was divided into daily seizures (at least once a day), weekly seizures (less than once daily and more than once a week), monthly (at least once a month but not more than once a week), seldom (less than once a month) and clusters (many seizures in clusters followed by seizure free periods). Information was taken from the medical records regarding status epilepticus which in most cases implied hospital care.

All results of EEGs were interpreted at the Department of Clinical Neurophysiology, Sahlgrenska University Hospital, Gothenburg. Results from the EEG recordings (performed before October 2015) were documented and reviewed together with an experienced clinical neurophysiologist. Epileptic discharges were divided into focal, multifocal, and generalized epileptic discharges. Information was obtained about the occurrence of hypsarrythmia and continuous spike-and-wave during sleep (CSWS), defined as an EEG pattern of almost continuous, slow (1.5–2 Hz) spike-wave during slow sleep.

Cognitive level was divided into normal (IQ > 70), mild intellectual disability (ID) (IQ 50–70) and severe ID (IQ < 50), based on neuropsychological assessment or in a few cases on clinical observation. Neuropsychiatric comorbidity referred to autism spectrum disorder (ASD) and attention-deficit/hyperactivity disorder (ADHD). In cases where diagnostic criteria were nor fulfilled, symptoms such as attention and concentration deficits, behavioural problems, routine dependency were also registered.

Statistical Analysis

We used descriptive statistics for the comparison of groups. The chi-square test for independence was used for the association between categorical variables; if more than two categories were present within an ordinal scale, the Cochran–Armitage chi-square test for trend was used. A *p*-value of less than 0.05 was regarded as statistically significant.

3. Results

In the total cohort, 60/140 (43%) had a diagnosis of epilepsy. At the review of the medical records in 2015 one child with epilepsy and one without epilepsy had died, leaving 138 children (60 girls and 78 boys), 59 children with epilepsy and 79 without epilepsy. Register data on the children with and without epilepsy are presented in Table 1.

Epilepsy was more common in children born at term ($\chi^2 = 6.24$; $p = 0.012$), compared to children born preterm. Children with epilepsy had more often peri/neonatal aetiology (61%; 36/59) compared to those without epilepsy (44%; 35/79). Prenatal aetiology was present in 32% (19/59) of children with epilepsy and 28% (22/79) of those without epilepsy, whereas unknown aetiology was found in 7% (4/59) and 28% (22/79), respectively.

An Apgar score < 5 at five minutes was associated with later epilepsy in term-born children ($\chi^2 = 6.07$; $p = 0.014$). Nearly two thirds of children with a history of neonatal seizures developed epilepsy compared to one third without neonatal seizures ($\chi^2 = 10.25$; $p = 0.001$). Most children (72%; 31/43) with neonatal seizures were born at term, and 24 of 31 developed epilepsy. A history of neonatal seizures was more frequent in children with dyskinetic CP (63%; 15/24) than in those with other types of CP ($\chi^2 = 13.30$; $p < 0.001$).

The most common neuroimaging finding in children with epilepsy was predominant grey matter injury (44%; 25/59), which was mostly seen in children born at term.

BSCP was the most common type of CP in children with epilepsy, while the children with dyskinetic CP had the highest occurrence of epilepsy.

A more severe motor impairment, i.e., wheelchair ambulation, was associated with more epilepsy (73%; 29/40) than preserved walking ability (31%; 30/98) ($\chi^2 = 20.36$; $p < 0.001$). Most children without epilepsy were at GMFCS levels I and II.

Table 1. Characteristics of children with cerebral palsy (CP) with and without epilepsy.

	CP with Epilepsy n = 59 (%)	CP without Epilepsy n = 79 (%)	Total n = 138
Sex			
female	28 (47)	32 (53)	60
male	31 (40)	47 (60)	78
Gestational age			
≤28 weeks	5 (33)	10 (67)	15
28–31 weeks	5 (29)	12 (71)	17
32–36 weeks	6 (27)	16 (73)	22
≥37 weeks	43 (51)	41 (49)	84
Apgar score < 5 at 5 min			
≤36 weeks	3 (38)	5 (62)	8
≥37 weeks	12 (80)	3 (20)	15
Neonatal seizures ≤ 72 h			
Yes	27 (63)	16 (37)	43
No	32 (34)	63 (66)	95
Neuroimaging			
A. Maldevelopments	7 (64)	4 (36)	11
B. Predominant white matter injury	15 (28)	39 (72)	54
C. Predominant grey matter injury	25 (58)	18 (42)	43
C1. Basal ganglia/thalamus lesions	13 (65)	7 (35)	20
C2. Cortical-subcortical lesions only	8 (67)	4 (33)	12
C3. Arterial infarctions	4 (36)	7 (64)	11
D. Miscellaneous	11 (100)	0	11
E. Normal	1 (8)	12 (92)	13
Normal CT	0	2 (100)	2
Not done	0	4 (100)	4
Type of cerebral palsy			
USCP	14 (26)	39 (74)	53
BSCP	24 (46)	28 (54)	52
Dyskinetic CP	17 (71)	7 (29)	24
Ataxic CP	4 (44)	5 (56)	9
GMFCS level			
I	15 (24)	47 (76)	62
II	6 (29)	15 (71)	21
III	9 (60)	6 (40)	15
IV	12 (57)	9 (43)	21
V	17 (89)	2 (11)	19

Data are n (%). USCP; unilateral spastic cerebral palsy. BSCP; bilateral spastic cerebral palsy. GMFCS; Gross Motor Function Classification System.

3.1. Epilepsy Characteristics

Many children (37%; 22/59) had epilepsy onset during the first year of life (Figure 1).

Most children (80%; 47/59) had an epilepsy diagnosis before five years, and by the age of ten all 59 had an epilepsy diagnosis. Age at onset varied by CP type. All six children with spastic tetraplegia had epilepsy onset before one year of age, while all four children with ataxic CP developed epilepsy at a later age.

Details on epilepsy in the 59 children, by CP type, are described in Table 2. In a few cases it was not possible to determine the frequency or detailed semiology of seizures due to lack of information in the medical records.

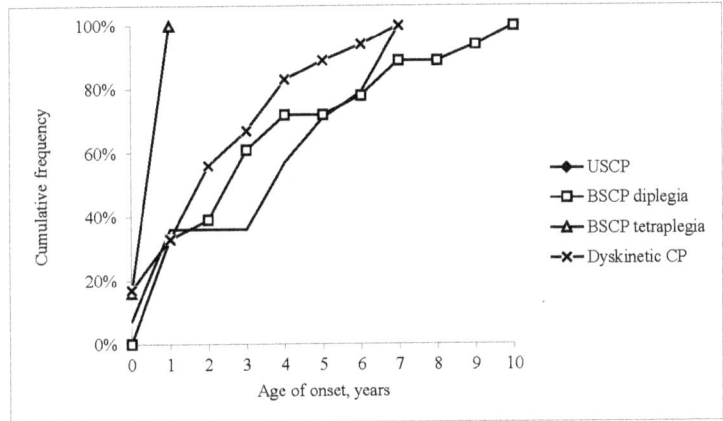

Figure 1. Cumulative frequency of epilepsy by age of onset (in years) in 59 children with epilepsy and unilateral spastic cerebral palsy (USCP), bilateral spastic cerebral palsy (BSCP; divided into diplegia and tetraplegia) and dyskinetic cerebral palsy.

Table 2. Characteristics of epilepsy in 59 children with cerebral palsy (CP).

	USCP n = 14	BSCP n = 24	Dyskinetic CP n = 17	Ataxic CP n = 4	Total n = 59 (%)
Type of seizures					
Focal	11	13	8	2	34 (57)
Generalized	1	3	1	2	7 (12)
Multiple types	2	8	7	0	17 (29)
Unknown	0	0	1	0	1 (2)
EEG: epileptic discharges (most recent EEG)					
Focal	10	15	8	1	34 (57)
Multifocal	1	7	7	1	16 (27)
Generalized	0	0	0	1	1 (2)
CSWS	1	0	0	0	1 (2)
Normal	2	2	2	1	7 (12)
Seizure frequency (last year)					
Seizure free	4	6	4	1	15 (25)
Seldom	7	4	5	1	17 (29)
Monthly	0	5	0	1	6 (10)
Weekly	0	1	1	0	2 (3)
Daily	1	5	2	0	8 (14)
Cluster	2	2	3	1	8 (14)
Unclear	0	1	2	0	3 (5)
Apgar score < 5 at 5 min	0	4	10	1	15 (25)
Neonatal seizures ≤ 72 h					
Yes	3	9	12	3	27 (46)
No	11	15	5	1	32 (54)
Infantile spasms					
Yes	0	2	6	0	8 (14)
No	14	22	11	4	51 (86)
Status epilepticus					
Yes	3	2	6	0	11 (19)
No	11	22	11	4	48 (81)
Antiseizure medication					
Monotherapy	5	13	7	2	27 (46)
Polytherapy	7	10	9	1	27 (46)
No ASM	2	1	1	1	5 (8)

Information is based on data obtained from medical records in 2015. n; number. CSWS; continuous spike-and-wave during sleep. ASM; antiseizure medication.

Focal seizures were the most common seizure type in all CP types (58%; 34/59), most prevalent in USCP (79%; 11/14).

Eight children had a history of infantile spasms, all with hypsarrhythmia on the EEG. The age of onset of infantile spasms varied between 2,5 and 16 months. Six of them had dyskinetic CP. Neuroimaging showed that four of the patients with infantile spasms had cortical/subcortical injury, two had predominant white matter injury, one had lesions in the basal ganglia, and one had miscellaneous findings. One child was at GMFCS level IV, and seven were at GMFCS level V. All except one had severe ID. Seven out of eight developed other types of seizures. One child had seizures seldom, one had seizures in clusters, two had weekly and three daily seizures. One child with dyskinetic CP with a history of infantile spasms, mild ID and predominant white matter injury was seizure free without medication.

Seizure frequency varied from daily seizures (14%; 8/59) to seizures occurring less than once a month (29%; 17/59), while 25% (15/59) of the children had been seizure free for one to six years, most of whom had a history of focal seizures (Table 3).

Table 3. Seizure frequency in 59 children with cerebral palsy and epilepsy at the age of 9–12 years (2015).

Type of Seizures	Seizure Free	Unclear	Seldom	Clusters	Monthly	Weekly	Daily	Total
Focal seizures	12	2	10	3	3	0	4	34
Generalised seizures	1	0	3	1	1	1	0	7
Multiple seizure types	1	1	4	4	2	1	4	17
Unknown	1	0	0	0	0	0	0	1
Total	15	3	17	8	6	2	8	59

Children with BSCP had the highest frequency of daily seizures (21%; 5/24); two of them had tetraplegia. (Table 2).

Nineteen per cent (11/59) of the children with epilepsy had a history of status epilepticus once or on several occasions: six of them had dyskinetic CP.

3.2. EEG Findings

Epileptic discharges were present in 88% of the latest EEGs and were mainly focal (58%) or multifocal (27%) (Table 2).

Eight children had one or several previous EEG recordings with CSWS. Five of them had dyskinetic CP and three had USCP. The neuroimaging findings were basal ganglia lesion in five children (four with dyskinetic CP and one with USCP), and cortical/subcortical injury, periventricular white matter injury and maldevelopment in one child each.

3.3. Epilepsy Treatment

Fifty-four of the 59 children with epilepsy had ASM in 2015 (92%). Out of 15 seizure free children, 13 were still on medication. Half of the children still on ASM had monotherapy and half had polytherapy: 17/54 (31%) had two, 9/54 (17%) three, and 1/54 (2%) four ASMs.

The most common drug used in monotherapy was valproate (14/27), followed by oxcarbazepine (6/27) and lamotrigine (5/27). There was a wide range of drug combinations as polytherapy. Valproate was also the most common drug used in combination with other drugs (18/27) such as lamotrigine, nitrazepam or levetiracetam, but many other combinations were also used. Levetiracetam was the second most used drug in polytherapy, used in different combinations in 12/27.

Valproate was a common drug in both sexes: 10/28 girls (36%) and 22/31 boys (71%) were on valproate.

Out of the 44 children who were not seizure free, nine had been referred for presurgical evaluation. Four children underwent epilepsy surgery between the age of 5 and 7 years, with different surgical procedures. At the 2-year follow-up after surgery, one was seizure free, and two had more than 75% reduction in seizure frequency. Five children had been referred for evaluation but were not accepted for surgery.

Two children had tried ketogenic diet without effect and the diet had been stopped. Vagus nerve stimulator had not been used in the studied group.

3.4. Follow-Up in 2019

Between 2015 and 2019 one child with USCP and epilepsy was lost to follow-up (moved abroad). There were no new cases of epilepsy, leaving 58 who were followed up.

Eleven children had become seizure free. Thus, 26 (17 girls and 9 boys) of 58 children were seizure free (45%) and had been so for 1–10 years. Nine of the 26 seizure free children were off medication. More girls than boys had become seizure free ($\chi^2 = 5.52$; $p = 0.019$). Children with predominant white matter injury had more often become seizure free (79%; 11/14) than children with other neuroimaging findings, distributed on all other groups ($\chi^2 = 8.50$; $p = 0.004$). Children with an early epilepsy onset (<2 years of age) were less likely to become seizure free than those with a later onset ($\chi^2 = 8.22$; $p = 0.004$). Seven of the 26 children had USCP, ten had BSCP, seven had dyskinetic CP while two had ataxic CP. Less severe motor impairment (GMFCS level I–III) was found in 17 (65%) while 9 (35%) used wheelchair ambulation. None of the 15 children at GMFCS level V and severe ID had become seizure free at follow-up.

At follow-up 48/58 (83%) were on ASM, 20 on monotherapy and 28 on polytherapy. Five out of six (83%) children with tetraplegia were on polytherapy. Valproate was still the most common drug used in monotherapy (9/20) followed by lamotrigine (5/20). The most common drug used in polytherapy was also valproate (19/28), followed by levetiracetam (13/28). Similar drug combinations were used as in 2015. Three out of 10 girls who had previously been on valproate had stopped medication and one had changed to levetiracetam, but six girls aged 13–16 years were still on valproate, in combination therapy in four and in monotherapy in two.

At follow-up at the age of 13–16 years, five more children, all with epilepsy, in total 84% (49/58) had a diagnosis of ID. The occurrence of epilepsy increased by ID ($\chi^2_{trend} = 48.05$, $p < 0.001$). All eight children with a history of infantile spasms had ID. Five with CSWS had severe ID, and two had a cognitive level within the normal range.

Autism was more common in children with epilepsy than in those without ($\chi^2 = 10.54$; $p = 0.001$), while there was no difference regarding ADHD ($\chi^2 = 1,79$; $p = 0.18$). Out of the seizure free children 73% (19/26) had ID, 10 with mild and 9 with severe ID, leaving seven (27%) with an intellectual level within the normal range. Eleven children had autism and 14 ADHD.

In children who were not seizure free, 94% (30/32) had ID, 4 with mild and 26 with severe ID. Eleven children had autism and six had ADHD.

4. Discussion

The prevalence of epilepsy in children with CP in this population-based cohort was 43% which is slightly higher than in an earlier Swedish study [18]. As previously described, the occurrence of epilepsy varied between different CP types [1], and it was more common in children with dyskinetic CP and less frequent in USCP [3].

Epilepsy in dyskinetic CP was associated with a more severe clinical picture, with infantile spasms and with CSWS. They had an early age of epilepsy onset, the highest frequency of status epilepticus, and many were on polytherapy. The occurrence of CSWS could be explained by the predominance of basal ganglia and thalamus lesions [19]. As reported previously, ID and more severe motor impairment were common [20]. Children with the most severe BSCP (tetraplegia) also had the highest seizure frequency and high use of polytherapy.

Neuroimaging findings depend on the timing of the brain insult [9]. The higher percentage of epilepsy seen in children born at term reflects their higher frequency of grey matter lesions, i.e., lesions acquired late in gestation. These results are in line with previous studies [21,22].

Both ID and more severe motor impairment were per se also associated with a higher frequency of epilepsy. A history of neonatal seizures, most common in dyskinetic CP, and the presence of severe ID and motor impairment represented a higher risk of developing epilepsy which is concurrent with other reports [23–26]. Symptomatic infantile spasms have been reported to be associated with a higher risk to develop other types of seizures and cognitive impairment [27]. Accordingly, almost all children with infantile spasms in our study developed other types of seizures and most had severe ID and motor impairment, related to the structural brain injury.

Epilepsy develops at an earlier age in children with CP compared to children without other neurological disorders [23]. In our study age at onset of epilepsy varied between the different CP types with earlier onset in children with the most severe BSCP, most likely due to more widespread brain pathology than in milder cases.

It is sometimes a challenge to differentiate epileptic seizures from other involuntary movements, especially in dyskinetic or ataxic CP [1]. Focal seizures were the most common seizure type in our cohort, but many children had multiple seizure types, especially those with dyskinetic CP and BSCP.

In our study the frequency of status epilepticus was 19% which was lower than in a previous Swedish study (47%) with children born 1987–1994 [18] which may be a result of improved treatment.

The most common finding on EEG was focal epileptic discharges also in children with generalized seizures. It is possible that some of these had a focal start although it had not been observed clinically. It is reasonable specifically to ask for a focal start in seizure semiology, as children with CP almost always have a structural cause of their epilepsy. Several children had multifocal epileptic discharges, most likely associated with the type and extent of underlying brain abnormality. Even though EEG is an important complement in the diagnosis of epilepsy it is important to remember that in children with CP, similar changes may be found even in the absence of clinical seizures [1].

The proportion of seizure free children had increased with age from 25% to 45% at the follow-up (at the age of 13–16 years), across all CP types. Similar findings have been reported by Tsubouchi et al. [7]. In the study by Tokatly Latzer et al. there was no difference in type of CP between the drug responsive or drug resistant epilepsy groups [6], while in another study remission rates varied by CP type, with the lowest remission rate in BSCP [28]. In our study, a better seizure outcome (seizure free for at least a year with or without ASM) was seen in girls, children with later epilepsy onset and predominant white matter injury, while children with epilepsy onset before 2 years of age, severe ID or severe motor impairment had a higher risk of persisting seizures. This is important to bear in mind when treating children with CP and epilepsy and when counselling their parents. There seemed to be a reluctance to discontinue ASM in seizure free children, probably due to the high risk of relapse, as reported by El Tantawi et al. [28]. However, we found that many children were on polytherapy despite seizure freedom for more than one year, often several years. We do not have the information if this was because attempts had been made to reduce ASM leading to relapses or if ASM was kept "to be on the safe side". It may well be that at least the number of ASM could be reduced to the benefit of the children's development, considering the possible side effects.

Valproate was the most common drug used in mono- and polytherapy and even if there was a slight decrease in its use in girls in 2019, there were still six girls in adolescence using valproate despite its known teratogenicity and risk for hormone abnormalities and polycystic ovarian syndrome [29].

Neuropsychiatric disorders such as ASD and ADHD are common in children with CP and are often associated with ID [8]. In this study we found an association between epilepsy and ASD but not with ADHD [30–32]. At the last follow-up we observed an increase in the diagnoses of both ID and ASD in children with CP and epilepsy but not in the group without epilepsy. This may be related to a negative impact of epilepsy and polytherapy on neurodevelopment as well as to the underlying brain impairment. In this cohort we have previously shown that the occurrence of intellectual disability, autism and ADHD increases with age as shown in repeated assessments [30]. Repeated assessments of cognitive function during childhood are important, in order to reveal these disabilities [33]. The background of the deterioration is probably multifactorial.

A strength of this study is the use of a population-based CP register including all children with CP born from 2003 to 2006 currently living in the county of Västra Götaland, Sweden, which eliminates selection bias. We reviewed all medical records from the paediatric clinics and habilitation centres comprising all possible places for the follow-up of children with CP.

The limitations of this study were its retrospective nature, and the fact that seizure semiology and frequency were not always well documented in the medical records.

5. Conclusions

In our population-based cohort of children with CP, 43% had epilepsy, all of them with onset before or at the age of 10 years. BSCP was the most common type of CP in children with epilepsy, while those with dyskinetic CP had the highest occurrence of epilepsy. Focal epilepsy dominated in all CP types. Epilepsy was associated with severe motor impairment, ID, and autism. Even if the epilepsy was often difficult to treat and many children were on polytherapy, 45% had been seizure free for more than one year by the age of 13–16 years. Prospective observational studies are warranted to identify cases who benefit from reduction or discontinuation of ASM.

Author Contributions: Conceptualization, A.D.S.R., K.H. and I.O.; methodology, A.D.S.R., M.P., K.H. and I.O.; formal analysis, A.D.S.R., M.P., K.H. and I.O.; investigation, A.D.S.R., M.P., K.H. and I.O.; writing—original draft preparation, A.D.S.R., K.H., I.O. and M.P.; writing—review and editing, A.D.S.R., M.P., K.H. and I.O.; visualization, A.D.S.R. and M.P.; supervision, K.H. and I.O.; funding acquisition, K.H. All authors have read and agreed to the published version of the manuscript.

Funding: The study was financed by grants from the Swedish state under the agreement between the Swedish government and the county councils, the ALF-agreement (ALFGBG-726001) and by grants from the Margarethahem Foundation.

Institutional Review Board Statement: The study was conducted in accordance with the Declaration of Helsinki, and approved by The Regional Ethical Review Board in Gothenburg (ref 145-07 and 398-12).

Informed Consent Statement: No informed consent was required for the register study. Informed consent was obtained for follow-up.

Data Availability Statement: The data presented in this study are available on reasonable request from the corresponding author.

Acknowledgments: We express our gratitude to Anders Hedström, at the Department of Clinical Neurophysiology, Sahlgrenska University Hospital, Gothenburg for reviewing the EEGs and valuable discussions about the EEG.

Conflicts of Interest: On behalf of all authors, the corresponding author states that there is no conflict of interest.

References

1. Wallace, S.J. Epilepsy in cerebral palsy. *Dev. Med. Child Neurol.* **2001**, *43*, 713–717. [CrossRef]
2. Camfield, P.; Camfield, C. Incidence, prevalence and aetiology of seizures and epilepsy in children. *Epileptic Disord.* **2015**, *17*, 117–123. [CrossRef] [PubMed]
3. Himmelmann, K.; Uvebrant, P. Function and neuroimaging in cerebral palsy: A population-based study. *Dev. Med. Child Neurol.* **2011**, *53*, 516–521. [CrossRef]
4. Kulak, W.; Sobaniec, W. Risk factors and prognosis of epilepsy in children with cerebral palsy in north-eastern Poland. *Brain Dev.* **2003**, *25*, 499–506. [CrossRef] [PubMed]
5. Zafeiriou, D.I.; Kontopoulos, E.E.; Tsikoulas, I. Characteristics and prognosis of epilepsy in children with cerebral palsy. *J. Child Neurol.* **1999**, *14*, 289–294. [CrossRef] [PubMed]

6. Latzer, I.T.; Blumovich, A.; Sagi, L.; Uliel-Sibony, S.; Fattal-Valevski, A. Prediction of Drug-Resistant Epilepsy in Children With Cerebral Palsy. *J. Child Neurol.* **2019**, *35*, 187–194. [CrossRef]
7. Tsubouchi, Y.; Tanabe, A.; Saito, Y.; Noma, H.; Maegaki, Y. Long-term prognosis of epilepsy in patients with cerebral palsy. *Dev. Med. Child Neurol.* **2019**, *61*, 1067–1073. [CrossRef]
8. Påhlman, M.; Gillberg, C.; Himmelmann, K. Autism and attention-deficit/hyperactivity disorder in children with cerebral palsy: High prevalence rates in a population-based study. *Dev. Med. Child Neurol.* **2020**, *63*, 320–327. [CrossRef]
9. Himmelmann, K.; Horber, V.; De La Cruz, J.; Horridge, K.; Mejaski-Bosnjak, V.; Hollody, K.; Krägeloh-Mann, I.; the SCPE Working Group. MRI classification system (MRICS) for children with cerebral palsy: Development, reliability, and recommendations. *Dev. Med. Child Neurol.* **2016**, *59*, 57–64. [CrossRef]
10. Himmelmann, K.; Uvebrant, P. The panorama of cerebral palsy in Sweden. XI. Changing patterns in the birth-year period 2003–2006. *Acta Paediatr.* **2014**, *103*, 618–624. [CrossRef]
11. Rosenbaum, P.; Paneth, N.; Leviton, A.; Goldstein, M.; Bax, M.; Damiano, D.; Dan, B.; Jacobsson, B. A report: The definition and classification of cerebral palsy April 2006. *Dev. Med. Child Neurol. Suppl.* **2007**, *109*, 8–14.
12. Cans, C. Surveillance of cerebral palsy in Europe: A collaboration of cerebral palsy surveys and registers. Surveillance of Cerebral Palsy in Europe (SCPE). *Dev. Med. Child Neurol.* **2000**, *42*, 816–824. [CrossRef]
13. Hagberg, B.; Hagberg, G.; Olow, I. The changing panorama of cerebral palsy in Sweden 1954-1970. I. Analysis of the general changes. *Acta Paediatr. Scand* **1975**, *64*, 187–192. [CrossRef] [PubMed]
14. Palisano, R.; Rosenbaum, P.; Walter, S.; Russell, D.; Wood, E.; Galuppi, B. Development and reliability of a system to classify gross motor function in children with cerebral palsy. *Dev. Med. Child Neurol.* **2008**, *39*, 214–223. [CrossRef]
15. Fisher, R.S.; Acevedo, C.; Arzimanoglou, A.; Bogacz, A.; Cross, J.H.; Elger, C.E.; Engel, J., Jr.; Forsgren, L.; French, J.A.; Glynn, M.; et al. ILAE Official Report: A practical clinical definition of epilepsy. *Epilepsia* **2014**, *55*, 475–482. [CrossRef] [PubMed]
16. Fisher, R.S.; Cross, J.H.; French, J.A.; Higurashi, N.; Hirsch, E.; Jansen, F.E.; Lagae, L.; Moshé, S.L.; Peltola, J.; Perez, E.R.; et al. Operational classification of seizure types by the International League Against Epilepsy: Position Paper of the ILAE Commission for Classification and Terminology. *Epilepsia* **2017**, *58*, 522–530. [CrossRef]
17. Aaberg, K.M.; Bakken, I.J.; Lossius, M.I.; Søraas, C.L.; Tallur, K.K.; Stoltenberg, C.; Chin, R.; Surén, P. Short-term Seizure Outcomes in Childhood Epilepsy. *Pediatrics* **2018**, *141*, e20174016. [CrossRef]
18. Carlsson, M.; Hagberg, G.; Olsson, I. Clinical and aetiological aspects of epilepsy in children with cerebral palsy. *Dev. Med. Child Neurol.* **2003**, *45*, 371–376. [CrossRef]
19. Monbaliu, E.; Himmelmann, K.; Lin, J.-P.; Ortibus, E.; Bonouvrié, L.; Feys, H.; Vermeulen, R.J.; Dan, B. Clinical presentation and management of dyskinetic cerebral palsy. *Lancet Neurol.* **2017**, *16*, 741–749. [CrossRef]
20. Ballester-Plané, J.; Laporta-Hoyos, O.; Macaya, A.; Póo, P.; Meléndez-Plumed, M.; Toro-Tamargo, E.; Gimeno, F.; Narberhaus, A.; Segarra, D.; Pueyo, R. Cognitive functioning in dyskinetic cerebral palsy: Its relation to motor function, communication and epilepsy. *Eur. J. Paediatr. Neurol.* **2017**, *22*, 102–112. [CrossRef]
21. Cooper, M.S.; Mackay, M.T.; Fahey, M.; Reddihough, D.; Reid, S.M.; Williams, K.; Harvey, A.S. Seizures in Children With Cerebral Palsy and White Matter Injury. *Pediatrics* **2017**, *139*, e20162975. [CrossRef] [PubMed]
22. Reid, S.M.; Dagia, C.D.; Ditchfield, M.R.; Reddihough, D.S. Grey matter injury patterns in cerebral palsy: Associations between structural involvement on MRI and clinical outcomes. *Dev. Med. Child Neurol.* **2015**, *57*, 1159–1167. [CrossRef]
23. Mert, G.G.; Incecik, F.; Altunbasak, S.; Herguner, O.; Mert, M.K.; Kiris, N.; Unal, I. Factors Affecting Epilepsy Development and Epilepsy Prognosis in Cerebral Palsy. *Pediatr. Neurol.* **2011**, *45*, 89–94. [CrossRef]
24. Pavone, P.; Gulizia, C.; Le Pira, A.; Greco, F.; Parisi, P.; Di Cara, G.; Falsaperla, R.; Lubrano, R.; Minardi, C.; Spalice, A.; et al. Cerebral Palsy and Epilepsy in Children: Clinical Perspectives on a Common Comorbidity. *Children* **2020**, *8*, 16. [CrossRef] [PubMed]
25. Sadowska, M.; Sarecka-Hujar, B.; Kopyta, I. Evaluation of Risk Factors for Epilepsy in Pediatric Patients with Cerebral Palsy. *Brain Sci.* **2020**, *10*, 481. [CrossRef]
26. Szpindel, A.; Myers, K.A.; Ng, P.; Dorais, M.; Koclas, L.; Pigeon, N.; Shevell, M.; Oskoui, M. Epilepsy in children with cerebral palsy: A data linkage study. *Dev. Med. Child Neurol.* **2021**, *64*, 259–265. [CrossRef]
27. Riikonen, R. Infantile Spasms: Outcome in Clinical Studies. *Pediatr. Neurol.* **2020**, *108*, 54–64. [CrossRef] [PubMed]
28. El Tantawi, N.T.; Elmegid, D.S.A.; Atef, E. Seizure outcome and epilepsy patterns in patients with cerebral palsy. *Seizure* **2019**, *65*, 166–171. [CrossRef]
29. Gotlib, D.; Ramaswamy, R.; Kurlander, J.E.; DeRiggi, A.; Riba, M. Valproic Acid in Women and Girls of Childbearing Age. *Curr. Psychiatry Rep.* **2017**, *19*, 58. [CrossRef]
30. Påhlman, M.; Gillberg, C.; Himmelmann, K. One-third of school-aged children with cerebral palsy have neuropsychiatric impairments in a population-based study. *Acta Paediatr.* **2019**, *108*, 2048–2055. [CrossRef]

31. Hanci, F.; Türay, S.; Dilek, M.; Kabakuş, N. Epilepsy and drug-resistant epilepsy in children with cerebral palsy: A retrospective observational study. *Epilepsy Behav.* **2020**, *112*, 107357. [CrossRef] [PubMed]
32. Reilly, C.; Atkinson, P.; Das, K.B.; Chin, R.F.; Aylett, S.E.; Burch, V.; Gillberg, C.; Scott, R.C.; Neville, B.G. Neurobehavioral Comorbidities in Children With Active Epilepsy: A Population-Based Study. *Pediatrics* **2014**, *133*, e1586–e1593. [CrossRef] [PubMed]
33. Stadskleiv, K. Cognitive functioning in children with cerebral palsy. *Dev. Med. Child Neurol.* **2020**, *62*, 283–289. [CrossRef] [PubMed]

Disclaimer/Publisher's Note: The statements, opinions and data contained in all publications are solely those of the individual author(s) and contributor(s) and not of MDPI and/or the editor(s). MDPI and/or the editor(s) disclaim responsibility for any injury to people or property resulting from any ideas, methods, instructions or products referred to in the content.

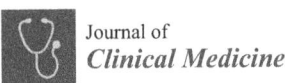

Article

Postoperative Airway Management after Submandibular Duct Relocation in 96 Drooling Children and Adolescents

Saskia E. Kok [1,*], Joris Lemson [2] and Frank J. A. van den Hoogen [1]

1. Department of Otolaryngology-Head and Neck Surgery, Radboud University Medical Center, P.O. Box 9101, 6500 HB Nijmegen, The Netherlands
2. Department of Paediatric Critical Care, Radboud University Medical Center, P.O. Box 9101, 6500 HB Nijmegen, The Netherlands
* Correspondence: saskia.kok@radboudumc.nl; Tel.: +31-(0)24-3614450

Abstract: The aim of this study was to evaluate our institutions airway management and complications after submandibular duct relocation (SMDR). We analysed a historic cohort of children and adolescents who were examined at the Multidisciplinary Saliva Control Centre between March 2005 and April 2016. Ninety-six patients underwent SMDR for excessive drooling. We studied details of the surgical procedure, postoperative swelling and other complications. Ninety-six patients, 62 males and 34 females, were treated consecutively by SMDR. Mean age at time of surgery was 14 years and 11 months. The ASA physical status was 2 in most patients. The majority of children were diagnosed with cerebral palsy (67.7%). Postoperative swelling of the floor of the mouth or tongue was reported in 31 patients (32.3%). The swelling was mild and transient in 22 patients (22.9%) but profound swelling was seen in nine patients (9.4%). In 4.2% of the patients the airway was compromised. In general, SMDR is a well-tolerated procedure, but we should be aware of swelling of the tongue and floor of the mouth. This may lead to a prolonged period of endotracheal intubation or a need for reintubation which can be challenging. After extensive intra-oral surgery such as SMDR we strongly recommend a extended perioperative intubation and extubation after the airway is checked and secure.

Keywords: Sialorrhea; cerebral palsy; submandibular duct relocation; postoperative management

1. Introduction

Drooling can be a serious problem in up to 58% of children and adolescents with cerebral palsy (CP) and other neurodevelopmental disabilities [1]. Unintentional loss of saliva may occur as a result of dysfunctional oral control, infrequent swallowing and diminished oral sensitivity [1]. This can cause physical discomfort (i.e., maceration of the skin) as well as emotional consequences (i.e., social isolation and lowered self-esteem). Different treatment options have been suggested in the past, such as oral motor therapy, behavioural treatment, systemic anticholinergic drugs, Botulinum Toxin injections and surgical treatments [1]. Although invasive, surgery is considered to be the most effective therapy to reduce drooling.

Submandibular duct relocation (SMDR) is a commonly performed procedure. During this procedure both submandibular ducts are relocated towards the base of the tongue and most often the sublingual glands are resected simultaneously. It involves relatively extensive floor of mouth surgery. Complications following this surgery may include postoperative pain, swelling of the submandibular gland, floor of the mouth and/or tongue, ranula formation, xerostomia, wound infection, inflammation of a salivary gland (sialadenitis), secondary bleeding or lingual nerve palsy [1–3]. Swelling of the floor of the mouth or tongue is a relatively common side effect reported by researchers, which could cause a life threatening airway obstruction in combination with difficult intubation conditions. Reintubation in an emergency setting is already challenging but in combination with severe swelling in the oral cavity and an often spastic, physically and mentally disabled child or young adult might make it impossible.

Although SMDR could cause a postoperative airway obstruction, most publications only briefly mention this potential life-threatening complication or do not describe it at all. A protocol of the postoperative period is rarely mentioned. To prevent airway obstruction in case of floor of the mouth swelling, children in our centre are admitted to a paediatric intensive care unit (PICU) and stay sedated and intubated for an extended period of time after surgery. Post-operative prolonged intubation protects the airway from obstruction to avoid potentially lethal respiratory problems in these already vulnerable children. Most children that we treat for drooling have physical and/or mental disabilities. They wake up after surgery and often do not understand what is happening. This could result in panic or distress, which may lead to increased movement and agitation. Manual manipulation of the intra-oral wounds or sutures may lead to haemorrhage. Disabilities of these children often make it difficult for them to follow our instructions.

The aim of this study is to investigate the complications of SMDR and evaluate if prolonged endotracheal intubation postoperatively is indicated to secure the airway.

2. Materials and Methods

2.1. Ethical Considerations

The present study was conducted in accordance with national and international ethical standards, and the Regional Committee on Research Involving Human Subjects approved the study. Before surgery informed consent was provided by caregivers for SMDR.

2.2. Patients

This study analysed a historic cohort of children and adolescents who were examined at the Multidisciplinary Saliva Control Centre of the Radboud university medical centre Nijmegen, the Netherlands, between March 2005 and April 2016. Ninety-nine patients had SMDR with simultaneous excision of the sublingual glands for excessive drooling. We excluded 3 patients because of their age (>24 years) [4]. All participants were considered to have a safe pharyngeal phase of swallowing. None of the children had previous surgical procedures of the floor of the mouth or for saliva control. Information was collected concerning age at time of surgery, duration of surgery, postoperative management, duration of intubation, and duration of hospital stay. Occurrence of tongue or floor of the mouth swelling, stridor, postoperative pneumonia and atelectasis were reviewed. Any other complications occurring during surgery or postoperatively were also identified. Co-morbidity was assessed preoperatively by an anaesthesiologist using the ASA physical status.

2.3. Procedure

All surgery were performed under general anaesthesia by the same surgeon. After the papillae of the submandibular ducts were located, the floor of the mouth was infiltrated with Xylocaine 2% with Epinephrine 1:80,000, and an incision was made to create two mucosal islands containing the papilla. The submandibular duct was freed from anterior to posterior, taking special care to prevent damage to the lingual nerve. The sublingual glands were resected bilaterally to prevent ranula formation. After submucosal re-routing of the submandibular ducts to the oropharynx, the papillae were sutured at the base of the tongue with a single stitch, posterior to the glossopharyngeal plica. Meticulous coagulation was performed. We routinely prescribed a 7-day postoperative course of antibiotics (amoxycilline/clavulanic acid) with 5 days of diclofenac for pain management [5].

Postoperative management changed in 2006. Before 2006 most patients returned to the ward after surgery. In 2005 a life-threatening complication occurred (airway obstruction due to postoperative haemorrhage), which led to a change in our standard protocol (meticulous bipolar coagulation, local anaesthetics with adrenalin, pre-emptive antibiotics and prolonged intubation with overnight PICU stay). Since 2006 patients were observed overnight at a PICU. Patients remained sedated and (endotracheally) intubated overnight.

The next day swelling of the floor of the mouth and tongue was evaluated by a resident ENT by intraoral assessment and in case of absent or minor swelling patients were extubated after weaning.

2.4. Statistical Analysis

Descriptive statistics were employed to summarize patient characteristics. All statistical analyses were performed using SPSS 20.0 for Windows (SPSS Inc, Chicago, IL, USA).

3. Results

Characteristics of the 96 patients included for analyses are shown in Table 1. The mean surgical time was 92 min (range 42–193 min), with a mean duration of hospital stay of 4 days (range 2–11 days). All patients were intubated using a nasotracheal cuffed tube. Sixty-two patients received pre-emptive steroids during or after surgery, of the remaining patients 30 did not receive steroids, and of four patients there were no records available. Ninety-three patients received antibiotic treatment during and after surgery, one patient did not receive antibiotics, and of two patients there are no records.

Table 1. Demographic data.

	No. Patients (Valid %) N = 96
Gender	
Male	62 (64.6%)
Female	34 (35.4%)
Age	
Mean (range)	14.9 (6–24)
Diagnosis	
Cerebral palsy [a]	
Bilateral paresis	61 (63.5%)
Unilateral paresis	4 (4.2%)
Other neurodevelopmental disabilities	31 (32.3%)
ASA grade	
1	11 (11.5%)
2	53 (55.2%)
3	30 (31.3%)
Unknown	2 (2.1%)
GMFCS level (N = 65)	
I	4 (6.2%)
II	8 (12.3%)
III	19 (29.2%)
IV	21 (32.3%)
V	13 (20.0%)
Epilepsy	
Controlled	43 (44.8%)
Intractable	15 (15.6%)
No epilepsy	38 (39.6%)
Developmental age	
<4 yrs	50 (52.1%)
4–6 yrs, IQ < 70	18 (18.8%)
4–6 yrs, IQ > 70	3 (3.1%)
>6 yrs	18 (18.8%)
Unknown	7 (7.3%)

[a] Confirmed by a paediatric neurologist. GMFCS = Gross Motor Function Classification System, only applicable for children with cerebral palsy; I = Able to walk, II = Difficulty with uneven surfaces, III = Walks with assistive mobility devices, IV = Walking ability severely limited with assistive devices, V = Impaired in all areas of motor function; IQ = Intelligence Quotient.

Six of the nine patients who had surgery in 2005, were extubated directly after surgery. Since January 2006 all children (N = 87) were admitted to an PICU with prolonged sedation and intubation after surgery. The mean duration of stay at the PICU was 33 h (range 8–148) with a mean duration of intubation of 24 h (range 3–96). One patient had an unplanned extubation, which was self-inflicted 3 h after surgery.

3.1. Complications concerning Airway Obstruction

A tree graph of complications is shown in Figure 1. Swelling of the floor of the mouth or tongue was reported in 31 patients (32.3%). The swelling was mild and transient in 22 patients (22.9%) and profound swelling was seen in nine patients (9.4%). Floor of the mouth swelling was mostly due to oedema. Haematoma was only reported in two patients. Minor bleeding occurred in one patient, which stopped spontaneously without swelling of the floor of the mouth. In one patient there were no records of swelling of the floor of the mouth. 9.7% of the patients who received pre-emptive steroid had profound swelling, 6.7% of the patients who did not receive pre-emptive steroids had profound swelling.

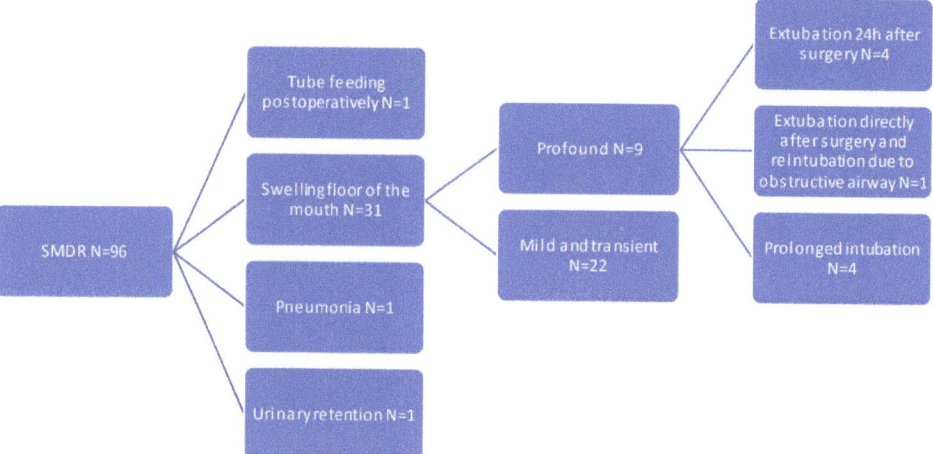

Figure 1. Complications. Tree graph of complications after SMDR.

In 2005 one of the patients, who was not admitted to a PICU immediately after surgery, developed profound swelling of the tongue and neck, stridor and increasing respiratory insufficiency within a few hours after surgery. The patient was rushed back to the OR, where an awake flexible nasotracheal intubation was performed and corticosteroids were given. The patient was admitted to the PICU, where he developed a pneumonia (possibly due to aspiration) and stayed on mechanical ventilation for five days. The intraoral swelling subsided and pneumonia was successfully treated with antibiotics. The patient left the hospital 7 days after surgery.

In four out of the nine patients with profound intraoral swelling, prolonged intubation was deemed necessary(4.2% of the 96 patients). These four patients were admitted to the PICU directly postoperatively according to protocol. Three patients had swelling of the floor of the mouth with tongue protrusion and were mechanically ventilated for 48 h, after which the swelling had decreased. During mechanical ventilation one of these patients developed a pneumonia, which was successfully treated with antibiotics. One patient had swelling of the neck and floor of the mouth with tongue protrusion due to a haematoma on the inferior part of the tongue and was mechanically ventilated for four days until the swelling subsided. No reintubations were necessary.

In four out of the nine patients with profound intraoral swelling, prolonged intubation was not deemed necessary (4.2% of the 96 patients). One patient had sufficient nasal flow/airway after extubation and was observed at the PICU for another 24 h, after which the swelling had settled. In three patients the swelling was more anterior or caudal and did not obstruct the airway.

3.2. Other Complications

Overall, patients experienced transient minor eating and drinking difficulties due to pain and discomfort after the surgery. One child had postoperative eating difficulties that necessitated tube feeding for three days. One child developed an atelectasis and postoperative pneumonia. One child experienced urinary retention one week postoperatively, which required suprapubic catheterization. None of the children suffered from ranulas or inflammation of the floor of the mouth. Four patients experienced transient minor nasal bleeding due to the nasotracheal intubation. One patient had a pressure ulcer located at the nose where the nasotracheal tube was positioned.

4. Discussion

SMDR is a well-tolerated procedure in children and adolescents. However, in our cohort almost 10% of these patients developed profound swelling of the tongue and floor of the mouth. In half of these cases a compromised airway was observed. Therefore, SMDR seems to justify prolonged postoperative intubation.

The strength of our study is the study sample size. Our study also has limitations, being the retrospective nature of the study, with a few missing data. We only provide descriptive statistics and did not have a control group. Our main goal of this study was to raise awareness of the risks involved in extensive floor of the mouth surgery related to postoperative airway control.

What is the role of SMDR in the broad spectrum of treatment options for excessive drooling? In our center a multidisciplinary team (a speech and language therapist, a psychologist, a paediatric neurologist, and an otorhinolaryngologist) evaluates all of these patients. In case of sufficient developmental age oral motor therapy and behavioral treatment could provide a good option. In young children who are not suitable for behavioral treatment with Botulinum Toxin injections can be effective. Botulinum Toxin injections reduce the amount of saliva by inhibiting the parasympathetic release of acetylcholine. This has shown to be effective in approximately 50% of children for 6–8 months. Although the effect is temporary, repeated injections are possible. If a more definitive solution is necessary surgery is an option. Our previous research showed that the effect of Botulinum Toxin injections is not a predictor for outcome of SMDR [6]. In our center children with safe oropharyngeal swallowing and non-progressive disease SMDR is the preferred surgical procedure. Due to the risk of aspiration in case of posterior drooling bilateral submandibular gland excision provides a good alternative [7]. If SMDR or submandibular gland excision have insufficient results, parotid duct ligation can be considered in addition.

Previous authors report that submandibular duct relocation with sublingual gland excision is a relatively safe procedure, though complications that could lead to airway obstruction are reported as well. Percentages reported of swelling of the floor of the mouth and airway obstruction vary between 1.4% and 25% [8–12]. Overall transient swelling of the tongue and floor of the mouth is mentioned by many authors. Although most studies describe the minor and major postoperative complications, preventions or treatment are scarcely mentioned.

Airway obstruction after floor of the mouth surgery can be a serious complication. PICU admittance with prolonged intubation and sedation prevents agitation in these children and can ease caregivers and surgeons'/anaesthesiologists' worries. Especially reintubation can be extremely difficult. With cerebral palsy being the leading diagnosis in this group of patients they already experience the effects of hypoxia on a daily basis.

On the other hand, prolonged intubation with or without mechanical ventilation has its disadvantages as well. Apart from the high costs associated with an overnight stay at a PICU ward, it also has an impact on parents and caregivers to see their child sedated and intubated on an PICU bed. Prolonged mechanical ventilation is mostly well tolerated, but has risks which could affect the health of the children. Mechanical ventilation could cause atelectasis, pulmonary oedema, pneumonia and (adult) respiratory distress syndrome [13]. With mechanical ventilation there is a need for sedation, which could cause withdrawal or delirium. It is important to avoid unnecessary mechanical ventilation. Also, there are sometimes a limited number of PICU beds available, which could result in OR planning problems or a need to reschedule surgery.

To date, no studies comparing postoperative PICU and non-PICU admission for SMDR have been performed. Without PICU admittance it is questionable where children after SMDR should be admitted. A child neurology ward has experience with these neurologically disabled children but has little knowledge of airway problems. An Ear, Nose, and Throat ward has knowledge about the procedure and airway problems but has little experience with these vulnerable children often requiring special care. Without a safe alternative, PICU admission might be the only option to maintain a safe airway postoperatively.

A relatively minor bleeding in the floor of the mouth could lead to substantial obstruction of the airway. In case of progressive swelling of the tongue or floor of the mouth a regular transoral intubation quickly becomes impossible. The remaining options in this case are awake flexible nasotracheal intubation or a challenging tracheotomy under local anaesthesia/anaesthetics. Both of these options are not desirable in neurologically disabled, often spastic, children. Cerebral palsy is often caused due to oxygen deprivation at birth. If awake flexible nasal intubation fails, there is a chance that an emergency tracheotomy has to be performed. A second time of oxygen deprivation should be avoided at all cost for both medical as well as emotional reasons.

The consequences if reintubation and a tracheotomy in a life-threatening situation fail are immense. There is no risk acceptable to possibly lose the life of one of these children. In our series it is reasonable to expect that the 4.2% that could not be extubated after prolonged intubation due to a compromised airway would have been candidates for a challenging reintubation in the event we had extubated them directly postoperatively. To lose a child with such a difficult airway in case reintubation fails is realistic and we can question whether it is justified to take such a risk.

Our study and the literature indicate that there is a reasonable risk of postoperative airway obstruction. In our view, the increased cost and added risk of minor complications associated with PICU admittance outweigh the risk of postoperative oral-oropharyngeal obstruction. As in most day-to-day situations, insurance against low-risk high-damage events is preferable over a higher risk of inconvenience. Therefore, we think postoperative PICU admittance is indicated.

Implications for Practice

SMDR is an effective treatment to decrease drooling in children and adolescents with developmental disabilities. However, our case series shows a significant risk of postoperative airway obstruction in 9.4% of the patients necessitating prolonged intubation in 4.2%. In order to prevent a life threatening airway compromise we recommend SMDR to be performed by an experienced surgeon with meticulous bipolar coagulation to prevent haemorrhage, local anaesthetics with adrenalin, pre-emptive antibiotics, overnight nasotracheal intubation and sedation. Only extubate the patient after the airway has been carefully checked. In case of profound swelling further prolonged intubation and treatment with steroids should be considered.

Author Contributions: S.E.K.: Design of the study, data acquisition and analysis, drafting and revising the article, final approval and agreement to be accountable. J.L.: Design of the study, interpretation of the analysis, revising the article critically, final approval and agreement to be accountable. F.J.A.v.d.H.: Design of the study, interpretation of the analysis, revising the article critically, final approval and agreement to be accountable. All authors have read and agreed to the published version of the manuscript.

Funding: This research received no external funding.

Institutional Review Board Statement: The study was conducted in accordance with the Declaration of Helsinki, and approved by the Institutional Review Board (or Ethics Committee) of Radboud University Nijmegen Medical Centre (protocol code 2022-16055 (25-11-2022).

Informed Consent Statement: Patient consent was waived due to the retrospective nature of the study and no patients can be identified.

Data Availability Statement: The data presented in this study are available on request from the corresponding author. The data are not publicly available due to privacy.

Conflicts of Interest: The authors declare no conflict of interest.

References

1. Walshe, M.; Smith, M.; Pennington, L. Interventions for drooling in children with cerebral palsy. *Cochrane Database Syst. Rev.* **2012**, *11*, CD008624. [PubMed]
2. Puraviappan, P.; Dass, D.; Narayanan, P. Efficacy of relocation of submandibular duct in cerebral palsy patients with drooling. *Asian J. Surg. /Asian Surg. Assoc.* **2007**, *30*, 209–215. [CrossRef] [PubMed]
3. ODwyer, T.P.; Conlon, B.J. The surgical management of drooling—A 15 year follow-up. *Clin. Otolaryngol.* **1997**, *22*, 284–287. [CrossRef] [PubMed]
4. Sawyer, S.M.; Azzopardi, P.S.; Wickremarathne, D.; Patton, G.C. The age of adolescence. *Lancet Child Adolesc. Health* **2018**, *2*, 223–228. [CrossRef] [PubMed]
5. Scheffer, A.R.; Erasmus, C.; VAN Hulst, K.; VAN Limbeek, J.; Rotteveel, J.J.; Jongerius, P.H.; Hoogen, F.J.V.D. Botulinum toxin versus submandibular duct relocation for severe drooling. *Dev. Med. Child Neurol.* **2010**, *52*, 1038–1042. [CrossRef] [PubMed]
6. Kok, S.E.; van Valenberg, H.F.J.P.; van Hulst, K.; Jongerius, P.; Erasmus, C.E.; van den Hoogen, F.J.A. Submandibular gland botulinum neurotoxin A injection for predicting the outcome of submandibular duct relocation in drooling: A retrospective cohort study. *Dev. Med. Child Neurol.* **2019**, *61*, 1323–1328. [CrossRef] [PubMed]
7. Delsing, C.P.; Cillessen, E.; Scheffer, A.; van Hulst, K.; Erasmus, C.E.; van den Hoogen, F.J. Bilateral submandibular gland excision for drooling: Our experience in twenty-six children and adolescents. *Clin. Otolaryngol.* **2015**, *40*, 285–290. [CrossRef] [PubMed]
8. Ethunandan, M.; Macpherson, D.W. Persistent drooling: Treatment by bilateral submandibular duct transposition and simultaneous sublingual gland excision. *Ann. R. Coll. Surg. Engl.* **1998**, *80*, 279–282. [PubMed]
9. Greensmith, A.L.; Johnstone, B.R.; Reid, S.; Hazard, C.J.; Johnson, H.M.; Reddihough, D.S. Prospective analysis of the outcome of surgical management of drooling in the pediatric population: A 10-year experience. *Plast. Reconstr. Surg.* **2005**, *116*, 1233–1242. [CrossRef] [PubMed]
10. Ekedahl, C.; Hallen, O. Quantitative Measurement of Drooling. *Acta Oto-Laryngol.* **1973**, *75*, 464–469. [CrossRef] [PubMed]
11. Webb, K.; Reddilwugh, D.S.; Johnson, H.; Bennett, C.S.; Byrt, T. Long-Term Outcome of Saliva-Control Surgery. *Dev. Med. Child Neurol.* **1995**, *37*, 755–762. [CrossRef] [PubMed]
12. Wilson, S.W.; Henderson, H.P. The surgical treatment of drooling in Leicester: 12 years experience. *Br. J. Plast. Surg.* **1999**, *52*, 335–338. [CrossRef] [PubMed]
13. Gajic, O.; Dara, S.I.; Mendez, J.L.; Adesanya, A.O.; Festic, E.; Caples, S.M.; Rana, R.; Sauver, J.S.; Lymp, J.F.; Afessa, B.; et al. Ventilator-associated lung injury in patients without acute lung injury at the onset of mechanical ventilation. *Crit. Care Med.* **2004**, *32*, 1817–1824. [CrossRef] [PubMed]

Disclaimer/Publisher's Note: The statements, opinions and data contained in all publications are solely those of the individual author(s) and contributor(s) and not of MDPI and/or the editor(s). MDPI and/or the editor(s) disclaim responsibility for any injury to people or property resulting from any ideas, methods, instructions or products referred to in the content.

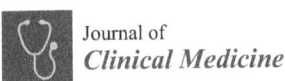

Journal of
Clinical Medicine

Article

Morphological Medial Gastrocnemius Muscle Growth in Ambulant Children with Spastic Cerebral Palsy: A Prospective Longitudinal Study

Nathalie De Beukelaer [1,*], Ines Vandekerckhove [1], Ester Huyghe [1], Geert Molenberghs [2,3], Nicky Peeters [1,4], Britta Hanssen [1,4], Els Ortibus [5], Anja Van Campenhout [6,7] and Kaat Desloovere [1,7]

1. Department of Rehabilitation Sciences, KU Leuven, 3000 Leuven, Belgium
2. Interuniversity Institute for Biostatistics and Statistical Bioinformatics (I-BIOSTAT), KU Leuven, 3000 Leuven, Belgium
3. Interuniversity Institute for Biostatistics and Statistical Bioinformatics (I-BIOSTAT), Data Science Institute, Hasselt University, 3590 Diepenbeek, Belgium
4. Department of Rehabilitation Sciences, Ghent University, 9000 Gent, Belgium
5. Department of Development and Regeneration, KU Leuven, 3000 Leuven, Belgium
6. Department of Orthopedics, University Hospitals Leuven, 3000 Leuven, Belgium
7. Clinical Motion Analysis Laboratory, University Hospitals Leuven, 3000 Leuven, Belgium
* Correspondence: nathalie.debeukelaer@kuleuven.be; Tel.: +32-474033110

Abstract: Only cross-sectional studies have demonstrated muscle deficits in children with spastic cerebral palsy (SCP). The impact of gross motor functional limitations on altered muscle growth remains unclear. This prospective longitudinal study modelled morphological muscle growth in 87 children with SCP (age range 6 months to 11 years, Gross Motor Function Classification System [GMFCS] level I/II/III = 47/22/18). Ultrasound assessments were performed during 2-year follow-up and repeated for a minimal interval of 6 months. Three-dimensional freehand ultrasound was applied to assess medial gastrocnemius muscle volume (MV), mid-belly cross-sectional area (CSA) and muscle belly length (ML). Non-linear mixed models compared trajectories of (normalized) muscle growth between GMFCS-I and GMFCS-II&III. MV and CSA growth trajectories showed a piecewise model with two breakpoints, with the highest growth before 2 years and negative growth rates after 6–9 years. Before 2 years, children with GMFCS-II&III already showed lower growth rates compared to GMFCS-I. From 2 to 9 years, the growth rates did not differ between GMFCS levels. After 9 years, a more pronounced reduction in normalized CSA was observed in GMFCS-II&III. Different trajectories in ML growth were shown between the GMFCS level subgroups. These longitudinal trajectories highlight monitoring of SCP muscle pathology from early ages and related to motor mobility. Treatment planning and goals should stimulate muscle growth.

Keywords: cerebral palsy; ultrasound; piecewise model; muscle volume; cross-sectional area; GMFCS

1. Introduction

Skeletal muscle changes are frequently manifested in children with spastic cerebral palsy (SCP) which interact with the neuromotor functioning throughout development [1–3]. However, the underlying mechanisms of this potential bilateral causations or associated presence remain unknown. Additionally, neuromotor impairments, such as spasticity and weakness, manifest from young ages, and result in heterogenous clinical presentations of children with SCP [1,4–7]. To classify the children based on functional abilities in daily life, the Gross Motor Function Classification System Expanded and Revised (GMFCS-E&R) is frequently used [8]. The 5 GMFCS levels are defined using standardized descriptions for which the lower levels indicate higher motor abilities. To reduce and manage the impact of neuromotor impairments on the daily motor functioning, children with SCP are frequently treated at the muscular level (e.g., botulinum neurotoxin injection or casting) from young ages [9].

In typical development, morphological muscle growth is triggered by body size increases and responds to the demands through protein synthesis [10–12]. However, for children with SCP, previous research highlighted lower increases in medial gastrocnemius (MG) muscle volume (MV) with increasing age, which was unrelated to the rate of skeletal growth and already presented at the age of 15 months [13]. Taking body length and mass into account, MVs were found to reduce by 3% over a 6-month follow-up period in 2–5 years old children with SCP [14]. Over the age ranges of 2 to 12 years, cross-sectional investigations identified normalized medial gastrocnemius MV deficits of 22–57% and shorter normalized muscle belly lengths (MLs) with deficits of 11–19% compared to age-matched typically developing (TD) children [15–19]. Since the muscle is a very plastic tissue, the observed muscular changes in SCP could reflect adaptations to the functional demands including altered muscle tone and limited motor functioning [12]. Indeed, previous cross-sectional studies demonstrated increasing muscle pathology, such as deficits in MV, anatomical cross-sectional area (CSA) and ML, in relation to higher GMFCS levels [8,13,18,20,21]. Yet, research to date has not determined the impact of the severity in motor impairments on the trajectory of altered muscle growth. Overall, these previous cross-sectional observations highlighted significant alterations in the SCP muscle from a young age, which were suggested to be multifactorial in origin, for example due to impaired neural activation, inflammation and altered or non-use of the muscle [3,12,22–24].

Up to now, cross-sectional investigations have already suggested altered associations between muscle morphology and age in SCP versus TD children [13,16]. These previous studies assumed a linear trajectory of morphological muscle growth with age. However, much uncertainty remains in the variability of the trajectories for altered muscle growth over the time-span from infancy to school ages and between different levels of severity in children with SCP [13,16,25]. Further, MV is frequently reported apart from the estimates of muscle growth in the cross-sectional dimension (e.g., CSA) and longitudinal dimension (e.g., ML). To delineate the muscle growth trajectories, repeated assessments over time per individual are required. These longitudinal datasets generate child-specific profiles per morphological measure. A better understanding of this time course may shed light on opportunities for the planning, development and promotion of muscle growth strategies, whether or not combined with the conventional therapeutic strategies.

The current prospective longitudinal study investigated morphological MG muscle growth over a wide age span, including infants (6 months–2 years), preschool (2–5 years) and school-aged SCP-children (6–11 years). The first objective was to model the muscle growth trajectory with respect to age by using repeated muscle assessments. Growth in the MG muscle morphology was expressed for different absolute and normalized outcomes. Second, we aimed to compare the trajectories in muscle growth between the GMFCS levels I and II–III. We hypothesized gradually increased morphological muscle outcomes (i.e., muscle volume, mid-belly cross-sectional area and belly length) with increasing age, with lower muscle growth rates in children of the higher GMFCS levels.

2. Materials and Methods

2.1. Study Design and Participants

This prospective, observational cohort study was designed with a prospective longitudinal research protocol of repeated assessments and was conducted between April 2018 and March 2022. Over a follow-up period of 2 years, predefined intervals of minimal 6 months up to 2 years were set between the repeated assessments. These intervals further depended on the timing of the regular clinical follow-up appointment during which the assessments were performed. As a result, the observational data was included with 2 to 5 assessments per child. Via the Clinical Motion Analysis Laboratory (CMAL-Pellenberg) and Cerebral Palsy Reference Center of the University Hospitals Leuven, children with a diagnosis of SCP confirmed by a paediatric neurologist, were recruited. SCP-children aged between 6 months and 9 years at baseline, with bi- or unilateral involvement and with GMFCS-E&R levels I to III, defined by the criteria per age-band [26], were included. Additionally, the following exclusion criteria were applied at baseline and during follow-up: (a) Botulinum neurotoxin type A (BoNT-A) treatment 10 months prior to the assessment (b) serial casting 3 months prior to assessment and (c) history of orthopedic and/or neurosurgery. Considering potential change in GMFCS level over time, which could be expected by consequence of motor development, especially at the youngest ages, the GMFCS level at the last assessment was used to define subgroups. These subgroups, i.e., GMFCS level I vs. level II & III, were selected to maximize the number of observations per group and to reduce heterogeneity [7,27]. For the latter, it has been described that children with GMFCS level I are more stable in motor function in comparison to children with levels II and III, and this stability is found to be already established by the age of four years [7,27]. To illustrate muscle deficits in the children with SCP, a retrospective dataset of cross-sectional assessments in age-matched TD children were selected from the established reference database at the CMAL-Pellenberg. This database included TD children with no history of neurological, neuromuscular or orthopedic disorders. Criteria for selecting the TD children for the current study were: (a) aged between 6 months and 9 years old and (b) assessments collected with similar measurement equipment and protocol as applied for the SCP participants. The study protocol was approved by the Ethical Commission UZ/KU Leuven, Leuven, Belgium (S59945, S62187, S62645) and registered (NCT05197764). Written informed consent was obtained for all participants.

2.2. Measurements

The three-dimensional freehand ultrasound (3DfUS), combining a conventional 2D US device and a motion tracking system, was used. This technique has proven to be valid and reliable for measuring healthy and pathological muscles, even from early ages [13,28–30]. The US device settings were kept constant throughout the study period. Details on the 3DfUS equipment and measurement protocol are given in previous studies [19,20]. While positioned in prone, the most affected leg was measured in all SCP participants, whereas a random leg was selected for TD children. The most affected leg was defined according to the MG spasticity and ankle joint range of motion (ROM) measured during a standardized clinical examination (Modified Ashworth Scale and goniometry, respectively) at the time of the baseline assessment [31]. The assessed leg remained the same for all follow-up assessments. Three experienced researchers were involved in the assessments with only 2 researchers for the same participant. Two of these researchers undertook the data processing, one of whom performed the data analysis. During the processing of the US images, the researchers were blinded to the GMFCS levels and timing of the assessment. All involved researchers were extensively trained in the CMAL research group and followed predefined guidelines and regular meetings to maximize similarities in the prescribed acquisition and processing workflow [32]. The inter-rater and intra-rater inter-session reliability was previously demonstrated with an intra-class correlation of minimal 0.95 [33]. Furthermore, the Portico (i.e., concave-shaped holder combined with concave gel pad) was used to minimize inter-acquire differences in probe pressure [34]. STRADWIN software (Version 6.0, Mechanical Engineering, Cambridge, UK) was used for both data acquisition and processing. MV (in mL) was defined by manually drawing muscle segmentations alongside the inner muscle border, starting from the medial femoral condyle until the last image of the muscle belly before approaching the muscle tendon junction. Subsequently, a cubic planimetry technique was applied for interpolation of the defined segmentations [35]. The mid-belly segmented anatomical CSA was extracted and is further referred to as the CSA (in mm^2). The ML of the MG muscle (in mm) was defined as the Euclidean distance between the muscle origin at the most superficial aspect of the medial femoral condyle and the muscle tendon junction. Accounting for inter-individual anthropometric variability and in line with previous studies, ratio scaling was applied for which the MV was normalized to the product of body mass and length (nMV, mL/(kg·m)), CSA to body mass (nCSA, mm^2/kg) and ML to body length (nML, %) [14,36].

2.3. Statistical Analysis

Participant characteristics and muscle outcomes at the baseline assessment were summarized by descriptive statistics reporting frequencies and median (interquartile ranges, IQ1-IQ3). Non-normality was confirmed with Shapiro–Wilk's test. Two subgroups considering the motor impairments were used: subgroup 1, GMFCS level I and subgroup 2, GMFCS level II & III. To model the change in muscle morphology with respect to age, non-linear mixed models were used [37,38]. These models accommodate (a) unbalanced longitudinal datasets, resulting from variable spacing of follow-up intervals and different numbers of follow-up assessments among the children with SCP, and (b) the correlation between the repeated assessments taking the variance between and within the children with SCP into account. Fixed effects were (a) the age (expressed in years) at the time of assessments within each child, representing the time-effect and (b) covariate, representing GMFCS with its specific subgroups to describe within-group and compare between-group changes in the muscle growth. Random intercepts were added to model the variability in the starting point between the children with SCP. To capture the changes in the trajectory of morphological muscle growth with age, piecewise models were allowed. The following workflow was used to construct these models: first, the average trend (i.e., mean structure) was explored by performing Loess regressions and by plotting the observed individual longitudinal trajectories. These explorations suggested piecewise trends, i.e., constatation of linear trends interrupted by breaking points. Second, residual trajectories calculated from the Loess regressions and the observed variance function (i.e., the change of the squared residuals over time) were explored, to define the random-effect structure. A random intercept was selected based on the exploration closely approaching a constant variance. Estimated starting values from the graphical explorations were used in the logistic piecewise models to obtain the predicted intercept, regression coefficients, breakpoints at specific ages, variance of the random intercept and measurement error.

The observed morphological outcomes included the MV, nMV, CSA, nCSA, ML and nML. The model with the jth observation in child i for GMFCS group g (GMFCS I = $_I$ and GMFCS II–III = $_{II-III}$ to estimate the response was described as follows:

$$\text{Respons}_{ijg} = (\alpha_0 g + a1i g) + \beta_1 g * age_{ijg} + \varepsilon_{(1)ijg} \qquad \text{if age} < c_1$$
$$\text{Respons}_{ijg} = (\alpha_0 g + a1i g) + c_1 g * (\beta_1 g - \beta_2 g) + \beta_2 g * age_{ijg} + \varepsilon_{(1)ijg} \qquad \text{if } c_1 \leq age < c_2$$
$$\text{Respons}_{ijg} = (\alpha_0 g + a1i g) + c_1 g * (\beta_1 g - \beta_2 g) + c_2 g * (\beta_2 g - \beta_3 g) + \beta_3 g * age_{ijg} + \varepsilon_{(1)ijg} \qquad \text{if age} \geq c_2$$

With α_0 = intercept; $a1i$ = random intercept; c_1 = first breakpoint; c_2 = second breakpoint; β_1 = regression coefficient of the slope before first breakpoint; β_2 = regression coefficient of the slope after first breakpoint and before second breakpoint; β_3 = regression coefficient of the slope after second breakpoint; $\varepsilon_{(1)ijg}$ = measurement error.

An F-test was used to test (a) if the slopes and the breakpoints differ from zero, and (b) if the slopes before and after the breakpoint differ from each other, confirming the non-linear trajectory. After formulating the piecewise regression model, so-called empirical Bayes estimates were calculated and used to assess the potential presence of outliers, i.e., patients with an "exceptional" starting point and evolution over time. Further, the F-test was used to compare the regression coefficients and breakpoints within and between the GMFCS groups. p-values were set at <0.05.

To enhance interpretation of the intercept, the age at all assessments was subtracted by 2 years, and therefore, the intercept represented the response's value at the age of 2 years. The regression coefficients of the slope represent the magnitude of response in morphological muscle growth per year. The observed individual outcomes, observed individual trajectories, predicted individual trajectories and predicted average trajectory per morphological muscle outcome were plotted. The observed individual trajectories were also presented per GMFCS level, providing descriptive results per GMFCS level (Figure S1). The individual observed outcomes of 102 TD children were visualized with grey dots combined with boxplots for median (interquartile ranges) per 1-year age groups, illustrating a cross-sectional reference dataset compared to the longitudinal trajectories of the SCP children. For the TD children, the median cross-sectional growth rate for a specific age range was calculated as the median of the muscle outcome divided by the median age. Illustrations of morphological growth trajectories in each GMFCS group of the children with SCP compared to a retrospective dataset of cross-sectional assessments in TD children were added in Figure S2 and Table S1. All analyses were performed in SAS® (Statistical Analysis Software version 9.4, SAS Institute Inc., Cary, NC, USA).

3. Results

Patient characteristics at the time of baseline assessment are summarized in Table 1. At the end of the follow-up, muscle data was collected until 10.3 years for GMFCS I and 11.1 years for GMFCS II–III (Figure 1). Only nine children changed from GMFCS level during the follow-up for which the re-classification was performed around 2–3 years of age. The study sample received standardized clinical care such as regular physical therapy, orthotic devices and medical and orthopedic services (e.g., serial casting and/or BoNT-A injections when indicated) within a multidisciplinary clinical setting (Table S2). The results of the piecewise models for the subgroups in GMFCS levels are summarized in Table 2, Figure 2 and Table S3. The comparisons of slopes and breakpoints between the groups are presented in Table 3.

Table 1. Participant characteristics of the children with SCP at baseline assessment.

Group	GMFCS I	GMFCS II–III
Participants	47	40
Observations	130	104
Sex (male/female)	25/22	21/19
GMFCS level (I/II/III)	47/0/0	0/22/18
Involvement (unilateral/bilateral)	37/10	14 (II, = 10 & III = 4)/26 (II = 12 & III = 14)
History of BoNT-A injection	11	7
Antropometric & muscle outcomes		
Age (y)	4.66 (2.25–6.83)	2.88 (1.47–4.81)
Body mass (kg)	18.0 (13.0–22.0)	12.5 (10.0–16.4)
Body length (cm)	104.7 (88.5–121.1)	90.0 (77.8–106.0)
MV (mL)	28.2 (16.7–38.4)	13.6 (7.4–25.5)
CSA (mm^2)	335.6 (260.1–392.1)	205.5 (162.3–285.8)
ML (mm)	127.1 (99.2–144.9)	96.0 (82.8–127.1)
nMV (mL/kg·m)	1.45 (1.26–1.58)	1.12 (0.92–1.39)
nCSA (mm^2/kg)	19.4 (16.1–22.1)	16.1 (13.8–19.0)
nML (%)	11.7 (11.3–12.6)	10.9 (9.8–11.9)

The frequencies are presented for the general characteristics. Anthropometric and muscle data are presented as median (interquartile 1–interquartile 3). SCP, spastic cerebral palsy; GMFCS, gross motor function classification system; BoNT-A, botulinum neurotoxin type A; y, years; kg, kilogram; cm, centimeter; MV, muscle volume; ml, milliliter; CSA, anatomical cross-sectional area; mm, millimeter; ML, muscle belly length; n, normalized; kg, kilogram; m, meter.

For the GMFCS Level I group, the MV increased with 12.8 mL/year (β_1, $p < 0.0001$) up to 2.1 years of age (c_1). After these infant ages, an MV increase of 5.7 mL/year was found until the age of 7.8 years (β_2, $p < 0.0001$ and c_2, respectively). From this second breakpoint at these older ages, a growth rate of 3.1 mL/year was found (β_3, $p = 0.0024$) which was significantly lower compared to growth rates for the younger ages (β_1 vs. β_3 and β_2 vs. β_3, $p < 0.05$, Table S3). On the other hand, after an increase in nMV of 0.83 mL/kg·m per year until 2.1 years, the nMV showed a non-significant rate of -0.03 mL/kg·m per year until the age of 8.0 years (β_2, $p = 0.0933$ and c_2). After this second breakpoint, a rate of -0.12 mL/kg·m per year was found (β_3, $p < 0.0001$) for which this linear trend showed significantly more decline compared to the muscle growth rates before 2 years and between 2 and 8 years old (β_1 vs. β_3 and β_2 vs. β_3, $p < 0.05$, Table S3). Similar to the growth rate in MV, the trajectory of CSA growth showed two breakpoints (age 2.2 years and 6.7 years, respectively) with only in the first and second linear trend, a significant yearly increase in CSA ($\beta_1 = 158.4$ mm^2/year, $p < 0.0001$; $\beta_2 = 37.0$ mm^2/year, $p < 0.0001$, respectively). The nCSA trajectory showed after an increase of 8.88 mm^2/kg per year only 1 breakpoint at the age of 2.1 years followed by decrease in nCSA per year (c_1 and $\beta_2 = -0.96$ mm^2/kg per year, $p < 0.0001$, respectively).

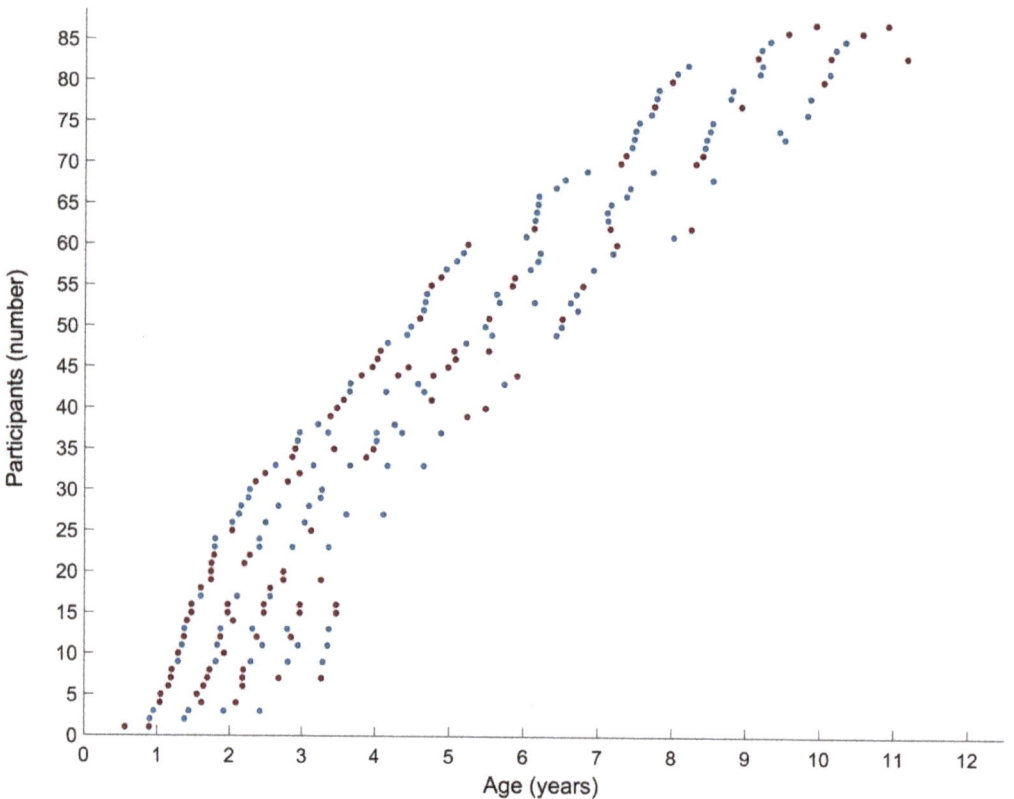

Figure 1. Representation of the number of the performed longitudinal assessments at the different ages for the group of children with spastic cerebral palsy (SCP) ($n = 87$) of gross motor function classification system level I (blue) versus levels II–III (red). The x-axis represents the ages at the time of the repeated assessment. On the y-axis, each participant is represented on one line, with each dot representing the performed assessments. The children were further ordered with increasing age. The group of GMFCS level I included 47 children with a total of 130 assessments (average (range) of 2.8 (2–5) assessments per child and average time of 10 months (4–25 months) between the assessments. The group of GMFCS level II–III included 40 children with a total of 104 assessments (average (range) of 2.6 (2–5) assessments per child and average time of 9 months (4–25 months) between the assessments).

Table 2. Fixed effects of the piecewise model for muscle morphology in GMFCS subgroups (level I, $n = 47$; levels II–III, $n = 40$).

Outcome	Participants	Intercept α_0	Regression Coefficients (β) and Breakpoints (c)				
			β_1 (CI) p-Value	c_1	β_2 (CI) p-Value	c_2	β_3 (CI) p-Value
MV	GMFCS I	13.2	12.8 (8.4–17.1) <0.0001	2.12 *	5.7 (4.6–6.7) <0.0001	7.82 *	3.1 (1.1–5.1) 0.0024
		α_0	β_1 (CI) p-value			c_1	β_2 (CI) p-value
	GMFCS II–III	11.1 *	4.5 (3.8–5.2) <0.0001			9.13 *	−0.8 (−5.1–3.5) 0.7154
		α_0	β_1 (CI) p-value	c_1	β_2 (CI) p-value	c_2	β_3 (CI) p-value
nMV	GMFCS I	1.57*	0.83 (0.55–1.11) <0.0001	2.11 *	−0.03 (−0.07–−0.01) 0.0933	8.04 *	−0.12 (−0.18–−0.06) <0.0001
		α_0	β_1 (CI) p-value	c_1	β_2 (CI) p-value		
	GMFCS II–III	1.25 *	0.28 (0.14–0.42) <0.0001	2.69 *	−0.07 (−0.10–−0.03) 0.0003		
		α_0	β_1 (CI) p-value	c_1	β_2 (CI) p-value	c_2	β_3 (CI) p-value
CSA	GMFCS I	241.1 *	158.4 (115.6–201.2) <0.0001	2.18 *	37.0 (23.1–50.9) <0.0001	6.71 *	6.96 (−8.35–22.3) 0.3688
	GMFCS II–III	209.5 *	88.6 (0.99–1.38) <0.0001	2.27	29.8 (4.62–6.80) <0.0001	9.13 *	−28.3 (−66.8–10.3) 0.1483
		α_0	β_1 (CI) p-value	c_1	β_2 (CI) p-value		
nCSA	GMFCS I	22.4 *	8.88 (5.42–12.3) <0.0001	2.09 *	−0.96 (−1.38–−0.54) <0.0001		
		α_0	β_1 (CI) p-value	c_1	β_2 (CI) p-value	c_2	β_3 (CI) p-value
	GMFCS II–III	18.4 *	2.70 (0.21–5.19) 0.0336	2.70 *	−0.86 (−3.89–−1.14) 0.0138	9.13 *	−2.52 (−3.89–−1.14) 0.0005
		α_0	β_1 (CI) p-value	c_1	β_2 (CI) p-value		
ML	GMFCS I	95.9 *	14.2 (12.2–16.3) <0.0001	5.11 *	6.80 (4.57–9.02) <0.0001		
	GMFCS II–III	91.3 *	18.8 (11.2–26.5) <0.0001	2.10 *	8.59 (7.56–9.62) <0.0001		
nML	GMFCS I	11.7 *	0.33 (0.07–0.58) 0.0125	5.13 *	−0.10 (−0.26–0.06) 0.1977		
			β_1 (CI) p-value				
	GMFCS II–III	10.8 *	0.12 (0.03–0.21) 0.0096				

The asterisks (*) indicate significance level at $p < 0.05$ for α and c. p-values in bold indicate significance level at $p < 0.05$. The following symbols represent: α = outcome at the age of 2 years, β = rate of change in muscle outcome per year, and c = age (years) of the breakpoint. The numbers (in subscript) associated with symbols β and c refer to the order of the observed growth ratio and breakpoint, respectively, e.g., β_1 as the first ratio before the c_1, the first breakpoint. SCP, spastic cerebral palsy; GMFCS, gross motor function classification system; n, number; CI 95% confidence interval; MV, muscle volume; n, normalized; CSA, anatomical cross-sectional area; ML, muscle belly length.

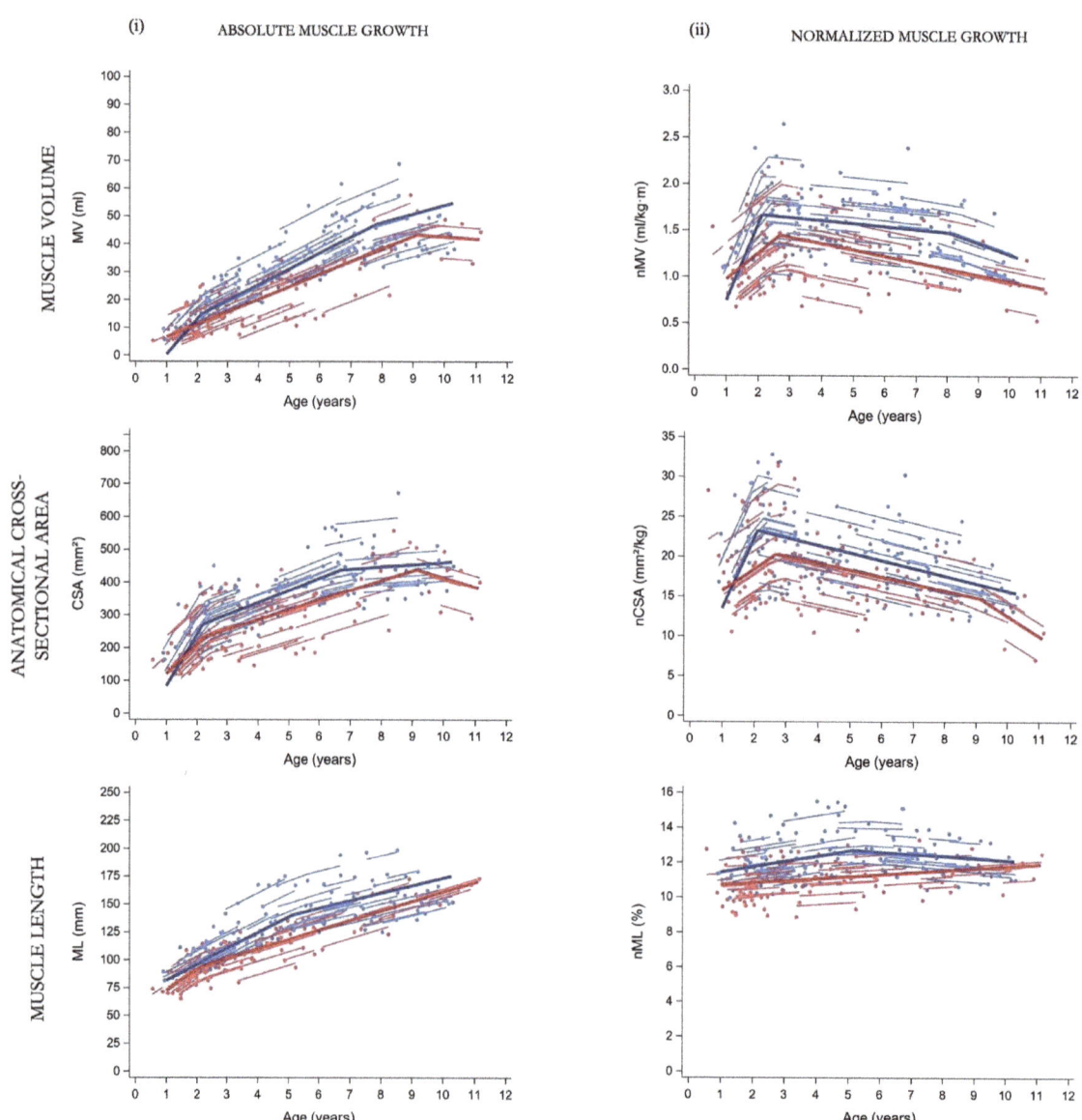

Figure 2. Predicted average trajectories (bold solid line) for the (**i**) absolute and (**ii**) normalized muscle morphology in SCP children with GMFCS level I (blue) and GMFCS level II–III (red). Observed outcomes (dots) and individual predicted trajectories (lines) are presented. SCP, spastic cerebral palsy; GMFCS, gross motor function classification system; MV, muscle volume; ml, milliliter; CSA, anatomical cross-sectional area; mm, millimeter; ML, muscle belly length; n, normalized; kg, kilogram; m, meters.

Table 3. Results of the comparison in slopes and breakpoints between the GMFCS subgroups.

Outcome	GMFCS I vs. II–III	Δ	p-Value
MV	$\beta_{1,I}$ vs. $\beta_{1,II-III}$	8.24	**0.0003**
	$\beta_{2,I}$ vs. $\beta_{1,II-III}$	1.16	0.0712
	$\beta_{3,I}$ vs. $\beta_{2,II-III}$	3.91	0.1069
	$c_{2,I}$ vs. $c_{1,II-III}$	1.31	**0.0326**
nMV	$\beta_{1,I}$ vs. $\beta_{1,II-III}$	0.55	**0.0007**
	$\beta_{2,I}$ vs. $\beta_{2,II-III}$	0.04	0.1710
	$\beta_{3,I}$ vs. $\beta_{2,II-III}$	0.05	0.1272
	$c_{1,I}$ vs. $c_{1,II-III}$	0.58	**0.0040**
	$\alpha_{1,I}$ vs. $\alpha_{1,II-III}$	0.32	**0.0056**
CSA	$\beta_{1,I}$ vs. $\beta_{1,II-III}$	69.8	**0.0112**
	$\beta_{2,I}$ vs. $\beta_{2,II-III}$	7.17	0.4328
	$\beta_{3,I}$ vs. $\beta_{3,II-III}$	35.2	0.0915
	$c_{1,I}$ vs. $c_{1,II-III}$	0.09	0.3783
	$c_{2,I}$ vs. $c_{2,II-III}$	2.66	**0.0033**
nCSA	$\beta_{1,I}$ vs. $\beta_{1,II-III}$	6.18	**0.0039**
	$\beta_{2,I}$ vs. $\beta_{2,II-III}$	−0.09	0.8168
	$\beta_{2,I}$ vs. $\beta_{3,II-III}$	1.56	**0.0334**
	$c_{1,I}$ vs. $c_{1,II-III}$	0.61	0.1152
	$\alpha_{0,I}$ vs. $\alpha_{0,II-III}$	3.97	**0.0063**
ML	$\beta_{1,I}$ vs. $\beta_{1,II-III}$	−4.61	0.2482
	$\beta_{2,I}$ vs. $\beta_{2,II-III}$	−1.79	0.1384
	$c_{1,I}$ vs. $c_{1,II-III}$	−3.01	**<0.001**
nML	$\beta_{1,I}$ vs. $\beta_{1,II-III}$	0.21	0.1311
	$\beta_{2,I}$ vs. $\beta_{1,II-III}$	−0.22	**0.0146**
	$\alpha_{0,I}$ vs. $\alpha_{0,II-III}$	0.91	**0.0024**

p-values in bold indicate significance level at $p < 0.05$. The following symbols represent: α = outcome at the age of 2 years, β = rate of change in muscle outcome per year, c = age (years) of the breakpoint, Δ = difference score, I = GMFCS level I and II–III = GMFCS level II & III. The numbers (in subscript) associated with symbols β and c refer to the order of the observed growth ratio and breakpoint, respectively, e.g., β_1 as the first ratio before the c_1, the first breakpoint; GMFCS, gross motor function classification system; MV, muscle volume; n, normalized; CSA, anatomical cross-sectional area; ML, muscle belly length.

After a significant MV increase with a rate of 4.5 mL/year (β_1, $p < 0.0001$), children in the GMFCS level II–III group showed only a breakpoint at the age of 9.1 years (c_1) which was followed by a rate of −0.8 mL/year (β_2, $p = 0.7154$). The nMV showed increases of 0.28 mL/kg·m per year until the breakpoint at the age of 2.7 years (c_1) and followed by decreases of 0.07 mL/kg·m per year (β_2, $p = 0.0003$). The trajectories for absolute and normalized CSA were modelled with two breakpoints, around approximately 2 and 9 years of age. During the (pre)school ages, nCSA decreased with significantly higher decline after the age of 9.1 years (β_2 vs. β_3, $p = 0.0424$, Table S3).

Before the age of 2 years, children with GMFCS level I showed significantly higher yearly increases for both absolute and normalized MV and CSA compared to level II–III ($\beta_{1, GMFCS-I}$ vs. $\beta_{1, GMFCS-II-III}$, Table 3, $p < 0.05$). After the age of 2 years, absolute MV and CSA were significantly increasing in both GMFCS subgroups until the age of 6–9 years old. However, GMFCS level I tended to have a higher absolute MV growth rate compared to GMFCS level II–III ($\beta_{2, GMFCS-I}$ vs. $\beta_{1, GMFCS-II-III}$ =1.16 mL/year, $p = 0.0712$). Despite the significant earlier second breakpoint for GMFCS levels I (Δ1.31 years for MV, $p = 0.0326$ and Δ2.66 years for CSA, $p = 0.0033$), no significant differences were found in the MV and CSA growth rate at these oldest ages between the GMFCS subgroups ($\beta_{3, GMFCS-I}$ vs. $\beta_{2, GMFCS-II-III}$, $p = 0.1069$ and $\beta_{3, GMFCS-I}$ vs. $\beta_{3, GMFCS-II-III}$, $p = 0.0915$, respectively). The trajectory for nMV and nCSA showed decreased rates from the age of 2 years in both GMFCS groups, with a significant higher decline in nCSA in children with GMFCS level II–III after the age of 6–9 years compared to level I ($\beta_{2, GMFCS-I}$ vs. $\beta_{3, GMFCS-II-III}$, $p = 0.0334$).

Absolute ML increased with age, with significantly lower ML growth rate after the age of 5.11 years in the GMFCS level I and after the age of 2.1 years in GMFCS levels II–III (β_1 vs. β_2, $p < 0.05$). Normalized ML showed significant different rates with increasing age between the GMFCS groups, for which the GMFCS levels I increased with 0.33%/year until 4.88 years (β_1, $p = 0.0125$) followed by a rate of -0.10%/year (β_2, $p = 0.1977$), whereas the levels II–III increased in nML with 0.12% per year from infancy to school ages, without a breakpoint (β_1, $p = 0.0096$).

4. Discussion

In this prospective longitudinal follow-up between 6 months and 11 years of age, the trajectory of morphological muscle growth for children with SCP was observed as piecewise profiles with increasing age, indicating linear trends interrupted with breakpoints. Therefore, our hypothesis of gradual increases in muscle morphology with increasing age could only be partially accepted as expressed by the changes in observed yearly muscle growth rates before and after the breakpoints. Indeed, MV and CSA significantly increased before the age of 2 years but this was followed by slower increases until the age of 6–7 years for GMFCS level I and 9 years for GMFCS level II–III. Normalized MV and CSA also increased during infancy but showed already reduced growth rates after the age of 2 years. Furthermore, from 8–9 years of age, both the absolute and normalized MV and CSA outcomes reduced per year, which is in contrast with the hypothesis of a linear trajectory of muscle growth with increasing age. Absolute ML increased over the entire age range with a breakpoint at the age of 5 years for GMFCS level I and 2 years for GMFCS level II–III, whereas nML showed less increase after this age for GMFCS level I. Lower muscle growth rates with increasing age in children of the higher GMFCS levels was hypothesized and was only confirmed for the absolute morphological growth before the age of 2 years and in teenagers. Next, the normalized MV and CSA outcomes reduced per year with a more pronounced decrease in CSA normalized to changes in body dimensions for GMFCS level II–III. Further, ML trajectories were different between the GMFCS levels and more specific, after normalization for skeletal growth.

These results revealed higher rate of muscle growth in early years of life, with lower growth rates for children with GMFCS level II–III compared to GMFCS level I. During these youngest ages, the current MV increased with 12.8 mL per year for GMFCS level I, which was slightly higher compared to the median growth rate of 10.3 mL per year. This growth rate is computed by dividing the average MV of 15.45 mL to the time period of 1.5 years to represent the 6 months to 2 years old TD children of our retrospective cross-sectional database (Figure S2 and Table S1). Only one previous study reported a cross-sectional growth rate for 8 months to 5-years-old children, with 8.16 mL/year for TD and 3.84 mL/year for CP children [13]. The latter is comparable to the growth rate of 4.5 mL/year in the current GMFCS level II–III children suggesting an early onset of more pronounced growth deficits in children with more severe impairments. Furthermore, the nMV rates of 0.83 mL/(kg·m) and 0.28 mL/(kg·m) per year were lower than our cross-sectional TD growth rate of 1.17 mL/(kg·m) per year. No growth rates for nMV during early ages have been previously reported. Nevertheless, growth rate calculated on cross-sectional datasets assumed linear growth, whereas the current results revealed non-linear trajectories of muscle growth with increasing age. However, caution is warranted with the interpretation of observed increases in normalized muscle data. In the case of optimal normalization for changes in body sizes, growth rates close to zero are expected, representing harmonization between muscle and anthropometric growth [39]. The validity of ratio-scaling in growing TD children, over a wide age range, has not yet been defined. The body composition in children is assumed to change with less amount of fat mass after the age of 2 years. Hence, normalization by taking body mass into account is considered invalid during infancy [40]. Further, significantly lower intercepts for nMV, nCSA and nML indicated that children with less motor abilities develop more muscle pathology already early in life (Table 3). These observations suggest early mechanisms hampering the muscle growth, such as the contribution of neural alterations as a result of the brain lesion as well as altered patterns of muscle use. However, limited muscle data on TD infants is available to compare the current suggestion of an early onset of muscle alterations, especially in GMFCS levels II–III. Further research also involving longitudinal assessments of TD infants is required to explore the impact of normalization techniques and provide valid references to investigate the onset and development of muscle alterations in infants with SCP.

Interestingly, from 2 years of age, similar muscle growth trajectories in (normalized) MV and CSA for the GMFCS subgroups were found. The average MV rates of 5.1 mL/year and 4.5 mL/year in GMFCS level I and level II–III, respectively, were comparable to earlier reported MV growth rates based on 6 months and 12 months follow-up studies in 2–5 years old children with SCP (6.0 mL/year and 6.6 mL/year, respectively) [14,41]. Furthermore, hampered morphological muscle growth is more clearly highlighted by investigating the changes in normalized MV and CSA compared to the investigation of the absolute parameters. It should be noted that altered anthropometric growth indicated by shorter body length and lower body mass, have already been shown in children with SCP compared to TD peers [42]. These growth deficits were found to be associated with increasing age, as well as with bilateral involvement and more severe gross motor impairments [43]. Although anthropometric growth in children with minor motor impairments is close to age-matched TD peers [42], the significant negative normalized muscle growth rates observed in the current study for the GMFCS level I group showed that the muscle growth was not in accordance with the skeletal growth. Since muscle morphological growth is assumed to be triggered by anthropometric growth and patterns of muscle use which might be defined by the gross motor functional abilities, the observed early presence of muscle pathology for GMFCS level II–III and increasing deficits after accounting for normalization to changes in body dimensions suggest that pathology-related biomechanical triggers contribute to hampered muscle growth.

From the age of 6–9 years, hampered muscle growth was presented in both GMFCS groups. Despite the lower number of data points at these older ages for children with GMFCS levels I, the level of gross motor mobility in daily life is suggested to further contribute to hampered growth as shown by the tendency of lower CSA growth and significantly lower nCSA growth for GMFCS level II–III compared to level I. These findings are in line with cross-sectional observations of significantly smaller MV and CSA in GMFCS levels II compared to level I for 5–12 years old children [18]. However, the current data set did not further distinguish the growth trajectories between GMFCS levels II and III for which the function level and severity of neuromotor impairments could be quite different. While the underlying mechanisms of these changes in trajectory between the GMFCS levels are currently unclear, they might be attributed to less weight bearing activities, reduced levels of physical activity, higher incidence of nutritional problems and increased (secondary) musculoskeletal alterations, especially from 6 to 9 years [11].

The current findings also suggested a different trajectory for the growth in cross-sectional and longitudinal dimension of the MG muscle, i.e., changes in CSA and ML, respectively. For CSA, a growth trajectory with an early breakpoint at 2 years of age was observed in both GMFCS groups, whereas the trajectory of ML showed a breakpoint at the age of 4–5 years in GMFCS level I and at the age of 2 years in GMFCS level II–III. The trajectories in CSA are aligned to the changes in MV, suggesting that alterations in cross-sectional MG muscle growth may be associated to the change in overall MG muscle size. This is in line with previous findings indicating that reduction in physiological CSA, a determinant for force generation, is determined by reduced MV rather than by changes in fascicle length [44,45]. Hence, clinical utility may be found in assessing only the mid-belly anatomical CSA as primary outcome for monitoring the muscle status and treatment follow-up.

With increasing age, evolution in neuromotor symptoms can be expected due to the natural history of SCP in children. Interestingly, breakpoint models describing changes in development at specific ages were already found in longitudinal follow-up studies for spasticity and lower limb ROM [5,6,46]. These previous studies showed that spasticity increases to the age of 4 years, followed by a decrease each year until the age of 12 year [6]. Decreasing ankle joint ROM was reported up to 5 years of age, followed by further decrease with age in GMFCS level I and II, while levels III showed increased ROM [5]. The current study showed similar non-linear models for the ML outcomes in GMFCS level I with a breakpoint at the age of 5.11 years. The nML changed from 0.33% per year to -0.10% per year for GMFCS level I, whereas a constant increase of 0.12%/year was presented for GMFCS level II–III. Therefore, the restricted ROM for GMFCS level I might result from reduced growth of muscle length. Furthermore, these similarities in longitudinal observations of neuromotor impairment and muscle development, including the breakpoint at 5 years, support the hypothesis that formation of contractures is triggered by different factors, of which spasticity is probably not the dominant one [46,47].

Over the last years, 3DfUS has already been extensively used mainly to describe muscle deficits in children with SCP compared to TD children [48]. These cross-sectional investigations included diverse age ranges and GMFCS levels resulting in variable results of deficits (for example 22% for the age range 2–5 years and 41% for 5–12 years old children) [16,19]. However, age-specific observations of hampered muscle growth for SCP children were missing in these previous studies. Our findings, derived from longitudinal models, emphasized the need for repeated assessments to accurately delineate muscle growth. Furthermore, the current muscle growth trajectories can be used to monitor the status of muscle pathology in individual children with SCP. The current results may support the clinical decision making of therapy selection, goals and planning at specific ages and for each GMFCS level with the aim of stimulating the muscle growth. For example, the application of strength training, considering the appropriate age and cognitive functioning, might be beneficial for maintaining the muscle size relative to the skeletal growth and might be further combined with age- and child-specific prescription of protein intake to increase the muscle size [49–51]. Beside interventions, the current observation of early muscle alterations for higher GMFCS levels and the breakpoint in growth trajectory at a very young age highlight the opportunity for prevention strategies aiming to maintain muscle size and lengths comparable to TD children and preserve muscle growth during childhood, e.g., intensive physical therapy with stimulation of lower leg movements and mechanical loading and a nutritional plan. Previous studies focusing already on the impact of BoNT-A injections, a frequently applied tone-reducing treatment, demonstrated hampered muscle growth in response to the first BoNT-A treatment [14,52]. This post-treatment effect on muscle growth was only assessed after 6 months for which the interference of BoNT-A injection with the trajectory of muscle changes is yet unclear. Future intervention studies could use the currently modelled muscle growth trajectories as a reference to assess the effect of treatment on muscle morphology and could fine tune the timing of treatment in relation to the potential hampered growth.

This study has some limitations to consider. First, the age-matched TD data could not be included in the models due to the lack of longitudinal assessments. Yet, visual inspection of cross-sectionally measured typical muscle morphology allowed one to judge the overall level of alterations in the data of children with SCP (Figure S2). We included children aged between 6 months and 9 years at baseline resulting in limited available data points at the beginning and end of the age range. More longitudinal data before and after this range is relevant to further enrich the muscle growth trajectories during the entire childhood. Combined with longitudinal data of TD children, a focused analysis of the muscle growth before 2 years of age and after 6 years of age would be interesting for future research. Second, this unique longitudinal database is limited to provide trajectories of medial gastrocnemius muscle growth for the specific diversity in SCP phenotypes such as the level of motor abilities and the topographic classes. In this study, only the GMFCS levels representing ambulant children with SCP were included. The GMFCS level II and III were merged to ensure sufficient power for the data analysis and to provide as much homogeneity as possible. By combining the data of children with GMFCS II and III across the broad age range from 6 months to 11 years, children who function at level II and use gait aids at younger ages when learning to walk, or walking longer distances, are included. This is distinct from children functioning at level I, who walk independently without the need for a gait aid. The current dataset was, however, limited in data points after the age of 6 years to describe the trajectories of muscle growth per GMFCS level. We only descriptively explored the muscle growth per GMFCS level with the individual observed profiles (Figure S1), indicating similar trajectories in morphological muscle growth. Nevertheless, it is important to further consider the potential heterogeneity in muscle growth based on the specificity in gross motor abilities and limitations through daily life per GMFCS level. Future studies should aim for more participants after the age of 6 years and with equally distributed number of children over each of the three ambulatory GMFCS levels in order to distinguish the models for muscle growth according to the GMFCS level. Next, the muscle growth associated with the SCP topography i.e., unilateral versus bilateral SCP was also not specifically investigated. However, further sub-analyses are important considerations due to the unbalanced number of participants between the topographic classes. Anthropometric growth, lower limb strength and gait were found to be less involved in unilateral compared to bilateral SCP, whereas only one investigation showed more muscle growth deficits for this SCP motor type [53,54]. These findings suggest the need to describe, in future research, separate muscle growth trajectories for the children with uni- and bilateral SCP in interaction with GMFCS level. As a first exploration, the observed individual trajectories per motor subtype for the current GMFCS subgroups are provided in Figure 3. Visual inspection suggests less muscle growth in children with bilateral SCP, especially for GMFCS level II–III of which 65% of the children were bilaterally involved.

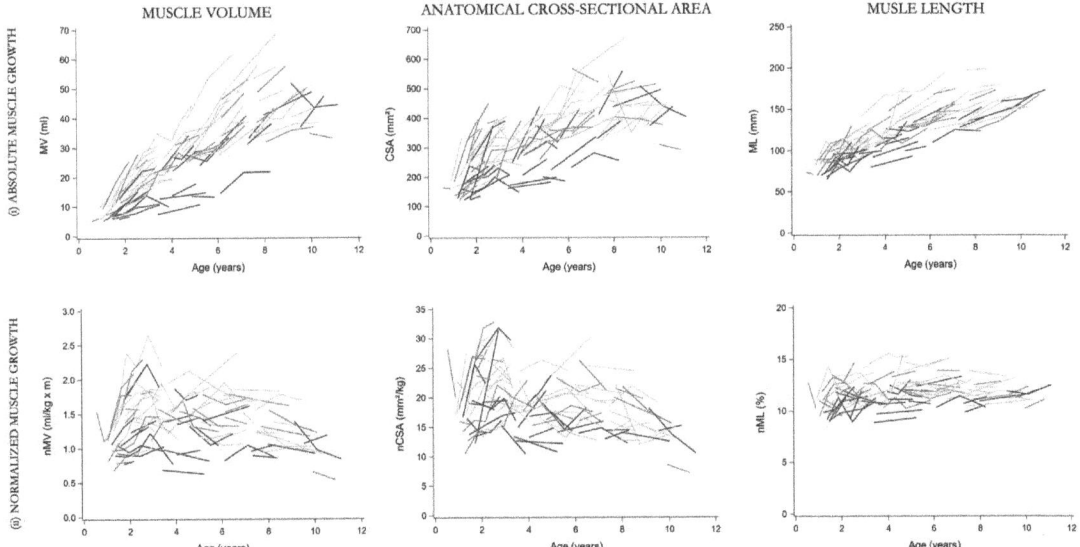

Figure 3. Observed individual trajectories for the (**i**) absolute and (**ii**) normalized muscle morphology for children with unilateral SCP (*n* = 51) (grey) and children with bilateral SCP (*n* = 36) (green), in GMFCS level I (light colors) and GMFCS level II–III (dark colors) group. GMFCS, gross motor function classification system; SCP, spastic cerebral palsy; n, number; MV, muscle volume; ml, milliliter; CSA, anatomical cross-sectional area; mm, millimeter; ML, muscle belly length; n, normalized.

Further, each muscle assessment during the follow-up was not accompanied with evaluation of motor impairments and functioning such as assessment of strength, spasticity and selective motor control as well as the gross motor function measure (GMFM). These clinical results combined with muscle growth data could create a comprehensive monitoring of SCP muscle pathology, which may help to understand the underlying mechanisms of altered muscle growth and eventually help to improve patient-specific treatment management. Of note, in the current study, children who received BoNT-treatment were allowed for further follow-up in cases when the BoNT-A treatment occurred minimal 10 months prior to the assessment. The current database included 24 children who received BoNT-A injection during the follow-up time. Our previous research highlighted that the muscle recovery is still ongoing at 6 months post BoNT-A injections [14]. Despite the 10-month interval between the BoNT-A treatment and muscle morphology assessments, which is already longer than the frequently used criteria of an interval of 6 months, there is no guarantee for full recovery of muscle growth at the follow-up assessment. Future studies should investigate the prolonged impact of treatments. Long-term follow-up assessments are essential to further understand if BoNT-A treatment is a confounding factor on the currently established trajectories of muscle growth.

5. Conclusions

To our knowledge, this was the first study that performed repeated muscle assessments over 2 years in an extended group of growing children with SCP and demonstrated piecewise model for MG muscle growth. The study sample is believed to be representative of the population of children receiving standardized clinical care in Belgium (Table S2). After high rates of muscle growth during the first 2 years of life, the trajectory of absolute MV and CSA changed, resulting in a slower gradual growth until 6–9 years, and subsequent reduction in muscle size growth after 9 years. With increasing age, normalized MV and mid-belly CSA represented a decrease in muscle morphology after approximately 2 years of age. Children with GMFCS level II–III showed more muscle growth reduction compared to children with level I. This lower growth rate started at a very young age. After infancy until approximately 9 years of age, the trajectory of muscle growth did not differ greatly between GMFCS levels. These longitudinal trajectories could be used to monitor the SCP muscle pathology during childhood and to optimize treatment planning and goals aiming to stimulate muscle growth.

Supplementary Materials: The following supporting information can be downloaded at: https://www.mdpi.com/article/10.3390/jcm12041564/s1, Figure S1: Observed individual profiles for the (A) absolute and (B) normalized muscle morphology for (i) the total group of children with SCP (blue = GMFCS level I, dark red = level II and pink = level III), (ii) children with GMFCS level I, (iii) children with GMFCS level II and (iv) children with GMFCS level III, Figure S2: A Reference dataset for absolute morphological muscle outcomes and B: Reference dataset for normalized morphological muscle outcomes, Table S1: Muscle morphology of retrospective cross-sectional dataset with TD children, Table S2: Standard clinical care of all SCP participants, Table S3: Fixed and random effects of the piecewise regressions for muscle morphology (GMFCS I n = 47 and GMFCS II–III n = 40) and results of the differences between slopes and breakpoints (GMFCS, I n = 47, and GMFCS II–III n = 40).

Author Contributions: Conceptualization, N.D.B., E.O., A.V.C. and K.D.; methodology, N.D.B., I.V., G.M. and K.D.; formal analysis, N.D.B., I.V. and G.M.; investigation, N.D.B., E.H., N.P. and B.H.; resources, E.O., A.V.C. and K.D.; data curation, N.D.B., E.H., N.P. and B.H.; writing—original draft preparation, N.D.B.; writing—review and editing, N.D.B., I.V., E.H., G.M., N.P., B.H., E.O., A.V.C. and K.D.; visualization, N.D.B., I.V. and G.M.; supervision, E.O., A.V.C. and K.D.; project administration, N.D.B. and K.D. All authors have read and agreed to the published version of the manuscript.

Funding: ND was funded by an internal KU Leuven grant, Belgium, 3D-MMAP-C24/18/103. This work was further supported by Internal funding of KU Leuven Biomedical Sciences Group: Fund for Translational Biomedical Research, Belgium, 2019 and the Research Foundation Flanders (FWO), Belgium, G0B4619N. BH and NP were funded by a TBM grant (TAMTA-T005416N). IV was funded through a research fellowship from FWO (1188921N).

Institutional Review Board Statement: The study was conducted in accordance with the Declaration of Helsinki, and approved by Ethical Committee of University Hospitals Leuven/KU Leuven (S59945, approved 18 July 2017; S62187, approved 8 February 2019 and S62645, approved 7 May 2019).

Informed Consent Statement: Informed consent was obtained from all subjects involved in the study.

Data Availability Statement: The raw data supporting the conclusions of this article will be made available by the authors via an online repository, without undue reservation.

Acknowledgments: The authors wish to thank Heidi Devolder and Julie Uytterhoeven for assistance in patient recruitment and planning of the follow-up appointments. We would like to thank Jorieke Deschrevel for the support during the data acquisition and Tijl Dewit for the support of 3DfUS measures and database management.

Conflicts of Interest: The authors declare no conflict of interest. The funders had no role in the design of the study; in the collection, analyses, or interpretation of data; in the writing of the manuscript; or in the decision to publish the results.

References

1. Graham, H.K.; Rosenbaum, P.; Paneth, N.; Dan, B.; Lin, J.-P.; Damiano, D.L.; Becher, J.G.; Gaebler-Spira, D.; Colver, A.; Reddihough, D.S.; et al. Cerebral Palsy. *Nat. Rev. Dis. Prim.* **2016**, *2*, 15082. [CrossRef] [PubMed]
2. Barrett, R.S.; Lichtwark, G.A. Gross Muscle Morphology and Structure in Spastic Cerebral Palsy: A Systematic Review. *Dev. Med. Child Neurol.* **2010**, *52*, 794–804. [CrossRef] [PubMed]
3. Schless, S.H.; Cenni, F.; Bar-On, L.; Hanssen, B.; Goudriaan, M.; Papageorgiou, E.; Aertbeliën, E.; Molenaers, G.; Desloovere, K. Combining Muscle Morphology and Neuromotor Symptoms to Explain Abnormal Gait at the Ankle Joint Level in Cerebral Palsy. *Gait Posture* **2019**, *68*, 531–537. [CrossRef] [PubMed]
4. Rosenbaum, P.L.; Walter, S.D.; Hanna, S.E.; Palisano, R.J.; Russell, D.J.; Raina, P.; Wood, E.; Bartlett, D.J.; Galuppi, B.E. Prognosis for Gross Motor Function in Cerebral Palsy Creation of Motor Development Curves. *JAMA* **2002**, *208*, 1357–1363. [CrossRef] [PubMed]
5. Nordmark, E.; Hägglund, G.; Lauge-Pedersen, H.; Wagner, P.; Westbom, L. Development of Lower Limb Range of Motion from Early Childhood to Adolescence in Cerebral Palsy: A Population-Based Study. *BMC Med.* **2009**, *7*, 65. [CrossRef]
6. Lindén, O.; Hägglund, G.; Rodby-Bousquet, E.; Wagner, P. The Development of Spasticity with Age in 4,162 Children with Cerebral Palsy: A Register-Based Prospective Cohort Study. *Acta Orthop.* **2019**, *90*, 286–291. [CrossRef]
7. Burgess, A.; Reedman, S.; Chatfield, M.D.; Ware, R.S.; Sakzewski, L.; Boyd, R.N. Development of Gross Motor Capacity and Mobility Performance in Children with Cerebral Palsy: A Longitudinal Study. *Dev. Med. Child Neurol.* **2022**, *64*, 578–585. [CrossRef]
8. Palisano, R.J.; Rosenbaum, P.; Bartlett, D.; Livingston, M.H. Content Validity of the Expanded and Revised Gross Motor Function Classification System. *Dev. Med. Child Neurol.* **2008**, *50*, 744–750. [CrossRef]
9. Molenaers, G.; Fagard, K.; Van Campenhout, A.; Desloovere, K. Botulinum Toxin A Treatment of the Lower Extremities in Children with Cerebral Palsy. *J. Child. Orthop.* **2013**, *7*, 383–387. [CrossRef]
10. Kruse, A.; Rivares, C.; Weide, G.; Tilp, M.; Jaspers, R.T. Stimuli for Adaptations in Muscle Length and the Length Range of Active Force Exertion—A Narrative Review. *Front. Physiol.* **2021**, *12*, 1677. [CrossRef]
11. Verschuren, O.; Smorenburg, A.R.P.; Luiking, Y.; Bell, K.; Barber, L.; Peterson, M.D. Determinants of Muscle Preservation in Individuals with Cerebral Palsy across the Lifespan: A Narrative Review of the Literature. *J. Cachexia. Sarcopenia Muscle* **2018**, *9*, 453–464. [CrossRef]
12. Gough, M.; Shortland, A.P. Early Muscle Development in Children with Cerebral Palsy: The Consequences for Further Muscle Growth, Muscle Function, and Long-Term Mobility. In *Cerebral Palsy in Infancy*; Churchill Livingstone: London, UK, 2014. [CrossRef]
13. Herskind, A.; Ritterband-Rosenbaum, A.; Willerslev-Olsen, M.; Lorentzen, J.; Hanson, L.; Lichtwark, G.; Nielsen, J.B. Muscle Growth Is Reduced in 15-Month-Old Children with Cerebral Palsy. *Dev. Med. Child Neurol.* **2016**, *58*, 485–491. [CrossRef] [PubMed]
14. De Beukelaer, N.; Weide, G.; Huyghe, E.; Vandekerckhove, I.; Hanssen, B.; Peeters, N.; Uytterhoeven, J.; Deschrevel, J.; Maes, K.; Corvelyn, M.; et al. Reduced Cross-Sectional Muscle Growth Six Months after Botulinum Toxin Type-A Injection in Children with Spastic Cerebral Palsy. *Toxins* **2022**, *14*, 139. [CrossRef] [PubMed]
15. Malaiya, R.; McNee, A.E.; Fry, N.R.; Eve, L.C.; Gough, M.; Shortland, A.P. The Morphology of the Medial Gastrocnemius in Typically Developing Children and Children with Spastic Hemiplegic Cerebral Palsy. *J. Electromyogr. Kinesiol.* **2007**, *17*, 657–663. [CrossRef] [PubMed]
16. Barber, L.; Hastings-Ison, T.; Baker, R.; Barrett, R.; Lichtwark, G. Medial Gastrocnemius Muscle Volume and Fascicle Length in Children Aged 2 to 5 Years with Cerebral Palsy. *Dev. Med. Child Neurol.* **2011**, *53*, 543–548. [CrossRef]
17. Oberhofer, K.; Stott, N.S.; Mithraratne, K.; Anderson, I.A. Subject-Specific Modelling of Lower Limb Muscles in Children with Cerebral Palsy. *Clin. Biomech.* **2010**, *25*, 88–94. [CrossRef]

18. Pitcher, C.A.; Elliott, C.M.; Valentine, J.P.; Stannage, K.; Williams, S.A.; Shipman, P.J.; Reid, S.L. Muscle Morphology of the Lower Leg in Ambulant Children with Spastic Cerebral Palsy. *Muscle Nerve* **2018**, *58*, 818–823. [CrossRef]
19. Hanssen, B.; Peeters, N.; Vandekerckhove, I.; De Beukelaer, N.; Bar-On, L.; Molenaers, G.; Van Campenhout, A.; Degelaen, M.; Van den Broeck, C.; Calders, P.; et al. The Contribution of Decreased Muscle Size to Muscle Weakness in Children With Spastic Cerebral Palsy. *Front. Neurol.* **2021**, *12*, 692582. [CrossRef]
20. Schless, S.H.; Cenni, F.; Bar-On, L.; Hanssen, B.; Kalkman, B.; O'brien, T.; Aertbeliën, E.; Van Campenhout, A.; Molenaers, G.; Desloovere, K. Medial Gastrocnemius Volume and Echo-Intensity after Botulinum Neurotoxin A Interventions in Children with Spastic Cerebral Palsy. *Dev. Med. Child Neurol.* **2018**, *61*, 783–790. [CrossRef]
21. Noble, J.J.; Chruscikowski, E.; Fry, N.R.D.; Lewis, A.P.; Gough, M.; Shortland, A.P. The Relationship between Lower Limb Muscle Volume and Body Mass in Ambulant Individuals with Bilateral Cerebral Palsy. *BMC Neurol.* **2017**, *17*, 223. [CrossRef]
22. Lieber, R.L.; Steinman, S.; Barash, I.A.; Chambers, H. Structural and Functional Changes in Spastic Skeletal Muscle. *Muscle Nerve* **2004**, *29*, 615–627. [CrossRef] [PubMed]
23. Gundersen, K. Excitation-Transcription Coupling in Skeletal Muscle: The Molecular Pathways of Exercise. *Biol. Rev. Camb. Philos. Soc.* **2011**, *86*, 564. [CrossRef] [PubMed]
24. Clowry, G.J. The Dependence of Spinal Cord Development on Corticospinal Input and Its Significance in Understanding and Treating Spastic Cerebral Palsy. *Neurosci. Biobehav. Rev.* **2007**, *31*, 1114–1124. [CrossRef] [PubMed]
25. Noble, J.J.; Fry, N.R.; Lewis, A.P.; Keevil, S.F.; Gough, M.; Shortland, A.P. Lower Limb Muscle Volumes in Bilateral Spastic Cerebral Palsy. *Brain Dev.* **2014**, *36*, 294–300. [CrossRef] [PubMed]
26. Gorter, J.W.; Van Tol, E.; Van Schie, P.; Ketelaar, M.; Palisano, R.; Rosenbaum, P.; Bartlett, D.; Livingston, M.; Palisano, R.; Rosenbaum, P.; et al. *GMFCS–E & R Gross Motor Function Classification System Expanded and Revised*; NetChild Network for Childhood Disability Research: Utrecht, The Netherlands, 2009; pp. 2007–2010.
27. Palisano, R.J.; Cameron, D.; Rosenbaum, P.L.; Walter, S.D.; Russell, D. Stability of the Gross Motor Function Classification System. *Dev. Med. Child Neurol.* **2006**, *48*, 424–428. [CrossRef]
28. Cenni, F.; Schless, S.H.; Bar-On, L.; Aertbeliën, E.; Bruyninckx, H.; Hanssen, B.; Desloovere, K. Reliability of a Clinical 3D Freehand Ultrasound Technique: Analyses on Healthy and Pathological Muscles. *Comput. Methods Programs Biomed.* **2018**, *156*, 97–103. [CrossRef]
29. Barber, L.; Alexander, C.; Shipman, P.; Boyd, R.; Reid, S.; Elliott, C. Validity and Reliability of a Freehand 3D Ultrasound System for the Determination of Triceps Surae Muscle Volume in Children with Cerebral Palsy. *J. Anat.* **2019**, *234*, 384–391. [CrossRef]
30. Williams, S.A.; Bell, M.; Kim, H.K.; Salim Al Masruri, G.; Stott, N.S.; Fernandez, J.; Mirjalili, S.A. The Reliability and Validity of Triceps Surae Muscle Volume Assessment Using Freehand Three-dimensional Ultrasound in Typically Developing Infants. *J. Anat.* **2021**, *240*, 567–578. [CrossRef]
31. Thomason, P.; Willoughby, K.; Graham, H.K. Orthopaedic Assessment. In *Cerebral Palsy: Science and Clinical Practice*; Mac Keith Press: London, UK, 2014.
32. Hanssen, B.; De Beukelaer, N.; Schless, S.H.; Cenni, F.; Bar-On, L.; Peeters, N.; Molenaers, G.; Van Campenhout, A.; Van den Broeck, C.; Desloovere, K. Reliability of Processing 3-D Freehand Ultrasound Data to Define Muscle Volume and Echo-Intensity in Pediatric Lower Limb Muscles with Typical Development or with Spasticity. *Ultrasound Med. Biol.* **2021**, *47*, 2702–2712. [CrossRef]
33. Hanssen, B. Muscle Structure, Weakness, and Strengthening: A Complex Triangle for Children with Spastic Cerebral Palsy. Doctoral Dissertation, KU Leuven, Leuven, Belgium, 2022.
34. Cenni, F.; Schless, S.H.; Monari, D.; Bar-On, L.; Aertbeliën, E.; Bruyninckx, H.; Hanssen, B.; Desloovere, K. An Innovative Solution to Reduce Muscle Deformation during Ultrasonography Data Collection. *J. Biomech.* **2018**, *77*, 194–200. [CrossRef]
35. Treece, G.; Prager, R.; Gee, A.; Berman, L. Fast Surface and Volume Estimation from Non-Parallel Cross-Sections, for Freehand Three-Dimensional Ultrasound. *Med. Image Anal.* **1999**, *3*, 141–173. [CrossRef] [PubMed]
36. Handsfield, G.G.; Meyer, C.H.; Hart, J.M.; Abel, M.F.; Blemker, S.S. Relationships of 35 Lower Limb Muscles to Height and Body Mass Quantified Using MRI. *J. Biomech.* **2014**, *47*, 631–638. [CrossRef] [PubMed]
37. Verbeke, G.; Molenberghs, G. *Linear Mixed Models in Practice: A SAS-Oriented Approach*; Springer: New York, NY, USA, 1997.
38. Molenberghs, G.; Verbeke, G. An Introduction to (Generalized) (Non-)Linear Mixed Models. In *Explantory im Respons Models: A Generalized Linear and Nonlinear Approach*; De Boeck, P., Wilson, M., Eds.; Springer: New York, NY, USA, 2004.
39. Jaric, S.; Mirkov, D.; Markovic, G. Normalizing Physical Performance Tests for Body Size: A Proposal for Standardization. *J. Strength Cond. Res.* **2005**, *19*, 467–474. [CrossRef]
40. Wells, J.C.K.; Davies, P.S.W.; Fewtrell, M.S.; Cole, T.J. Body Composition Reference Charts for UK Infants and Children Aged 6 Weeks to 5 Years Based on Measurement of Total Body Water by Isotope Dilution. *Eur. J. Clin. Nutr.* **2020**, *74*, 141–148. [CrossRef] [PubMed]
41. Barber, L.; Hastings-Ison, T.; Baker, R.; Kerr Graham, H.; Barrett, R.; Lichtwark, G. The Effects of Botulinum Toxin Injection Frequency on Calf Muscle Growth in Young Children with Spastic Cerebral Palsy: A 12-Month Prospective Study. *J. Child. Orthop.* **2013**, *7*, 425–433. [CrossRef]
42. Day, S.M.; Strauss, D.J.; Vachon, P.J.; Rosenbloom, L.; Shavelle, R.M.; Wu, Y.W. Growth Patterns in a Population of Children and Adolescents with Cerebral Palsy. *Dev. Med. Child Neurol.* **2007**, *49*, 167–171. [CrossRef]
43. de las Mercedes Ruiz Brunner, M.; Cuestas, E.; Heinen, F.; Schroeder, A.S. Growth in Infants, Children and Adolescents with Unilateral and Bilateral Cerebral Palsy. *Sci. Rep.* **2022**, *12*, 1879. [CrossRef] [PubMed]

44. Bénard, M.R.; Harlaar, J.; Becher, J.G.; Huijing, P.A.; Jaspers, R.T. Effects of Growth on Geometry of Gastrocnemius Muscle in Children: A Three-Dimensional Ultrasound Analysis. *J. Anat.* **2011**, *219*, 388–402. [CrossRef]
45. Lieber, R.L.; Fridén, J. Functional and Clinical Significance of Skeletal Muscle Architecture. *Muscle Nerve* **2000**, *23*, 1647–1666. [CrossRef]
46. Hägglund, G.; Wagner, P. Spasticity of the Gastrosoleus Muscle Is Related to the Development of Reduced Passive Dorsiflexion of the Ankle in Children with Cerebral Palsy: A Registry Analysis of 2,796 Examinations in 355 Children. *Acta Orthop.* **2011**, *82*, 744–748. [CrossRef]
47. Mathewson, M.A.; Lieber, R.L. Pathophysiology of Muscle Contractures in Cerebral Palsy. *Phys. Med. Rehabil. Clin. N. Am.* **2015**, *26*, 57–67. [CrossRef] [PubMed]
48. Williams, I.; Reid, L.; Stott, N.S.; Valentine, J.; Elliott, C. Measuring Skeletal Muscle Morphology and Architecture with Imaging Modalities in Children with Cerebral Palsy: A Scoping Review. *Dev. Med. Child Neurol.* **2020**, *63*, 263–273. [CrossRef] [PubMed]
49. Park, E.-Y.; Kim, W.-H. Meta-Analysis of the Effect of Strengthening Interventions in Individuals with Cerebral Palsy. *Res. Dev. Disabil.* **2014**, *35*, 239–249. [CrossRef] [PubMed]
50. Anker–van der Wel, I.; Smorenburg, A.R.P.; de Roos, N.M.; Verschuren, O. Dose, Timing, and Source of Protein Intake of Young People with Spastic Cerebral Palsy. *Disabil. Rehabil.* **2020**, *42*, 2192–2197. [CrossRef] [PubMed]
51. Hanssen, B.; Peeters, N.; De Beukelaer, N.; Vannerom, A.; Peeters, L.; Molenaers, G.; Van Campenhout, A.; Deschepper, E.; Van den Broeck, C.; Desloovere, K. Progressive Resistance Training for Children with Cerebral Palsy: A Randomized Controlled Trial Evaluating the Effects on Muscle Strength and Morphology. *Front. Physiol.* **2022**, *13*, 1678. [CrossRef] [PubMed]
52. Alexander, C.; Elliott, C.; Valentine, J.; Stannage, K.; Bear, N.; Donnelly, C.J.; Shipman, P.; Reid, S. Muscle Volume Alterations after First Botulinum Neurotoxin A Treatment in Children with Cerebral Palsy: A 6-Month Prospective Cohort Study. *Dev. Med. Child Neurol.* **2018**, *60*, 1165–1171. [CrossRef]
53. Damiano, D.; Abel, M.; Romness, M.; Oeffinger, D.; Tylkowski, C.; Gorton, G.; Bagley, A.; Nicholson, D.; Barnes, D.; Calmes, J.; et al. Comparing Functional Profiles of Children with Hemiplegic and Diplegic Cerebral Palsy in GMFCS Levels I and II: Are Separate Classifications Needed? *Dev. Med. Child Neurol.* **2006**, *48*, 797–803. [CrossRef]
54. Barber, L.A.; Read, F.; Lovatt Stern, J.; Lichtwark, G.; Boyd, R.N. Medial Gastrocnemius Muscle Volume in Ambulant Children with Unilateral and Bilateral Cerebral Palsy Aged 2 to 9 Years. *Dev. Med. Child Neurol.* **2016**, *58*, 1146–1152. [CrossRef]

Disclaimer/Publisher's Note: The statements, opinions and data contained in all publications are solely those of the individual author(s) and contributor(s) and not of MDPI and/or the editor(s). MDPI and/or the editor(s) disclaim responsibility for any injury to people or property resulting from any ideas, methods, instructions or products referred to in the content.

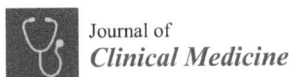

Article

The Effect of Bimanual Intensive Functional Training on Somatosensory Hand Function in Children with Unilateral Spastic Cerebral Palsy: An Observational Study

Catherine V. M. Steinbusch [1,2,*], Anke Defesche [1], Bertie van der Leij [1], Eugene A. A. Rameckers [2,3,4], Annemarie C. S. Knijnenburg [5,6], Jeroen R. J. Vermeulen [5,6] and Yvonne J. M. Janssen-Potten [2,3]

1. Adelante Rehabilitation Centre, 6301 KA Valkenburg, The Netherlands
2. Research School CAPHRI, Department of Rehabilitation Medicine, Maastricht University, 6229 ER Maastricht, The Netherlands
3. Adelante Centre of Expertise in Rehabilitation and Audiology, 6432 CC Hoensbroek, The Netherlands
4. Paediatric Rehabilitation, Biomed, Faculty of Medicine & Health Science, Hasselt University, 3500 Hasselt, Belgium
5. Department of Neurology, Maastricht University Medical Centre+, 6229 ER Maastricht, The Netherlands
6. Research School Mental Health and NeuroScience, Maastricht University Medical Centre+, 6229 ER Maastricht, The Netherlands
* Correspondence: catherine.steinbusch@adelantegroep.nl

Abstract: (1) Background: Next to motor impairments, children with unilateral spastic cerebral palsy (CP) often experience sensory impairments. Intensive bimanual training is well known for improving motor abilities, though its effect on sensory impairments is less known. (2) Objective: To investigate whether bimanual intensive functional therapy without using enriched sensory materials improves somatosensory hand function. (3) Methods: A total of twenty-four participants with CP (12–17 years of age) received 80–90 h of intensive functional training aimed at improving bimanual performance in daily life. Somatosensory hand function was measured before training, directly after training, and at six months follow-up. Outcome measures were: proprioception, measured by thumb and wrist position tasks and thumb localization tasks; vibration sensation; tactile perception; and stereognosis. (4) Results: Next to improving on their individual treatment goals, after training, participants also showed significant improvements in the perception of thumb and wrist position, vibration sensation, tactile perception, and stereognosis of the more affected hand. Improvements were retained at six months follow-up. Conversely, proprioception measured by the thumb localization tasks did not improve after training. (5) Conclusions: Intensive functional bimanual training without environmental tactile enrichment may improve the somatosensory function of the more affected hand in children with unilateral spastic CP.

Keywords: cerebral palsy; upper limb; sensory function; bimanual intensive functional therapy; hand function

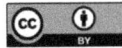

1. Introduction

Children with cerebral palsy (CP) often have motor and sensory impairments which negatively impact upper limb function, causing limitations in daily activity and participation [1–4]. Intensive goal-oriented upper limb therapies are effective in promoting bimanual performance and daily functioning [5,6]. These rehabilitation approaches mainly focused on motor deficits. These days, however, there is increased attention on sensory impairments because of the clear link between somatosensory impairment and poor hand function in children with CP [7]. Conversely, the effects of rehabilitation interventions on changes in somatosensory hand function in children with CP are relatively understudied [8]. The studies that have been published show varying effects. Charles et al. [9] reported an improvement in two-point discrimination after constrain-induced movement therapy (CIMT) in three children with unilateral spastic CP. The less affected upper extremities of these children were constrained six hours daily for 14 consecutive days. Charles and colleagues attributed this improvement in tactile discrimination to an increase in tactile input and its subsequent change in cortical receptor fields for the fingers. Matusz et al. [10] studied the effect of hybrid CIMT on somatosensory hand function in ten children with CP. Their intervention encompassed 120 h of CIMT, 22 h of goal-directed training and shaping, and 10 h of fine motor activities that involved sensory feedback components such as temperature, texture, light and deep pressure, and vibration. Reliable differences in stereognosis, grip, and pinch tests were revealed between the more affected and less affected hands before but also after CIMT. However, only grip strength in the more affected hand was influenced by CIMT. Another study on the effects of hybrid CIMT is the study of Jobst et al. [11]. To optimize potential changes in somatosensory function, somatosensory activities were enhanced within the CIMT protocol, focusing on tactile, stereognosis, and proprioceptive modalities. They detected a significant change in tactile registration in the affected hand, but not in other aspects of clinical sensory functioning, i.e., 2-point discrimination, proprioception, and kinesthesia. Maitre and colleagues [12] reported on the effects of a multi-component intervention in infants (n = 37) aged 6 to 24 months. They studied somatosensory processing using cortical event-related potential (ERP) responses for tactile stimulation of the more affected hand at the contralateral and ipsilateral frontal scalp regions. Their intervention improved somatosensory processing. Kuo et al. [13] investigated the effect of a 90 h standardized hand-arm bimanual training program (HABIT), with and without tactile training, in twenty children with unilateral spastic CP. They concluded that tactile spatial resolution can improve after bimanual training and that intensive bimanual training alone, or with the incorporation of materials with a diversity of shapes/textures, may drive these changes. An intensive motor skill learning intervention involving both the upper- and lower-extremities (HABIT-ILE), without a sensory enriched environment, showed an improvement in stereognosis in the more affected hand in CP subjects, but no significant change in tactile spatial discrimination [14].

In the present study, the effectiveness of a 15-day functional, intensive, goal-oriented, clinical therapy program, focused on improving bimanual performance in daily activities in children and adolescents with CP, aged between 11–20 years, on somatosensory performance is investigated. We hypothesize that somatosensory function may improve after intensive training, even without the addition of sensory-enriched material.

2. Materials and Methods

2.1. Patients

A convenience sample of children and adolescents, diagnosed with CP, who participated in a bimanual intensive functional training (BIMT) program for the first time between 2017 and 2021, was used. Inclusion criteria were: Gross Motor Function Classification System (GMFCS) I-IV (able to stand/transfer independently), Manual Ability Classification System (MACS) I-III (able to perform, at least partially independent, on manual tasks), between 11–20 years of age, unilateral or asymmetric bilateral CP (spastic/dyskinetic/ataxic), and having clear treatment goals regarding bimanual performance tasks. Exclusion criteria were: unable to sleep over at Adelante Paediatric Rehabilitation Centre for 15 days and severe cognitive impairments that hinder active participation in the program. Inclusion for BIMT was performed by a rehabilitation physician and his/her rehabilitation team.

We tried to retrospectively collect the brain MRI of each participant because children with periventricular leukomalacia (PVL) lesions have significantly better hand function and sensation scores than children with cortical-subcortical/middle cerebral artery (MCA) lesions [15]. For the classification of the type of lesion, we used the classification introduced by Himmelmann et al. [16]. Informed consent from parents and participants was obtained.

2.2. Bimanual Intensive Functional Training

The BIMT program is a 15-day clinical intervention for children and adolescents, developed by researchers and clinical staff of Adelante Paediatric Rehabilitation Centre in Houthem, the Netherlands. All the staff have over seven years of experience working with children with unilateral spastic CP and are specialized in hand function problems in these children. The program is based on motor learning principles and functional therapy, according to the (inter)national guidelines in CP, i.e., the therapy is goal-directed, using a context-based approach, aimed at the active participation of the child, focusing on activity and participation, and incorporating parent involvement. The program focuses on using both hands in numerous everyday two-handed skills. The affected hand is considered the assisting hand in a stabilizing or supporting role. Potential candidates are extensively screened before participation by members of our expert team. During this screening, every participant formulated their treatment goals and needs. Together with the therapist and parents, these goals were ranked in the top three. The performance of these three goals was assessed, and after a task analysis, they were translated into individualized goal-directed therapy sessions by experienced therapists. All training was performed on-site. To encourage training intensity, all participants were paired with a personal buddy who continuously prompted the participant to use both hands when performing activities throughout the day. These buddies were interns in occupational therapy, movement sciences, medicine, or sports training who followed a one-day training program by experienced therapists. During the program, the students were supervised by experienced therapists. In terms of manpower, one healthcare professional supervised three participants.

Therapy starts from the moment of waking up, when self-care activities such as dressing and grooming are practiced. As for breakfast activities, participants have to set the table, prepare their breakfast, and clean up afterwards. All breakfast items are chosen in such a way that two hands are needed to spread the bread, pour the milk, or get the yogurt out of the package, for example. The breakfast session is followed by a therapy block of 90–120 min in which the specific personal treatment goals are trained. In the afternoon, activities that specifically focus on personal goals are alternated with group activities (survival, sports, bimanual gaming, and recreational activities). The participants are also involved in preparing lunch and dinner. To improve retention of the trained skills in the home environment after the therapy program, in the intervening weekend, participants train on personal goals together with their caregivers. This way, participants receive a daily total of 6–7 h of intensive therapy, totaling 80–90 h for the entire program.

Before participating in this clinical BIMT program, these children received therapy as usual. According to the Dutch guidelines for the treatment of children with CP, this amounts to 30 min of therapy once or twice a week. Treatment is given based on requests for help from the parents and/or the children themselves, or is based on the rehabilitation team's findings during regular examinations.

2.3. Somatosensory Function Testing

The tactile perception was measured using a monofilament task (MFT): We used the 6.65 Semmes-Weinstein monofilament (SWM) [17] and tested nine palmar areas of the affected hand in random order, with vision blocked. Participants were asked if they felt the monofilament by saying 'yes', and, subsequently, to point out the location of touch with their less affected hand while vision was restored. We chose to only use the 6.65 monofilament to reduce testing time and the burden to the participant. With this, we deviated from the original protocol as described by Bell-Krotoski [18]. When participants were able to identify the monofilament touch within a range of two centimeters, the score was 1; when identified over two centimeters from the tested site, the score was 2. Participants scored 3 if no administered stimulus was identified. A few practice trials were given on the less affected hand until the procedure was understood. The MFT can be reliably performed in the vast majority of children aged four years and above [19] and is recommended for assessing tactile function in children with cerebral palsy [20].

Vibration sense was measured using a vibration task (VT): A 128 Hz tuning fork was placed on 18 areas of the affected hand. Participants had to report whether a vibration was recognized in these 18 areas. The number of reported areas resulted in a final score (i.e., score 0–18) [21].

Stereognosis was measured using a stereognosis task (SGT): Participants were asked to identify three familiar items (marble, button, key) without vision after the assessor had placed the item in the affected hand. If these three items were correctly identified, an extra 10 items were added (clothespin, comb, dice, screw, bolt, paperclip, rubber band, pen, pencil, coin). The Jamar® Stereognosis Kit was used, including matching cards featuring a drawing of the item to point at the item recognized, as recommended [20,22]. The total number of correctly identified items was the final score (i.e., score 0–13).

Proprioception was measured using a thumb-wrist-position task (TWPT): The therapist passively moved the participant's wrist into dorsal or palmar flexion and the MCP joint into extension or flexion with the participant's vision blocked. Subjects were required to verbally indicate the end joint position. Outcomes were rated as 1 (unable), 2 (unable to identify either wrist or thumb end position), or 3 (able to correctly identify end position of both thumb and wrist).

In addition to the TWPT used, proprioception was also measured using a thumb localization task (TLT): With the participant's vision blocked, the therapist passively moved the participant's non-dominant upper limb laterally from the midline. The participant was asked to pinch the thumb of the non-dominant hand with the thumb and index finger of their dominant hand [23]. The task was scored as 1 (unable to locate thumb position), 2 (difficulty locating thumb position), or 3 (no difficulty locating thumb position).

Data were collected at three different time points. Baseline measurements were collected 14 days before the initial start of the therapy program (PRE). Post-intervention measurements were taken on the last day of the program (POST). Follow-up measurements were taken at six months follow-up (FOLLOW-UP). At all three measurement times, the child was assessed by the same therapist, not the child's own therapist. Therapists were not blinded to the time of measurement.

2.4. Secondary Outcome Measures

Goal Attainment Scaling (GAS) is an evaluative tool to assess individual treatment and/or intervention goals achieved during/after an intervention. The GAS consists of a 6-point scale, ranging from −3 to +2. A score of −2 represents the participant's performance at baseline, and improvements in the performance of the goal are scored ranging from −1 to +2, where the 0 score corresponds to the expected outcome and a score of −3 reflects deterioration [24]. GAS has shown to be a sensitive and valid method for defining motor function goals and shows excellent intra- and inter-rater reliability [25,26]. Changes of two points or more are defined as a clinically relevant difference [27]. For each participant, the most important rehabilitation goal was translated into a GAS by the participant's assigned therapist from Adelante. Predetermined criteria for the progress towards that specific rehabilitation goal were defined. The individual's performance of this goal was filmed and scored by therapists who have vast expertise in working with children with unilateral spastic CP and who are specialized in hand function problems in children. The video recordings of one participant were scored by the same therapist, not the child's own therapist, on all three measurement time points. Therapists were not blinded to previous outcomes.

Canadian Occupational Performance Measure (COPM) is a semi-structured interview in which participants identify and rank their perceived hand function problems in everyday bimanual activities. The approach of this measure corresponds to the goal-oriented approach of the therapy program. The primary problem corresponds to the most important rehabilitation goal. Participants were asked to rate their performance and satisfaction for each problem on a 10-point scale, resulting in a mean total performance and satisfaction score. The COPM has good construct, content, and criterion validity. Test-retest reliability is high (0.76–0.89), and other ICC values of reliability remain to be tested in this population [28]. COPM performance and satisfaction were scored by the participants. Changes of two points or more were classified as a clinically relevant difference [29].

Assisting Hand Assessment (AHA) is an evaluative tool to rate bimanual performance. The AHA assesses the spontaneous use of the impaired hand in bimanual activities during a semi-structured activity session, which is video recorded. Afterwards, 22 items describing object-related hand actions were scored and converted to 0–100 logit-based AHA units [30]. We used the AHA 18–18 'Go-with-the-Floe' board game in most cases, and in some participants, the Present task. A change of ±5 AHA units is considered the smallest detectable difference [30,31]. The video recordings of the participant's performance on the AHA were scored by a selected group of therapists trained in the scoring of these videos. AHA scores of one participant were scored by the same therapist, not the child's own therapist, on all three measurement time points. Therapists were not blinded to previous outcomes.

2.5. Data Analyses

Non-parametric statistics were used. To test overall improvement, a one-way analysis of variance by ranks (Friedman) was applied with post hoc Wilcoxon analyses when a significant effect was found. Data were analyzed using IBM SPSS Statistics version 27 (IBM SPSS Statistics, IBM Inc., New York, NY, USA). Statistical significance was set at $\alpha = 0.05$. Multiple comparisons included the Bonferroni correction to avoid spurious false positives.

3. Results

3.1. Participants

Twenty-four children, 14 boys (58.3%) and 10 girls (41.7%), were analyzed. In 2017, seven participants were included, five in 2018, five in 2019, three in 2020, and four participants in 2021. The mean age at baseline was 14.21 years (±1.62), ranging from 12 to 17 years. Based on MRI data, we were able to perform a classification of 22 of the participants. Patient characteristics of the study sample are presented in Table 1.

Table 1. Descriptive data of participants ($n = 24$).

Characteristics	Group
Age (years) (mean, SD)	14.21 (±1.62)
Gender (n (%))	
Male	14 (58.3)
Female	10 (41.7)
Type of CP (n (%))	
Unilateral spastic	23 (95.8)
Bilateral spastic	1 (4.2)
MACS (n (%))	
I	9 (37.5)
II	12 (50)
III	3 (12.5)
GMFCS (n (%))	
I	20 (83.3)
II	4 (16.7)
Paretic hand (n (%))	

Table 1. *Cont.*

Characteristics	Group
Right	15 (62.5)
Left	9 (37.5)
Lesion type (*n* (%))	
WMI	8 (33.3)
CM	5 (20.8)
GMI	9 (37.5)
Unknown	2 (8.3)

Abbreviations used: MACS = Manual Ability Classification System; GMFCS = Gross Motor Function Classification System; GMI = Gray matter injury; WMI = white matter injury; CM = cortical malformation.

3.2. Error Analysis

Post-intervention measurements were taken on the last day of the program so participants did not have to return to the rehabilitation center, especially for this. In some cases, however, this led to time constraints for the therapists, which meant they had to make choices about which test could be taken and which could not. This led to missing values (time). A COVID infection in two children at follow-up also caused missing data (COVID). One participant was hospitalized at follow-up (hospital). The reason for hospitalization was not related to arm-hand function impairments or participation in our program. An overview of the number of missing values per test on each of the three measurement points is given in Table 2.

Table 2. The number of missing values per test, per measurement point.

	PRE *n* Missings	POST *n* Missings	FOLLOW-UP *n* Missings
TLT	1→1 (time)	1→1 (time)	4→1 (time) 2 (COVID) 1 (hospital)
SGT	0	0	3→2 (COVID) 1 (hospital)
MFT	0	0	3→2 (COVID) 1 (hospital)
TWPT	1→1 (time)	1→1 (time)	4→1 (time) 2 (COVID) 1 (hospital)
VT	1→1 (time)	0	3→2 (COVID) 1 (hospital)
GAS	0	0	3→2 (COVID) 1 (hospital)
COPM	0	0	3→2 (COVID) 1 (hospital)
AHA	0	0	3→2 (COVID) 1 (hospital)

Abbreviations used: TLT = thumb localization task; SGT = stereognosis task; MFT = monofilament task; TWPT = thumb wrist position task; VT = vibration task; GAS = Goal Attainment Scaling; COPM = Canadian Occupational Performance Measure; AHA = Assisted Hand Assessment.

3.3. Somatosensory Function

Changes in clinical somatosensory outcomes are summarized in Table 3.

Table 3. Number and percentage of participants and their test scores at baseline, directly after BIMT, and six months follow-up.

	Score	PRE n (%)	POST n (%)	FU n (%)	Overall Difference p	PRE-POST Bonferroni Difference p	POST-FU Bonferroni Difference p	PRE-FU Bonferroni Difference p
TLT	1	3 (13)	3 (13)	2 (10)	0.076	0.317	0.180	0.059
	2	3 (13)	1 (4.3)	0 (0)				
	3	17 (74)	19 (82.7)	18 (90)				
SGT	0	13 (54.2)	7 (29.2)	7 (33.3)	0.018 *	<0.001 *	0.411	0.009 *
	1–3	7 (29.1)	9 (37.4)	5 (23.8)				
	≥4	4 (16.7)	8 (33.3)	9 (42.9)				
MFT	1	7 (29.2)	16 (66.7)	14 (66.7)	<0.001 *	<0.001 *	0.317	<0.001 *
	2	11 (45.8)	8 (33.3)	7 (33.3)				
	3	6 (25)	0 (0)	0 (0)				
TWPT	1	3 (13)	1 (4.3)	1 (5)	<0.001 *	0.059	1.00	0.059
	2	2 (8.7)	1 (4.3)	1 (5)				
	3	18 (78.3)	21 (91.3)	18 (90)				
VT	0	3 (13)	0 (0)	0 (0)	<0.001 *	0.003 *	0.180	0.007 *
	1–10	5 (21.7)	0 (0)	1 (4.7)				
	11–18	15 (65.3)	24 (100)	20 (95.3)				

Abbreviations used: TLT = thumb localization task; SGT = stereognosis task; MFT = monofilament task; TWPT = Thumb wrist position task; VT = vibration task; PRE = baseline; POST = directly after the program; FU = Follow-up six months after the program; * significant difference.

The participants showed increased scores on the somatosensory function tests over time ($p < 0.001$), except for the thumb localization task. Multiple comparisons showed that participants scored significantly better on the stereognosis task, monofilament task, and vibration task between the PRE and POST measurements and between the PRE and FOLLOW-UP measurements. Differences between POST and FOLLOW-UP scores were not statistically significant.

3.4. GAS

GAS scores on the most important treatment goal, post-intervention and at follow-up, are shown in Figure 1.

Overall, participants showed a better GAS score on the primary treatment goal over time ($p < 0.001$). All participants, except one, exceeded the minimal clinical important difference (MCID) of 2 points. Post hoc pairwise comparisons revealed a significant difference between baseline and post-intervention ($p < 0.001$) and between baseline and follow-up ($p < 0.001$). The difference in GAS scores between post-intervention and follow-up was not significant ($p = 0.480$).

A list of the individual treatment goals for all participants is provided as supplementary information.

3.5. COPM

In total, 113 rehabilitation goals ($17 \times 5 + 7 \times 4$) were formulated using the COPM. Seventeen participants formulated five goals, whereas seven participants formulated four goals. The median and inter-quartile ranges of the weighted average COPM performance and satisfaction scores, for all time points, are depicted in Figures 2 and 3. It should be noted here that not all children were able to score their satisfaction with the achievement of their treatment goal at baseline ($n = 6$).

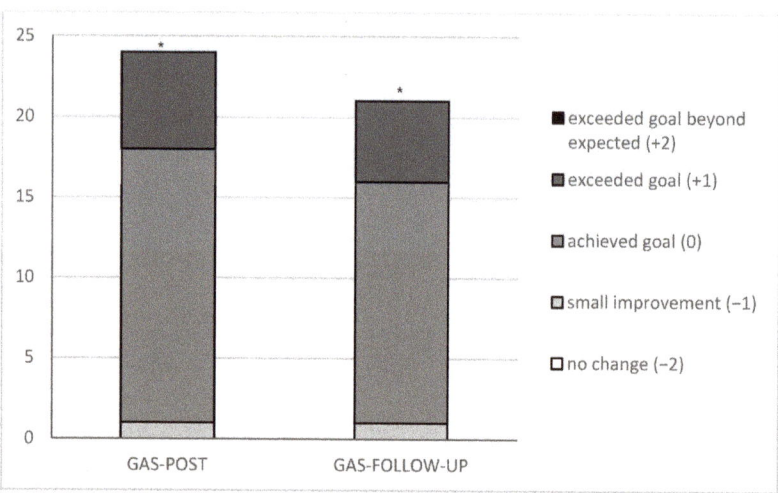

Figure 1. GAS score POST intervention and at FOLLOW-UP. Abbreviations: GAS = Goal Attainment Scaling; POST = directly after the program; FOLLOW-UP = six months after the program; * = significant difference $p < 0.016$ (Wilcoxon signed-rank test).

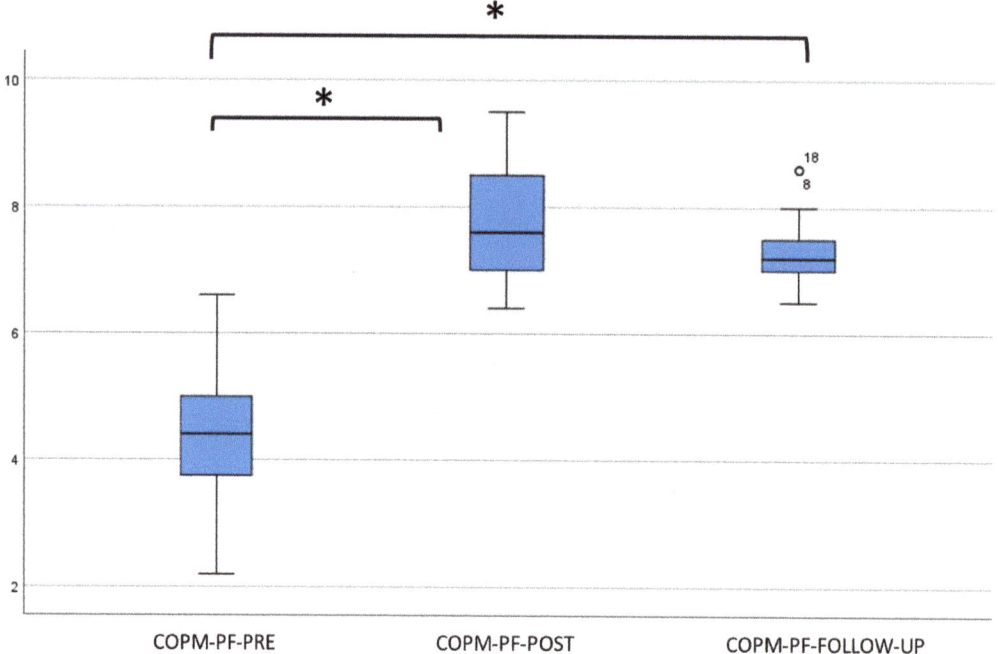

Figure 2. Boxplot of the weighted mean COPM performance score at baseline, post-intervention, and follow-up. Abbreviations used: COPM = Canadian Occupational Performance Measure; PF = Performance; PRE = baseline measurements; POST = directly after the program; FOLLOW-UP = six months after the program; * = significant difference $p < 0.016$ compared to baseline (Wilcoxon signed-rank test); circle identifies ouliers.

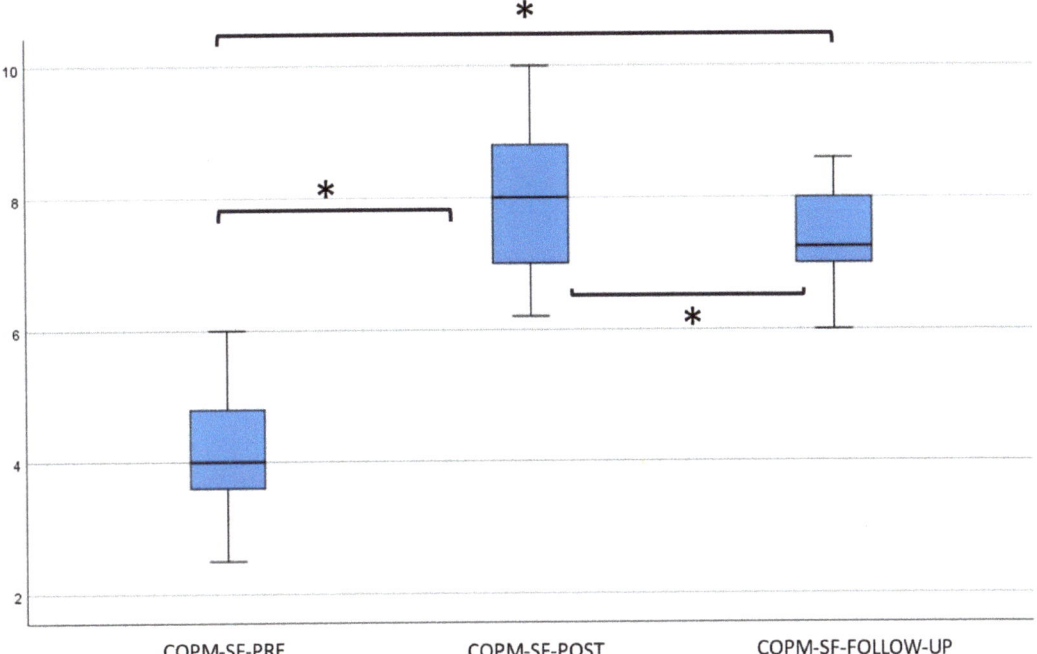

Figure 3. Boxplot of the weighted mean COPM satisfaction score at baseline, post-intervention, and follow-up. Abbreviations used: COPM = Canadian Occupational Performance Measure; SF = Satisfaction; PRE = baseline measurements; POST = directly after the program; FOLLOW-UP = six months after the program; * = significant difference $p < 0.016$ compared to baseline (Wilcoxon signed-rank test).

Participants gave better COPM performance scores over time ($p < 0.001$). Post hoc pairwise comparisons revealed a significant difference between pre- and post-intervention ($p < 0.001$) and between pre-intervention and follow-up ($p < 0.001$). The difference between post-intervention and follow-up was not significant ($p = 0.064$).

COPM satisfaction scores were significantly better over time ($p < 0.001$). Post hoc analysis showed a significant increase in COPM satisfaction between PRE and POST scores, as well as between PRE and FOLLOW-UP scores ($p < 0.001$). COPM satisfaction scores between POST and FOLLOW-UP reveal a significant decrease ($p = 0.007$).

3.6. AHA

The unit scores on the AHA over time are shown in Figure 4.

Participants showed better AHA unit scores over time ($p < 0.001$). Post-intervention, 17/24 participants improved clinically meaningfully on the AHA with five or over five units, and 7/24 improved, but under five units. Multiple comparisons showed an increase in AHA scores between pre- and post-intervention ($p < 0.001$) and between pre-intervention and follow-up ($p < 0.001$). The difference in AHA scores between post-intervention and follow-up was not significant ($p = 0.050$).

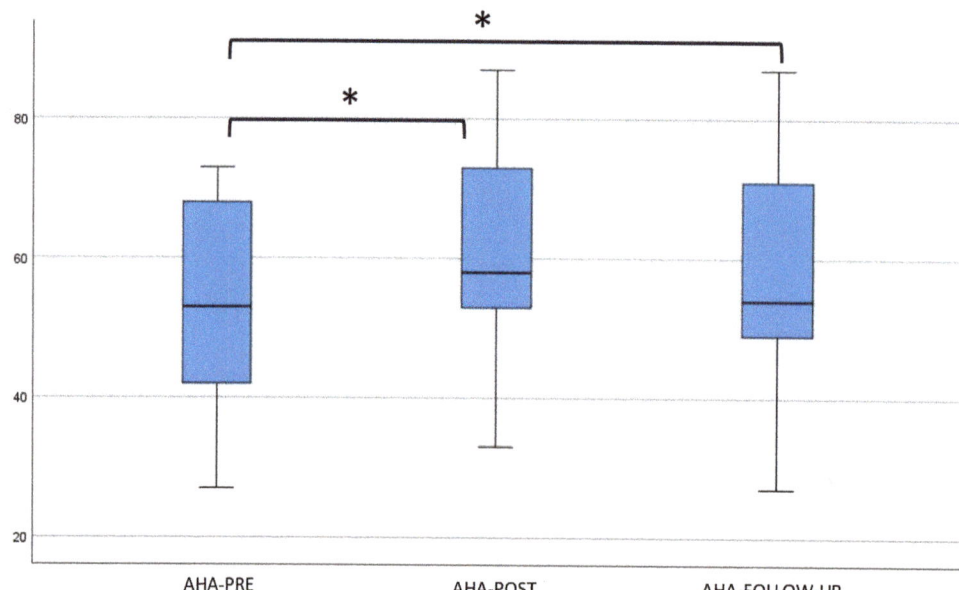

Figure 4. AHA unit scores at baseline, post-intervention, and follow-up. Abbreviations used: AHA = Assisting Hand Assessment; PRE = baseline measurements; POST = directly after the program; FOLLOW-UP = six months after the program; * = significant difference $p < 0.016$ (Wilcoxon signed-rank test).

4. Discussion

Although the somatosensory function is important for motor output, changes in somatosensory function associated with rehabilitation interventions have been understudied. The current study aimed to assess the effectiveness of a 15-day intensive functional clinical therapy program on somatosensory function. This program was focused on improving individual bimanual goals in children and adolescents with CP, GMFCS classification I-IV, MACS I-III, aged between 11–20 years, unilateral or asymmetric bilateral CP, and clear treatment goals on bimanual performance tasks. A significant improvement in personal goals and a significant improvement in the AHA were found, suggesting improved hand use of the more affected hand during bimanual task performance. Our results are consistent with the findings in the literature, indicating that intensive bimanual therapy leads to improvements in the bimanual performance of children and adolescents with USCP [32]. However, more importantly, somatosensory hand function also appears to improve as a result of this type of intervention. Even though no tactile-directed training nor exposure to special tactile-enriched materials were given during the intervention period, significant improvements were observed on all but one somatosensory test.

4.1. Improvements in Primary and Secondary Outcome Measures

Vibration sense, tactile perception (measured by a modified version of the monofilament test), stereognosis, and proprioception (measured by the thumb-wrist position task) improved during the program. This effect was retained at six months follow-up. Regarding proprioception, only a main effect of the intervention was found. Proprioception, as measured with the thumb localization task, showed no significant improvement. It is worthwhile noticing that at baseline, 74% of the participants already performed at the maximum level on this task. In hindsight, the thumb localization test may be less appropriate to investigate possible impairments in proprioception in children with CP. These clinical tools to quantify proprioception are known to lack sensitivity to small changes, offer poor reliability, and carry the potential for examiner bias [33].

The improvements in tactile perception and stereognosis, however, are promising findings, as they are essential for the dexterous manipulation of objects [7,34] and activities of daily life [35]. Somatosensory contributions to motor control in children with CP have been investigated [36–38], and it is acknowledged that somatosensory impairment has an effect on motor impairments in children with CP [7]. As mentioned before, studies on the effects of rehabilitation interventions on somatosensory hand function in children with CP are scarce and reveal varying results. In terms of intervention dose and content, our clinical program is most similar to the HABIT program, studied by Kuo and colleagues [13]. In their study, twenty children with USCP were randomized to receive either bimanual therapy (HABIT) or HABIT plus tactile training using tactile stimulating materials without vision. The HABIT group received the same dosage of training with the same material, but without specific tactile-directed training, i.e., standardized HABIT-full vision. Both groups improved on the grating orientation task, while stereognosis of the more-affected hand tended to improve, and no changes were found in the two-point discrimination task and monofilaments. Saussez et al. [14] investigated a similar intervention also involving the lower-extremities (HABIT-ILE) and without sensory enriched environment. They showed an improvement in stereognosis in the more affected hand in CP subjects, but no significant change in tactile spatial discrimination. Even though no additional sensory-enriched material or specific tactile training was used in our program, changes in tactile perception were found in addition to the improvement in stereognosis. These findings may be explained by the fact that participants were trained extensively in sensorimotor integration rather than just in sensory abilities. After all, goal-directed movements of the hand, which are necessary to perform most tasks of daily living, involve interacting with and manipulating objects in the environment and rely on sensorimotor integration. Intensive hand therapy is known to induce neuroplastic changes. Functional Magnetic Resonance Imaging (fMRI) or magnetoencephalography (MEG) after CIMT [39] or HABIT [40] demonstrated increased activation in the primary somatosensory cortex and an increase in the activation and size of the motor areas controlling the affected hand. Jobst et al. [11] were the first to demonstrate simultaneous improvement in sensory tactile registration in the affected hand and enhanced sensory processing in the contralateral primary somatosensory cortex after CIMT in children with hemiplegic CP.

In addition to improvement in somatosensory hand function, intensive bimanual training resulted in improvements in performance of personal treatment goals, as reflected by a higher GAS score, indicating a better execution of these activities in daily life. Most participants reached or exceeded their expected performance level, and the effect was retained at follow-up. Similar effects were observed regarding personal rehabilitation goals, as gauged using the COPM [41,42]. This finding is promising, since the improvement in the execution of activities in daily life settings results in an increase in independence, benefitting participation and quality of life. We assume that training and focusing on improving child-specific functional goals enhances the performance of these tasks in daily life. The satisfaction scores of the COPM increased significantly immediately after BIMT, though a slight decrease was observed at six months follow-up. A recent report by Figueiredo et al. [43] showed similar results in a group of children with bilateral CP participating in an intensive 90 h bimanual training program called HABIT. The group that performed the program exhibited greater improvements in performance and satisfaction with the performance of functional goals and functional skills than children who maintained their customary care routines and are following the results found by Bleyenheuft et al. [44]. It is acknowledged that targeting daily activities in individuals with CP is important [45,46]. Caregivers' priorities of children with CP report on activities of daily living, especially self-care, to be the most frequent functional priority [46,47], while children's ability to perform self-care activities facilitates socialization with peers, participation in community activities, and transition to independent living, as well as a reduction in caregiver's burden [46]. Intensive goal-oriented bimanual training of participants, with the engagement of their caregivers, may play an important role in addressing this outcome.

Spontaneous use of the affected hand in bimanual performance tasks (AHA) improved to a clinically important difference after the program, and this effect was retained at follow-up. These findings are in line with the findings of the above-mentioned study by Kuo et al. [13].

4.2. Limitations

Direct comparison of our study results with the literature is difficult because of the large variability in study design, patient characteristics, and sensory assessment methods used. Even when the same sensory test is used, the method of administration and/or the method of scoring may differ. To improve our understanding of somatosensory hand function, we advocate for an international consensus on a clinically relevant core set with uniformity in methodology and scoring.

In our study group, 20.8% of participants have cortical malformation, which is known to result in less severe hand impairments than white or grey matter damage [48]. White matter lesions, in turn, lead to less severe hand function problems than grey matter lesions [15]. Participants with white matter damage and grey matter damage were approximately equally distributed in our study group. However, the relatively small number of participants does not allow for an extensive multivariate analysis to look for group differences.

Our study is a non-blinded observational cohort study, lacking a formal control group. Therefore, the level of evidence of the efficacy of our program is limited (level III on the Oxford levels of evidence). However, studies reporting on the efficacy of intensive bimanual training on sensory function in children and adolescents with CP are limited. Therefore, this study adds to the evidence that functional, intensive, goal-directed therapy may be effective in improving somatosensory hand function. Future studies including a larger number of participants and a control condition (e.g., waiting list control group) are needed to show the efficacy at a higher level of evidence, though complete blinded randomization can never be accomplished due to the nature of the intervention.

Finally, we used a clinical measurement protocol to measure somatosensory hand function. This protocol takes into account the testing time and burden for the participants, because motor outcome measures at the ICF activity level were recorded in addition to somatosensory measures. The advantage of this protocol is that it allows for proper assessment of the participant's hand function, and a disadvantage is that it deviates slightly from the original protocol, especially regarding the Semmes-Weinstein monofilament test. The fact that we asked the participants to point to the location of touch may have influenced the reliability of the test [18].

5. Conclusions

Somatosensory function, including tactile perception, vibration sense, stereognosis, and position sense of the more affected hand in children and adolescents with unilateral spastic CP may improve after bimanual intensive functional training, without environmental tactile enrichment. A possible explanation for this might be that goal-directed training enhances sensorimotor integration.

Supplementary Materials: The following supporting information can be downloaded at: https://www.mdpi.com/article/10.3390/jcm12041595/s1, File S1: Intervention description of the BIMT program according to the TIDieR guideline; File S2: list of individual treatment goals for all participants.

Author Contributions: Conceptualization, A.D. and B.v.d.L.; Investigation, A.C.S.K.; Writing—original draft, C.V.M.S.; Writing—review & editing, E.A.A.R., J.R.J.V. and Y.J.M.J.-P. All authors have read and agreed to the published version of the manuscript.

Funding: We thank the Stichting Vooruit for the financial support of this study.

Informed Consent Statement: Informed consent was obtained from all subjects involved in the study.

Data Availability Statement: The data are not publicly available due to privacy restrictions. The data presented in this study are available on request from the corresponding author.

Conflicts of Interest: The authors declare no conflict of interest.

References

1. Klevberg, G.L.; Østensjø, S.; Krumlinde-Sundholm, L.; Elkjær, S.; Jahnsen, R.B. Hand Function in a Population-Based Sample of Young Children with Unilateral or Bilateral Cerebral Palsy. *Phys. Occup. Ther. Pediatr.* **2017**, *37*, 528–540. [CrossRef]
2. Öhrvall, A.-M.; Eliasson, A.-C.; Löwing, K.; Ödman, P.; Krumlinde-Sundholm, L. Self-care and mobility skills in children with cerebral palsy, related to their manual ability and gross motor function classifications. *Dev. Med. Child. Neurol.* **2010**, *52*, 1048–1055. [CrossRef]
3. Arner, M.; Eliasson, A.-C.; Nicklasson, S.; Sommerstein, K.; Hägglund, G. Hand function in cerebral palsy. Report of 367 children in a population-based longitudinal health care program. *J. Hand Surg. Am.* **2008**, *33*, 1337–1347. [CrossRef]
4. Brun, C.; Traverse, É.; Granger, É.; Mercier, C. Somatosensory deficits and neural correlates in cerebral palsy: A scoping review. *Dev. Med. Child. Neurol.* **2021**, *63*, 1382–1393. [CrossRef]
5. Novak, I.; Honan, I. Effectiveness of paediatric occupational therapy for children with disabilities: A systematic review. *Aust. Occup. Ther. J.* **2019**, *66*, 258–273. [CrossRef]
6. Novak, I. Evidence-based diagnosis, health care, and rehabilitation for children with cerebral palsy. *J. Child. Neurol.* **2014**, *29*, 1141–1156. [CrossRef]
7. Bleyenheuft, Y.; Gordon, A.M. Precision grip control, sensory impairments and their interactions in children with hemiplegic cerebral palsy: A systematic review. *Res. Dev. Disabil.* **2013**, *34*, 3014–3028. [CrossRef]
8. Auld, M.L.; Russo, R.; Moseley, L.; Johnston, L.M. Determination of interventions for upper extremity tactile impairment in children with cerebral palsy: A systematic review. *Dev. Med. Child. Neurol.* **2014**, *56*, 815–832. [CrossRef]
9. Charles, J.; Lavinder, G.; Gordon, A. Effects of constraint-induced therapy on hand function in children with hemiplegic cerebral palsy. *Pediatr. Phys. Ther.* **2001**, *13*, 68–76. [CrossRef]
10. Matusz, P.J.; Key, A.P.; Gogliotti, S.; Pearson, J.; Auld, M.; Murray, M.M.; Maitre, N. Somatosensory Plasticity in Pediatric Cerebral Palsy following Constraint-Induced Movement Therapy. *Neural. Plast.* **2018**, *2018*, 1891978. [CrossRef]
11. Jobst, C.; D'Souza, S.J.; Causton, N.; Master, S.; Switzer, L.; Cheyne, D.; Fehlings, D. Somatosensory Plasticity in Hemiplegic Cerebral Palsy Following Constraint Induced Movement Therapy. *Pediatr. Neurol.* **2022**, *126*, 80–88. [CrossRef]
12. Maitre, N.L.; Jeanvoine, A.; Yoder, P.J.; Key, A.P.; Slaughter, J.C.; Carey, H.; Needham, A.; Murray, M.M.; Heathcock, J.; Burkhardt, S.; et al. Kinematic and Somatosensory Gains in Infants with Cerebral Palsy After a Multi-Component Upper-Extremity Intervention: A Randomized Controlled Trial. *Brain Topogr.* **2020**, *33*, 751–766. [CrossRef]
13. Kuo, H.C.; Gordon, A.M.; Henrionnet, A.; Hautfenne, S.; Friel, K.M.; Bleyenheuft, Y. The effects of intensive bimanual training with and without tactile training on tactile function in children with unilateral spastic cerebral palsy: A pilot study. *Res. Dev. Disabil.* **2016**, *49–50*, 129–139. [CrossRef]
14. Saussez, G.; Van Laethem, M.; Bleyenheuft, Y. Changes in Tactile Function During Intensive Bimanual Training in Children With Unilateral Spastic Cerebral Palsy. *J. Child. Neurol.* **2018**, *33*, 260–268. [CrossRef]
15. Knijnenburg, A.C.S. Determinants of sensory problems in children with unilateral cerebral palsy; a systematic review. *Front. Rehabil. Sci.* **2022**, Submitted.
16. Himmelmann, K.; Horber, V.; Sellier, E.; De la Cruz, J.; Papavasiliou, A.; Krägeloh-Mann, I. Neuroimaging Patterns and Function in Cerebral Palsy-Application of an MRI Classification. *Front. Neurol.* **2020**, *11*, 617740. [CrossRef]
17. Weinstein, S. Fifty years of somatosensory research: From the Semmes-Weinstein monofilaments to the Weinstein Enhanced Sensory Test. *J. Hand Ther.* **1993**, *6*, 11–22; Discussion 50. [CrossRef]
18. Bell-Krotoski, J.; Weinstein, S.; Weinstein, C. Testing sensibility, including touch-pressure, two-point discrimination, point localization, and vibration. *J. Hand Ther.* **1993**, *6*, 114–123. [CrossRef]
19. Dua, K.; Lancaster, T.; Abzug, J. Age-dependent Reliability of Semmes-Weinstein and 2-Point Discrimination Tests in Children. *J. Pediatr. Orthop.* **2019**, *39*, 98–103. [CrossRef]
20. Auld, M.L.; Boyd, R.N.; Moseley, G.L.; Johnston, L.M. Tactile assessment in children with cerebral palsy: A clinimetric review. *Phys. Occup. Ther. Pediatr.* **2011**, *31*, 413–439. [CrossRef]
21. Pestronk, A.; Florence, J.; Levine, T.; Al-Lozi, M.T.; Lopate, G.; Miller, T.; Ramneantu, I.; Waheed, W.; Stambuk, M. Sensory exam with a quantitative tuning fork: Rapid, sensitive and predictive of SNAP amplitude. *Neurology* **2004**, *62*, 461–464.
22. Klingels, K.; De Cock, P.; Molenaers, G.; Desloovere, K.; Huenaerts, C.; Jaspers, E.; Feys, H. Upper limb motor and sensory impairments in children with hemiplegic cerebral palsy. Can They be measured reliably? *Disabil. Rehabil.* **2010**, *32*, 409–416.
23. Hirayama, K.; Fukutake, T.; Kawamura, M. 'Thumb localizing test' for detecting a lesion in the posterior column-medial lemniscal system. *J. Neurol. Sci.* **1999**, *167*, 45–49. [CrossRef]
24. Kiresuk, T.J.; Sherman, R.E. Goal attainment scaling: A general method for evaluating comprehensive community mental health programs. *Community Ment. Health J.* **1968**, *4*, 443–453. [CrossRef]
25. Cusick, A.; McIntyre, S.; Novak, I.; Lannin, N.; Lowe, K. A comparison of goal attainment scaling and the Canadian Occupational Performance Measure for paediatric rehabilitation research. *Pediatr. Rehabil.* **2006**, *9*, 149–157.
26. Steenbeek, D.; Ketelaar, M.; Lindeman, E.; Galama, K.; Gorter, J.W. Interrater reliability of goal attainment scaling in rehabilitation of children with cerebral palsy. *Arch. Phys. Med. Rehabil.* **2010**, *91*, 429–435.

27. Steenbeek, D.; Meester-Delver, A.; Becher, J.G.; Lankhorst, G.J. The effect of botulinum toxin type A treatment of the lower extremity on the level of functional abilities in children with cerebral palsy: Evaluation with goal attainment scaling. *Clin. Rehabil.* **2005**, *19*, 274–282. [CrossRef]
28. Sakzewski, L.; Boyd, R.; Ziviani, J. Clinimetric properties of participation measures for 5- to 13-year-old children with cerebral palsy: A systematic review. *Dev. Med. Child. Neurol.* **2007**, *49*, 232–240.
29. Cusick, A.; Lannin, N.; Lowe, K. Adapting the Canadian Occupational Performance Measure for use in a paediatric clinical trial. *Disabil. Rehabil.* **2007**, *29*, 761–766. [CrossRef]
30. Krumlinde-Sundholm, L.; Lindkvist, B.; Plantin, J.; Hoare, B. Development of the assisting hand assessment for adults following stroke: A Rasch-built bimanual performance measure. *Disabil. Rehabil.* **2019**, *41*, 472–480. [CrossRef]
31. Krumlinde-Sundholm, L.; Holmefur, M.; Kottorp, A.; Eliasson, A.-C. The Assisting Hand Assessment: Current evidence of validity, reliability, and responsiveness to change. *Dev. Med. Child. Neurol.* **2007**, *49*, 259–264. [CrossRef]
32. Novak, I.; Morgan, C.; Fahey, M.; Finch-Edmondson, M.; Galea, C.; Hines, A.; Langdon, K.; Mc Namara, M.; Paton, M.C.; Popat, H.; et al. State of the Evidence Traffic Lights 2019: Systematic Review of Interventions for Preventing and Treating Children with Cerebral Palsy. *Curr. Neurol. Neurosci. Rep.* **2020**, *20*, 3. [CrossRef]
33. Kuczynski, A.M.; Carlson, H.L.; Lebel, C.; Hodge, J.A.; Dukelow, S.P.; Semrau, J.A.; Kirton, A. Sensory tractography and robot-quantified proprioception in hemiparetic children with perinatal stroke. *Hum. Brain Mapp.* **2017**, *38*, 2424–2440. [CrossRef]
34. Gordon, A.M.; Duff, S.V. Relation between clinical measures and fine manipulative control in children with hemiplegic cerebral palsy. *Dev. Med. Child. Neurol.* **1999**, *41*, 586–591. [CrossRef]
35. Auld, M.L.; Boyd, R.N.; Moseley, L.; Ware, R.; Johnston, L.M. Tactile function in children with unilateral cerebral palsy compared to typically developing children. *Disabil. Rehabil.* **2012**, *34*, 1488–1494. [CrossRef]
36. Auld, M.L.; Boyd, R.N.; Moseley, L.; Ware, R.; Johnston, L.M. Impact of tactile dysfunction on upper-limb motor performance in children with unilateral cerebral palsy. *Arch. Phys. Med. Rehabil.* **2012**, *93*, 696–702. [CrossRef]
37. Cooper, J.; Majnemer, A.; Rosenblatt, B.; Birnbaum, R. The determination of sensory deficits in children with hemiplegic cerebral palsy. *J. Child. Neurol.* **1995**, *10*, 300–309. [CrossRef]
38. Arnould, C.; Penta, M.; Thonnard, J. Hand impairments and their relationship with manual ability in children with cerebral palsy. *J. Rehabil. Med.* **2007**, *39*, 708–714. [CrossRef]
39. Juenger, H.; Kuhnke, N.; Braun, C.; Ummenhofer, F.; Wilke, M.; Walther, M.; Koerte, I.; Delvendahl, I.; Jung, N.H.; Berweck, S.; et al. Two types of exercise-induced neuroplasticity in congenital hemiparesis: A transcranial magnetic stimulation, functional MRI, and magnetoencephalography study. *Dev. Med. Child. Neurol.* **2013**, *55*, 941–951. [CrossRef]
40. Bleyenheuft, Y.; Dricot, L.; Gilis, N.; Kuo, H.-C.; Grandin, C.; Bleyenheuft, C.; Gordon, A.M.; Friel, K.M. Capturing neuroplastic changes after bimanual intensive rehabilitation in children with unilateral spastic cerebral palsy: A combined DTI, TMS and fMRI pilot study. *Res. Dev. Disabil.* **2015**, *43–44*, 136–149. [CrossRef]
41. Law, M.; Baptiste, S.; McColl, M.; Opzoomer, A.; Polatajko, H.; Pollock, N. The Canadian occupational performance measure: An outcome measure for occupational therapy. *Can. J. Occup. Ther.* **1990**, *57*, 82–87. [CrossRef] [PubMed]
42. Verkerk, G.J.Q.; Wolf, M.J.M.A.G.; Louwers, A.M.; Meester-Delver, A.; Nollet, F. The reproducibility and validity of the Canadian Occupational Performance Measure in parents of children with disabilities. *Clin. Rehabil.* **2006**, *20*, 980–988. [CrossRef] [PubMed]
43. Figueiredo, P.R.P.; Mancini, M.C.; Feitosa, A.M.; Teixeira, C.M.M.F.; Guerzoni, V.P.D.; Elvrum, A.G.; Ferre, C.L.; Gordon, A.M.; Brandão, M.B. Hand-arm bimanual intensive therapy and daily functioning of children with bilateral cerebral palsy: A randomized controlled trial. *Dev. Med. Child. Neurol.* **2020**, *62*, 1274–1282. [CrossRef] [PubMed]
44. Bleyenheuft, Y.; Ebner-Karestinos, D.; Surana, B.; Paradis, J.; Sidiropoulos, A.; Renders, A.; Friel, K.M.; Brandao, M.; Rameckers, E.; Gordon, A.M. Intensive upper- and lower-extremity training for children with bilateral cerebral palsy: A quasi-randomized trial. *Dev. Med. Child. Neurol.* **2017**, *59*, 625–633. [CrossRef]
45. Bergqvist, L.; Öhrvall, A.-M.; Himmelmann, K.; Peny-Dahlstrand, M. When I do, I become someone: Experiences of occupational performance in young adults with cerebral palsy. *Disabil. Rehabil.* **2019**, *41*, 341–347. [CrossRef]
46. Chiarello, L.A.; Palisano, R.J.; Maggs, J.M.; Orlin, M.N.; Almasri, N.; Kang, L.-J.; Chang, H.-J. Family priorities for activity and participation of children and youth with cerebral palsy. *Phys. Ther.* **2010**, *90*, 1254–1264. [CrossRef]
47. Brandão, M.B.; Oliveira, R.; Mancini, M. Functional priorities reported by parents of children with cerebral palsy: Contribution to the pediatric rehabilitation process. *Braz J. Phys. Ther.* **2014**, *18*, 563–571. [CrossRef]
48. Gordon, A.; Bleyenheuft, Y.; Steenbergen, B. Pathophysiology of impaired hand function in children with unilateral cerebral palsy. *Dev. Med. Child. Neurol.* **2013**, *55* (Suppl. 4), 32–37. [CrossRef]

Disclaimer/Publisher's Note: The statements, opinions and data contained in all publications are solely those of the individual author(s) and contributor(s) and not of MDPI and/or the editor(s). MDPI and/or the editor(s) disclaim responsibility for any injury to people or property resulting from any ideas, methods, instructions or products referred to in the content.

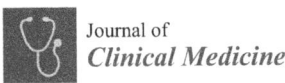

Article

Associated Impairments among Children with Cerebral Palsy in Rural Bangladesh—Findings from the Bangladesh Cerebral Palsy Register

Aditya Narayan [1], Mohammad Muhit [2,3], John Whitehall [1], Iskander Hossain [2], Nadia Badawi [4,5], Gulam Khandaker [3,6,7,8,*] and Israt Jahan [2,3,6,8]

1. School of Medicine, Western Sydney University, Penrith, NSW 2751, Australia
2. CSF Global, Dhaka 1213, Bangladesh
3. Asian Institute of Disability and Development (AIDD), University of South Asia, Dhaka 1213, Bangladesh
4. Cerebral Palsy Alliance Research Institute, Specialty of Child and Adolescent Health, Sydney Medical School, Faculty of Medicine and Health, The University of Sydney, Sydney, NSW 2006, Australia
5. Grace Centre for Newborn Intensive Care, The Children's Hospital, Westmead, Sydney, NSW 2145, Australia
6. School of Health, Medical and Applied Sciences, Central Queensland University, Rockhampton, QLD 4701, Australia
7. Discipline of Child and Adolescent Health, Sydney Medical School, The University of Sydney, Sydney, NSW 2006, Australia
8. Central Queensland Public Health Unit, Central Queensland Hospital and Health Service, Rockhampton, QLD 4700, Australia
* Correspondence: gulam.khandaker@health.qld.gov.au

Abstract: Background: We aimed to describe the burden, severity, and underlying factors of associated impairments among children with cerebral palsy (CP) in rural Bangladesh. Methods: This study reports findings from the Bangladesh Cerebral Palsy Register—the first population-based surveillance of children with CP in any LMIC, where children with confirmed CP aged < 18 years are registered by a multidisciplinary team following a standard protocol. Associated impairments were documented based on clinical assessment, available medical records, and a detailed clinical history provided by the primary caregivers. Descriptive analysis, as well as unadjusted and adjusted logistic regression, were completed using R. Results: Between January 2015 and February 2022, 3820 children with CP were registered (mean (SD) age at assessment: 7.6 (5.0) y; 39% female). Overall, 81% of children had ≥1 associated impairment; hearing: 18%, speech: 74%, intellectual: 40%, visual: 14%, epilepsy: 33%. The presence of a history of CP acquired post-neonatally and having a gross motor function classification system levels III–V significantly increased the odds of different types of associated impairments in these children. Most of the children had never received any rehabilitation services and were not enrolled in any mainstream or special education system. Conclusions: The burden of associated impairments was high among children with CP, with comparatively low receipt of rehabilitation and educational services in rural Bangladesh. Comprehensive intervention could improve their functional outcome, participation, and quality of life.

Keywords: associated impairment; comorbidities; register; children; cerebral palsy; low- and middle-income country

1. Introduction

Cerebral palsy (CP) refers to a heterogeneous group of disorders, characterized by motor deficits and functional difficulties such as sensory and cognitive impairment, caused by non-progressive but permanent insults to the developing brain [1]. In the past few years, data from CP registers in low- and middle-income countries (LMICs) have improved the understanding of the epidemiology of CP in LMICs [2,3]. The limited available evidence indicates that the burden of CP is high in LMICs, and most children have severe functional impairment with relatively low access to any rehabilitation services or assistive devices [2–4].

Data from high-income countries suggest that children with CP often present with associated impairments [5,6]. In a recent study using data from the Norwegian Patient Registry, it was reported that 95% of children with CP in Norway had at least one comorbidity [5]. A similarly high burden was reported in Australia [6]. Data from the Australian CP Register (ACPR) show that 48% of children with CP had an intellectual impairment, 61% had speech impairment, 12% had hearing impairment, 36% had visual impairment, and 28% had epilepsy [6]. The authors also reported a higher prevalence of associated impairments among children with more severe gross motor function limitations [6]. Although it is expected that the condition among children with CP in LMICs is likely to be worse due to a lack of early intervention and rehabilitation services, there is limited data available on the burden of associated impairments among children with CP in low-resource settings [7,8].

In 2015, the Bangladesh CP Register (BCPR: the first population-based surveillance of children with CP in any LMIC) was established in rural Bangladesh [9]. The BCPR enabled the first population-based estimation of the prevalence of CP (i.e., 3.4 per 1000 children) and provided an understanding of the epidemiology of CP among children in Bangladesh [10]. Furthermore, the data enabled the team to tailor need-based services for children with CP in the country [11–14].

The presence of associated impairments can complicate the management of children with CP, especially in LMICs, which often lack the necessary resources required to adequately manage the additional burden of disease, leading to negative impacts on health and functional outcome. Estimation of the burden of associated impairments and identification of children more vulnerable to associated impairments could support the development of comprehensive programs and guide adequate resource allocation/mobilization and needs-based service provision for children with CP in LMICs. In this study, we aimed to describe the burden, severity, and underlying factors of associated impairments among children with CP in rural Bangladesh.

2. Materials and Methods

The BCPR is an ongoing population-based surveillance of children with CP living in rural areas of Bangladesh [9,10].

2.1. Study Participants and Study Area

The study participants are children with confirmed CP aged < 18 years, registered in the BCPR as per the strict clinical definition adopted from the Surveillance of Cerebral Palsy in Europe (SCPE) and Australian Cerebral Palsy Register (ACPR), and a standard protocol published previously [9,15,16]. Children included in this study were recruited from 18 sub-districts of Bangladesh. The study area covers approximately 803,320 households, with an approximate total population of 3,492,088 and a child population of 1,416,254 [17].

2.2. Screening and Identification of Children with CP from Community

BCPR uses the key informant method (KIM) to identify children with suspected CP from the community [9,10]. KIM is a valid and widely practiced method that involves the capacity development of local community volunteers known as key informants (KIs) to identify children with suspected CP in their communities via structured training [18]. Following training, the KIs are given 4–6 weeks to identify and list children with suspected CP in their communities [18]. Once identified, the KIs with support from the community mobilizers (paid project staff) invite/bring these children with their caregivers/families to the nearest medical assessment camps for a confirmed diagnosis, registration in the BCPR and services [9,10,18]. More details are available in our previous publications [9,10]. Since its establishment, the BCPR team has trained over 2000 KIs in the surveillance area.

2.3. Multi-Disciplinary Medical Assessment

Children with suspected CP identified by the KIs underwent a thorough neurodevelopmental assessment, performed by a multidisciplinary medical assessment team comprising of a paediatrician, a physiotherapist, a counsellor, and a nutritionist. Detailed information about socio-demographic characteristics, pre-, peri and postnatal characteristics, clinical characteristics, nutritional status, rehabilitation, and educational status were documented using the BCPR registration form. The detailed medical assessment procedure is available in our previous publications [9,10] and has been briefly discussed in the subsequent sections.

2.3.1. Socio-Demographic Characteristics

The mothers or primary caregivers accompanying children with CP were interviewed, and the responses were documented following standard reporting guidelines of the census and the demographic and health survey in Bangladesh [17,19].

2.3.2. Known Risk Factors

Data on selected known risk factors of CP were documented by reviewing available medical records and obtaining a detailed clinical history provided by the mothers/caregivers. The components of a pre- and perinatal history such as antenatal care practices (ANC), gestational age, birth weight, attendant of childbirth, history of any complications during delivery, history of febrile illness during pregnancy or labour, history of intrapartum-related neonatal respiratory depression (IPR NRD), and early feeding difficulties were documented following the standard guideline. A child was considered preterm if born before 37 weeks of gestation and was considered to have low birthweight if the birthweight was <2500 g [20]. A child was classified as having a history of intrapartum-related neonatal respiratory depression if they failed to cry at the time of birth, experienced delayed onset of breathing (>1 min), or required assistance to initiate breathing (ranging from drying, stimulation, milking the umbilical cord, or mouth-to-mouth breaths) following birth [21]. Probable intrapartum-related neonatal respiratory depression was defined as neonatal respiratory depression among infants born at term without congenital malformations [21].

2.3.3. Predominant Motor Type, Topography, and Motor Impairment Severity

The predominant motor type of CP and topography were assessed at the time of registration following the ACPR and SCPE classification [15,16]. Gross Motor Function Classification System (GMFCS) level and Manual Ability Classification System (MACS) level were used to document motor impairment severity using standard guidelines [22,23].

2.3.4. Associated Impairments and Epilepsy

The presence and severity of associated impairments (i.e., visual, hearing, speech, and intellectual impairments) and epilepsy were primarily documented based on clinical assessment by the paediatrician and review of any previous medical records and a detailed clinical history provided by the caregivers in the absence of medical records as described in the subsequent sections.

Visual impairment: The presence of visual impairment was recorded based on the assessment of visual acuity and functional vision (including counting fingers, perceiving hand motions, and light perception). In addition, the available medical records were reviewed, and a clinical history was obtained from the primary caregivers. The severity of visual impairment was documented as "some impairment" or "functionally blind" [10].

Hearing impairment: Physical examination (both naked eye examination of the external ear and otoscopic examination) was performed to identify any signs of ear discharge, visual identification of any structural defects, impacted cerumen or foreign objects, perforation, or any other abnormalities of the tympanic membrane and for any conditions that may be contributing to hearing loss requiring further evaluation and treatment. Furthermore, distraction testing was performed to identify signs of hearing impairment among young children and a whispered voice test was performed for children who could communicate to identify signs of any hearing loss [24,25]. The child's response to name calls and perception of other sounds (e.g., loud noises, clapping) was also observed during the assessment. Any previous history of infection and conditions (e.g., pain, drainage) of the ear and use of any hearing loss intervention were assessed thoroughly by asking the primary caregiver and reviewing available medical records. The severity of hearing impairment was further classified as "some impairment" or "bilateral deafness" [10].

Speech impairment: The presence of speech impairment was documented based on speech and language assessment, review of medical records, and clinical history provided by the primary caregivers of children. Receptive and expressive language, conversational speech quality, and naming quality of the children were evaluated. The severity of speech impairment was classified as "some impairment" or "non-verbal" [10].

Intellectual impairment: The presence and severity of intellectual impairment was determined following the definitions/criteria of the Diagnostic and Statistical Manual of Mental Disorders, 5th Edition (DSM-5) [26], which places emphasis on a child's adaptive functioning and their performance in daily activities/usual life skills. The assessor interviewed the caregivers to determine if the child had any difficulties in adaptive behaviour, conceptualization, daily communication and comprehension, concentration on daily tasks, learning new skills, relationships, and other practical areas of living [26]. If the caregiver responded yes, then the severity of intellectual impairment was documented as follows: (i) mild— "Can live independently with minimum levels of support", (ii) moderate—"Independent living may be achieved with moderate levels of support, such as those available in group homes", and (iii) severe/profound—"Requires daily assistance with self-care activities and safety supervision/requires 24-hour care" [26]. Relevant medical records were also reviewed if available [10].

Epilepsy: Diagnosis of epilepsy was made based on the history of tonic–clonic seizures by interviewing the primary caregivers and reviewing available medical records. In consultation with a paediatric neurologist, a child was documented as having active epilepsy if s/he presented with a history of one or more unprovoked seizures in the preceding three months of data collection at medical assessment camps and after the neonatal period [10,13].

2.4. Data Management and Analysis

Data management and analyses were completed using R (version 4.2.1). Descriptive (such as mean, standard deviation, proportions with 95% confidence intervals; CI) and bivariate analysis (cross-tabulation with chi-square and Fisher's exact test as appropriate) were completed to describe the socio-demographic characteristics, the burden of different impairments, and the potential underlying factors of different types of impairments among children with CP in Bangladesh. Unadjusted and adjusted logistic regression (OR and aOR respectively) were completed to control potential confounding factors and identify the predictors of different forms of associated impairments among children with CP in Bangladesh.

2.5. Ethical Considerations

Ethics approval for BCPR was obtained from the Human Research Ethics Committee of Bangladesh Medical Research Council (BMRC) (southasia-irb-2014-I-01), Cerebral Palsy Alliance (EC00402; ref no. 2015-03-02), and the Asian Institute of Disability and Development (AIDD) (southasia-irb-2014-I-01). Informed written consent was obtained from the primary caregiver/parents of the children prior to registration in the BCPR. A participant information sheet written in the Bengali language was provided to each of the primary caregivers/parents of children with CP registered in the BCPR.

3. Results

Between January 2015 and February 2022, 3820 children with clinically confirmed CP were registered in the BCPR. The mean (SD) age at assessment was 7.6 (5.0) y and 39% female.

3.1. Cohort Profile

3.1.1. Socio-Demographic Characteristics

Most children were aged below 10 years (69.4%) at the time of registration into the BCPR. The majority of their parents had received at least some formal schooling (76% of the mothers and 67% of the fathers). Of all, 92% of families had a monthly income less than 15,000 BDT (~146 USD) (mean (SD) monthly family income: 9953 (7301) BDT ~68 (71) USD). Only 29% of the families were living in semi-permanent or permanent houses. Although 98% of the household had access to tube wells for collecting drinking water, nearly half (43%) did not have any access to sanitary toilets. (Table 1).

Table 1. Cohort profile (socio-demographic characteristics, predominant motor type, topography, and GMFCS level).

Characteristics	n (%), N = 3820
Age in years, n = 3809 [1]	
0–4	1412 (37.1)
5–9	1231 (32.3)
10–14	836 (21.9)
15–18	339 (8.7)
Gender, n = 3820	
Female	1485 (38.9)
Male	2335 (61.1)
Maternal literacy, n = 3813 [1]	
No formal schooling	915 (24.0)
Literate	2898 (76.0)
Paternal literacy, n = 3793 [1]	
No formal schooling	1242 (32.7)
Literate	2551 (67.3)
Monthly family income, BDT (~ USD), n = 3787 [1,2]	
<15,000 (~<146)	3475 (91.8)
15,000–25,000 (~146–243)	234 (6.2)
>25,000 (~>243)	78 (2.1)
Accommodation type, n = 3764 [1]	
Temporary shelter (jhupri)	17 (0.5)
Non-permanent (kutcha) house	2654 (70.5)
Semi-permanent (semi-pucca) house	868 (23.1)
Permanent brick (pucca) house	225 (6.0)
Source of drinking water, n = 3809 [1]	
Other sources	5 (0.1)
Tap water	79 (2.1)
Tube well	3725 (97.8)
Access to sanitation, n = 3758 [1]	
No toilet facility	68 (1.8)
Non-sanitary latrine	1551 (41.3)
Sanitary latrine	2139 (56.9)

Table 1. Cont.

Characteristics	n (%), N = 3820
Predominant motor type, n = 3820	
Spastic	3059 (80.1)
Dyskinesia	244 (6.4)
Ataxia	184 (4.8)
Hypotonia	333 (8.7)
Spastic topography, n = 3059	
Unilateral	854 (27.9)
Bilateral	2205 (72.1)
GMFCS level, n = 3782 [1]	
I–II	1097 (29.0)
III–V	2685 (71.0)

[1] Missing data; [2] 1 USD ~ 103 BDT.

3.1.2. Predominant Motor Type, Topography and GMFCS Level

Most children in our cohort had spastic CP (80%) and more than two-thirds of them (72%) had spastic bilateral CP. The majority of children also represented severe functional impairment; 71% of children had GMFCS level III–V (Table 1).

3.2. Presence of Associated Impairments

Table 2 summarizes the presence of different forms of associated impairments among participating children. Overall, 82% [95% CI 80.5, 82.9] had at least one type of associated impairment. Hearing impairment was documented in 18% [95% CI 17.2, 19.7] children; of them 4% [95% CI 3.5, 4.8] had bilateral deafness. Speech impairment was identified in 74% [95% CI 73.1, 75.8] of children and 41% [95% CI 39.2, 42.3] of them were non-verbal. Overall, 40% [95% CI 38.5, 41.7] of children had confirmed intellectual impairment, and of them, 8% [95% CI 7.5, 9.3] had severe intellectual impairment. Visual impairment was identified in 14% of the children, including 5% [95% CI 4.7, 5.4] of children with functional blindness. Epilepsy was present in 33% [95% CI 31.3, 34.3] of the children and was reported to have resolved by the age of 5 in 9% [95% CI 8.3, 10.2] of children.

Table 2. Presence of associated impairments among children with CP in Bangladesh.

Associated Impairment	n	% [95% CI]
Number of associated impairments, n = 3820		
None	697	18.2 [17.0, 19.5]
1–2	2658	69.6 [68.1, 71.0]
≥3	465	12.2 [11.2, 13.2]
Hearing impairment, n = 3811 [1]		
None	3109	81.6 [80.3, 82.8]
Some impairment	529	13.9 [12.8, 15.0]
Bilateral deafness	156	4.1 [3.5, 4.8]
Unknown	17	0.4 [0.3, 0.7]
Speech impairment, n = 3818 [1]		
None	974	25.5 [24.1, 26.9]
Some impairment	1263	33.1 [31.6, 34.6]
Nonverbal	1557	40.8 [39.2, 42.3]
Unknown	24	0.6 [0.4, 0.9]
Visual impairment, n = 3786 [1]		
None	3219	85.0 [83.8, 86.1]
Some impairment	355	9.4 [8.5, 10.3]
Functionally blind	178	4.7 [4.7, 5.4]
Unknown	34	0.9 [0.6, 1.2]

Table 2. Cont.

Associated Impairment	n	% [95% CI]
Intellectual impairment, n = 3629 [1]		
None	1193	32.9 [31.3, 34.4]
Mild	418	11.5 [10.5, 12.6]
Moderate	735	20.3 [19.0, 21.6]
Severe	302	8.3 [7.5, 9.3]
Unconfirmed/unknown	981	27.0 [25.6, 28.5]
Epilepsy, n = 3812 [1]		
No	2187	57.4 [55.8, 58.9]
Currently present	1251	32.8 [31.3, 34.3]
Resolved by age 5 years	351	9.0 [8.3, 10.2]
Unknown	23	0.6 [0.4, 0.9]

[1] Missing data.

3.3. Relationship between Predominant Motor Type and Topography of CP, GMFCS Level, and Associated Impairments

Hearing impairment is significantly ($p < 0.001$) higher among children with Ataxia (29%) compared to other predominant motor types (10% among unilateral spastic CP, 21% among bilateral spastic CP, 19% among dyskinetic CP, and 15% among hypotonic CP). The proportion of speech impairment ranges between 73% and 80% among children with bilateral spastic CP, dyskinesia, ataxia, and hypotonia, and is significantly ($p < 0.001$) lower among children with unilateral CP (56%). Visual impairment is present in 17% of children with bilateral spastic CP and 13% of children with dyskinesia. Intellectual impairment is more common among children with bilateral spastic CP (62%), dyskinesia (63%), and ataxia (63%). Furthermore, 39% of children with ataxia and 37% of children with bilateral spastic CP have epilepsy.

All types of associated impairments are more common among children with GMFCS level III–V compared to children with GMFCS level I–II. Among children with GMFCS level I, 7% have hearing impairment, 58% have speech impairment, 5% have visual impairment, 34% have intellectual impairment, and 20% have epilepsy, whereas these percentages are 28%, 91%, 24%, 78%, and 49% ($p < 0.001$) among children with GMFCS level V, respectively. (Figure S1).

3.4. Predictors of Associated Impairments

Tables S1 and 3 show findings from unadjusted and adjusted logistic regression.

3.4.1. Hearing Impairment

The odds of hearing impairment are significantly higher among children who acquired CP post-neonatally (aOR, 95% CI: 2.96 (2.33–3.74)), ataxic children (aOR, 95% CI: 2.48 (1.60–3.82)), and children with GMFCS level III–V (aOR, 95% CI: 2.64 (2.01–3.50)) when adjusted for antenatal care visits, birth attendants, and history of IPR NRD.

3.4.2. Speech Impairment

The odds of speech impairment are significantly higher among children who have a history of IPR NRD (aOR, 95% CI: 2.31 (1.93–2.77)), acquired CP post-neonatally (aOR, 95% CI: 1.43 (1.11–1.86)), and have GMFCS level III–V (aOR, 95% CI: 2.51 (2.07–3.04)). Furthermore, compared to unilateral spastic CP, children with bilateral spastic CP, dyskinesia CP, ataxia, and hypotonic have significantly higher odds of speech impairment when adjusted for other factors.

3.4.3. Visual Impairment

Unskilled birth attendants (aOR, 95% CI: 1.90 (1.43–2.51)), history of IPR NRD (aOR, 95% CI: 1.38 (1.09–1.77)), post-neonatally acquired CP (aOR, 95% CI: 2.27 (1.74–2.94)), and GMFCS level III–V (aOR, 95% CI: 2.58 (1.90–3.55)) are significant predictors of visual impairment among children with CP in the cohort when adjusted for antenatal care visits and predominant motor type or topography.

Table 3. Predictors of associated impairments among children with CP in rural Bangladesh.

Factors	Hearing	Speech	Visual	Intellectual	Epilepsy
Antenatal care visits					
Adequate	Ref	Ref	Ref	Ref	Ref
Inadequate	0.41 (0.34–0.50)	0.94 (0.78–1.13)	0.46 (0.37–0.57)	0.87 (0.72–1.06)	0.95 (0.81–1.12)
Childbirth attended by					
Doctor/midwife	Ref	Ref	Ref	Ref	Ref
Skilled birth attendant/TBA	0.98 (0.79–1.21)	1.34 (1.12–1.61)	0.88 (0.70–1.11)	1.04 (0.86–1.26)	0.67 (0.56–0.79)
Family members	2.09 (1.61–2.71)	1.15 (0.89–1.49)	1.90 (1.43–2.51)	1.80 (1.39–2.35)	1.09 (0.88–1.36)
History of birth-related complications					
No	N/A	Ref	N/A	Ref	Ref
Yes	N/A	1.17 (0.98–1.39)	N/A	1.14 (0.95–1.37)	1.17 (1.00–1.37)
History of IPR NRD					
No	Ref	Ref	Ref	Ref	Ref
Yes	1.13 (0.91–1.41)	2.31 (1.93–2.77)	1.38 (1.09–1.77)	2.01 (1.64–2.47)	1.47 (1.23–1.77)
Timing of brain injury					
Pre and perinatal	Ref	Ref	Ref	Ref	Ref
Postnatal	2.96 (2.33–3.74)	1.43 (1.11–1.86)	2.27 (1.74–2.94)	3.26 (2.48–4.33)	1.73 (1.39–2.14)
Predominant motor type and topography					
Spastic—Unilateral	Ref	Ref	Ref	Ref	Ref
Spastic—Bilateral	1.30 (0.97–1.75)	1.87 (1.51–2.31)	1.30 (0.95–1.79)	1.84 (1.45–2.33)	1.28 (1.03–1.58)
Dyskinesia	1.43 (0.92–2.20)	4.43 (2.87–7.07)	1.16 (0.71–1.88)	2.30 (1.52–3.53)	1.62 (1.16–2.26)
Ataxia	2.48 (1.60–3.82)	1.91 (1.31–2.84)	0.93 (0.52–1.59)	2.01 (1.35–3.01)	1.01 (0.69–1.47)
Hypotonia	1.03 (0.66–1.57)	1.59 (1.16–2.19)	1.30 (0.83–2.03)	1.25 (0.87–1.79)	1.11 (0.80–1.51)
GMFCS level					
I–II	Ref	Ref	Ref	Ref	Ref
III–V	2.64 (2.01–3.50)	2.51 (2.07–3.04)	2.58 (1.90–3.55)	2.00 (1.62–2.46)	1.95 (1.60–2.38)

3.4.4. Intellectual Impairment

Similar to visual impairment, unskilled birth attendants (aOR, 95% CI: 1.80 (1.39–2.35)), history of IPR NRD (aOR, 95% CI: 2.01 (1.64–2.47)), CP acquired post-neonatally (aOR, 95% CI: 3.26 (2.48–4.33)), and GMFCS level III–V (aOR, 95% CI: 2.00 (1.62–2.46)) are significant predictors of intellectual impairment among children with CP in the BCPR cohort. Additionally, when adjusted for other factors, the odds of intellectual impairment are 1.8 times higher among children with bilateral spastic CP, 2.3 times higher among children with dyskinesia, and 2.0 times higher among children with ataxia than children with unilateral CP.

3.4.5. Epilepsy

The odds of epilepsy are significantly higher among children with a history of IPR NRD (aOR, 95% CI: 1.47 (1.23–1.77)), CP acquired post-neonatally (aOR, 95% CI: 1.73

(1.39–2.14)), have bilateral spastic CP (aOR, 95% CI: 1.28 (1.03–1.59)), dyskinetic CP (aOR, 95% CI: 1.63 (1.16–2.26)), and GMFCS level III–V (aOR, 95% CI: 1.95 (1.60–2.38)).

3.5. Rehabilitation and Education Status of Children with CP According to the Presence of Different Associated Impairments

More than half (54.3%) of the children with at least one or more associated impairments have never received any rehabilitation. The proportion of children who have ever received any rehabilitation is lowest among children with hearing impairment and is highest among children with epilepsy. Furthermore, among school-aged children, only 6.2% with hearing impairment, 9.7% with speech impairment, 7.5% with visual impairment, 12% with intellectual impairment, and 9.2% with epilepsy are enrolled in any mainstream or special education schools (Table 4).

Table 4. Rehabilitation and education status of children with different forms of associated impairments.

Rehabilitation and Education Status	Hearing		Speech		Visual		Intellectual		Epilepsy	
	No	Yes	No	Yes	No	Yes	No	Yes	No	Yes
N	3109	685	974	2820	3219	533	1193	1455	2538	1251
Ever received rehabilitation services	1776 (58%)	273 (40%)	525 (54%)	1522 (54%)	1770 (55%)	251 (48%)	667 (56%)	749 (52%)	1341 (53%)	705 (57%)
p-value	<0.001		>0.9		<0.001		0.03		0.044	
Enrolled in mainstream/special schools	534 (19%)	40 (6.2%)	324 (37%)	251 (9.7%)	532 (18%)	38 (7.5%)	339 (31%)	156 (12%)	468 (20%)	106 (9.2%)
p-value [1]	<0.001		<0.001		<0.001		<0.001		<0.001	

[1] Pearson's chi-squared test.

4. Discussion

In this study, we reported population-based data on the frequency and severity of associated impairments among children with CP in rural Bangladesh. We found a substantially high burden of associated impairments among participating children. We also identified several factors that increased the odds of different types of associated impairments among children with CP registered in the BCPR. Unfortunately, the majority of the children with mild to severe associated impairments never received any rehabilitation services and the school enrolment rate was also low among those with multiple associated impairments compared to children with no associated impairments registered in the BCPR.

Speech impairment is the most common form of associated impairment among children with CP registered in the BCPR, followed by intellectual impairment and epilepsy. The findings are consistent with previously reported data from both LMICs and HICs [6,8,27–29]. In a population-based study in Uganda, intellectual impairment and epilepsy were reported among 75% and 45% of children in the cohort, respectively [27]. A few other studies in Vietnam, Moldova, and Ethiopia also reported a similarly high burden of speech and intellectual impairments among children with CP, however, those studies were conducted in hospital-based settings [8,28,29]. When compared to other HICs (such as west Sweden, Norway, and Australia), the proportion of severe intellectual impairment is slightly higher in Bangladesh (29%) compared to west Sweden (21–26%) and Australia (22%), but is similar to Norway (31%) [6,30,31]. The proportion of epilepsy observed among children with CP in Bangladesh (33%) is also similar to that reported in western Sweden (33–34%), Norway (28%), and Australia (28%) [6,30,31]. Interestingly, the proportion of severe speech impairment/non-verbal among children with CP is substantially higher in Bangladesh (41%) compared to Australia (24%) or Norway (28%) [6,30,31]. These differences could be attributed to the differences observed in functional impairment severity, motor type, etiology, diagnosis age, and rehabilitation status of children with CP in these countries.

Nevertheless, caution should be taken when comparing or interpreting these findings from different countries and regions due to the differences in data collection methods and study populations. More research is required to understand the regional similarities and differences in the profile of associated impairments among children with CP in LMICs such as Bangladesh.

The presence and severity of different types of associated impairments among children in our cohort vary according to their predominant motor type and topography. Speech, intellectual impairments, and epilepsy are more prevalent among children with bilateral spastic CP and dyskinetic CP, whereas hearing impairment is more common among children with ataxic CP. Similar findings were reported in Uganda (an LMIC) [27], Canada, and Sweden (HICs) [32,33], However, in Australia, speech and hearing impairment, and epilepsy were more common among children with dyskinetic CP, as well as among children with bilateral spastic CP [6].

All types of associated impairments are significantly higher among children with GMFCS level III to V. The findings are consistent with population-based data from Australia (i.e., ACPR), Sweden, and Uganda [6,27,33]. One possible explanation for this is that children with more severe motor impairment have suffered a more severe insult to the developing brain, resulting in a higher degree of brain injury that leads to more extensive disruption of white matter pathways, causing an increased number of associated impairments [34].

A positive relationship is observed between the presence of intellectual impairment or epilepsy and a history of IPR NRD in a child registered in the BCPR. History of IPR NRD is a strong indicator for adverse peri/neonatal events such as hypoxic–ischaemic encephalopathy (HIE) in newborns, and the risk is even higher in LMICs such as Bangladesh where homebirths in the absence of medical professionals are commonly observed. A positive relationship between a history of such adverse peri/neonatal events and gross motor function limitation, as well as a high burden of associated impairments, was previously reported in Sweden [33]. However we could not establish this causal relationship in this study and need further exploration.

Interestingly, the odds of different associated impairments, including hearing impairment, are significantly higher among children with postnatally acquired CP. One possible explanation for this may be that the auditory system is less susceptible than the brain to damage from perinatal hypoxia in the absence of associated ischemia. However, such ischemia is likely to be a complication of postnatal insults to the brain, such as cardiovascular instability due to sepsis, or repeated respiratory failures, thus, ensuring a greater association with hearing loss [35].

Our data show that nearly half of our study participants have never received any rehabilitation services. Developing needs-based rehabilitation services (including assistive devices) could improve the functional outcome and participation of these children (i.e., children with CP and other associated impairments) in daily activities. The very low school enrolment rate in this cohort is likely to be attributed to the limited functional capacity and lack of inclusive education system in the country. Similar findings were reported in other LMICs [2]. Such inequality in meeting the basic needs, e.g., health care, education, and inclusiveness, eventually makes these children vulnerable to falling into the vicious cycle of poverty, disability, and inequity in low-resource settings of LMICs.

Despite our considerable effort, the study has several limitations. Firstly, with the absence of adequate medical records and access to advanced diagnostic tools/equipment, it is difficult to apply the adopted case definitions and documentation of severity in a consistent manner for all children, especially for those with severe motor impairment and clinical complications. This may also have led to an underestimation of the true burden and misclassification of severity in very young children or children with severe intellectual impairments. Second, we used the key informant method to identify children with suspected CP from the community. Although KIM is a cost-effective method compared to door-to-door surveys, it is possible that due to a lack of expertise, the KIs may have missed a few milder cases of CP. This may also slightly influence the proportion of gross motor function limitation levels and severity of different associated impairments among registered children. Third, in the absence of medical records, we had to mostly rely on mother/caregiver-reported clinical history to determine the aetiology, timing, and potential causes of the brain injury that led to CP. As a result, we could not establish the confirmed underlying causes of different types of associated impairments among children with CP registered in the BCPR. Finally, as mentioned in the methods, the BCPR is an ongoing surveillance, and we have not achieved complete case ascertainment in some of the surveillance sites. Hence, we could not report the population-based prevalence of different associated impairments among children with CP in rural Bangladesh.

5. Conclusions

Associated impairments are commonly observed among children with CP in rural Bangladesh. The presence and severity of different associated impairments are also influenced by the motor and clinical characteristics of CP among children. It is therefore important to undertake a comprehensive approach for early intervention and rehabilitation services to address the needs for both motor function as well as associated impairments among children with CP. Unfortunately, the lack of service provision delays the initiation of early intervention and limits the opportunity of improving the functional capacity of these children and the scope for their participation in daily activities. Capacity development of mid-level rehabilitation workers, innovations to improve accessibility to assistive devices, and undertaking a community-based approach are some potential strategies to improve the situation in the country.

Supplementary Materials: The following supporting information can be downloaded at: https://www.mdpi.com/article/10.3390/jcm12041597/s1, Figure S1: Presence of associated impairment among children with CP according to their predominant motor type, topography, and GMFCS level; Table S1: Predictors of different types of associated impairment among children with CP in rural Bangladesh (unadjusted analysis).

Author Contributions: Conceptualization, M.M., G.K. and N.B.; methodology, M.M., G.K. and N.B.; software, I.J., I.H. and A.N.; validation, G.K. and I.J.; formal analysis, G.K., I.J., I.H. and A.N.; investigation, G.K.; resources, G.K.; data curation, G.K., I.J. and I.H.; writing—original draft preparation, A.N.; writing—review and editing, M.M., J.W., I.H., N.B, G.K. and I.J.; visualization, I.J., A.N. and G.K.; supervision, G.K., J.W. and I.J.; project administration, G.K. and M.M.; funding acquisition, G.K., N.B. and M.M. All authors have read and agreed to the published version of the manuscript.

Funding: The Bangladesh CP Register is funded by the Cerebral Palsy Alliance Research Foundation (PG4314—Bangladesh CP Register), Sydney Medical School Foundation of the University of Sydney, and internally from CSF Global. GK is supported by NHMRC Investigator Grant (APP2009873), and IJ is supported by Cerebral Palsy Alliance Research Foundation Emerging Researcher Grant (ERG02021).

Institutional Review Board Statement: Ethics approval for BCPR was obtained from the Human Research Ethics Committee of Bangladesh Medical Research Council (BMRC) (southasia-irb-2014-l-01), Cerebral Palsy Alliance (EC00402; ref no. 2015-03-02), and the Asian Institute of Disability and Development (AIDD) (southasia-irb-2014-l-01).

Informed Consent Statement: Informed written consent was obtained from all caregivers of children with CP prior to registration into the BCPR.

Data Availability Statement: The data presented in this study are available on request from the corresponding author. The data are not publicly available due to ethical considerations.

Acknowledgments: We thank all children with CP registered in the BCPR, and their family members for their valuable time, participation, and the information provided. We thank the CSF Global team in Bangladesh who support and work closely with children with CP and their families.

Conflicts of Interest: The authors declare no conflict of interest.

References

1. Rosenbaum, P.; Paneth, N.; Leviton, A.; Goldstein, M.; Bax, M.; Damiano, D.; Dan, B.; Jacobsson, B. A report: The definition and classifi-cation of cerebral palsy April 2006. *Dev. Med. Child Neurol.* **2007**, *49*, 8–14.
2. Jahan, I.; Muhit, M.; Hardianto, D.; Laryea, F.; Chhetri, A.B.; Smithers-Sheedy, H.; McIntyre, S.; Badawi, N.; Khandaker, G. Epidemiology of cerebral palsy in low- and middle-income countries: Preliminary findings from an international multi-centre cerebral palsy register. *Dev. Med. Child Neurol.* **2021**, *63*, 1327–1336. [CrossRef]
3. McIntyre, S.; Goldsmith, S.; Webb, A.; Ehlinger, V.; Hollung, S.J.; McConnell, K.; Arnaud, C.; Smithers-Sheedy, H.; Oskoui, M.; Khandaker, G.; et al. Global prevalence of cerebral palsy: A systematic analysis. *Dev. Med. Child Neurol.* **2022**, *64*, 1494–1506. [CrossRef]
4. Kakooza-Mwesige, A.; Andrews, C.; Peterson, S.; Mangen, F.W.; Eliasson, A.C.; Forssberg, H. Prevalence of cerebral palsy in Uganda: A population-based study. *Lancet Glob. Health* **2017**, *5*, e1275–e1282. [CrossRef]
5. Hollung, S.J.; Bakken, I.J.; Vik, T.; Lydersen, S.; Wiik, R.; Aaberg, K.M.; Andersen, G.L. Comorbidities in cerebral palsy: A patient registry study. *Dev. Med. Child Neurol.* **2020**, *62*, 97–103. [CrossRef]
6. Delacy, M.J.; Reid, S.M. The Australian cerebral palsy register group Profile of associated impairments at age 5 years in Australia by cerebral palsy subtype and Gross Motor Function Classification System level for birth years 1996 to 2005. *Dev. Med. Child Neurol.* **2016**, *58*, 50–56. [CrossRef]
7. Jahan, I.; Al Imam, M.H.; Karim, T.; Muhit, M.; Hardianto, D.; Das, M.C.; Smithers-Sheedy, H.; Badawi, N.; Khandaker, G. Epidemiology of cerebral palsy in Sumba Island, Indonesia. *Dev. Med. Child Neurol.* **2020**, *62*, 1414–1422. [CrossRef]
8. Karim, T.; Dossetor, R.; Huong Giang, N.T.; Dung, T.Q.; Son, T.V.; Hoa, N.X.; Tuyet, N.H.; Van Anh, N.T.; Chau, C.M.; Bang, N.V.; et al. Data on cerebral palsy in Vietnam will inform clinical practice and policy in low and mid-dle-income countries. *Disabil. Rehabil.* **2022**, *44*, 3081–3088. [CrossRef]
9. Khandaker, G.; Smithers-Sheedy, H.; Islam, J.; Alam, M.; Jung, J.; Novak, I.; Booy, R.; Jones, C.; Badawi, N.; Muhit, M. Bang-ladesh Cerebral Palsy Register (BCPR): A pilot study to develop a national cerebral palsy (CP) register with sur-veillance of children for CP. *BMC Neurol.* 2015 *15*, 173.
10. Khandaker, G.; Muhit, M.; Karim, T.; Smithers-Sheedy, H.; Novak, I.; Jones, C.; Badawi, N. Epidemiology of cerebral palsy in Bangladesh: A population-based surveillance study. *Dev. Med. Child Neurol.* **2019**, *61*, 601–609. [CrossRef]
11. Al Imam, M.H.; Jahan, I.; Muhit, M.; Das, M.C.; Power, R.; Khan, A.; Akbar, D.; Badawi, N.; Khandaker, G. Supporting Ul-tra Poor People with Rehabilitation and Therapy among families of children with Cerebral Palsy in rural Bangla-desh (SUPPORT CP): Protocol of a randomised controlled trial. *PLoS ONE* **2021**, *16*, e0261148. [CrossRef]
12. Jahan, I.; Al Imam, M.H.; Muhit, M.; Akbar, D.; Bashar, K.; Khandaker, G. Effectiveness of a Sustainable Model of eARly Intervention and Tele-Rehabilitation Service to Increase Early Intervention and Rehabilitation Service Uptake among Children with Cerebral Palsy in rural Bangladesh (SMART CP)—A Cluster Randomized Controlled Trial. Trial ID: ACTRN12622000396729. 2022. Available online: https://www.anzctr.org.au (accessed on 4 February 2023).
13. Karim, T.; Das, M.C.; Muhit, M.; Badawi, N.; Khandaker, G.; Mohammad, S.S. Improving epilepsy control among children with cerebral palsy in rural Bangladesh: A prospective cohort-based study. *BMJ Open* **2022**, *12*, e052578. [CrossRef]
14. Karim, T.; Muhit, M.; Jahan, I.; Galea, C.; Morgan, C.; Smithers-Sheedy, H.; Badawi, N.; Khandaker, G. Outcome of Community-Based Early Intervention and Rehabilitation for Children with Cerebral Palsy in Rural Bangladesh: A Quasi-Experimental Study. *Brain Sci.* **2021**, *11*, 1189. [CrossRef]
15. Smithers-Sheedy, H.; Waight, E.; Goldsmith, S.; Reid, S.; Gibson, C.; Watson, L.; Auld, M.; Badawi, N.; Webb, A.; Diviney, L.; et al. Declining trends in birth prevalence and severity of singletons with cerebral palsy of prenatal or perinatal origin in Australia: A population-based observational study. *Dev. Med. Child Neurol.* **2022**, *64*, 1114–1122. [CrossRef]
16. Cans, C. Surveillance of cerebral palsy in Europe: A collaboration of cerebral palsy surveys and registers. *Dev. Med. Child Neurol.* **2000**, *42*, 816–824. [CrossRef]
17. Bangladesh Bureau of Statistics. Population and Housing Census 2022 (National Volume 2: Union Statistics). 2014. Available on-line: http://203.112.218.65:8008/WebTestApplication/userfiles/Image/National%20Reports/Union%20Statistics.pdf (accessed on 4 February 2023).
18. Mackey, S.; Murthy, G.V.; Muhit, M.A.; Islam, J.J.; Foster, A. Validation of the key informant method to identify chil-dren with disabilities: Methods and results from a pilot study in Bangladesh. *J. Trop. Pediatr.* **2012**, *58*, 269–274. [CrossRef]
19. National Institute of Population Research and Training (NIPORT); ICF. Bangladesh Demographic and Health Survey 2017–2018. Dhaka, Bangladesh, and Rockville, Maryland, USA: NIPORT and ICF. 2020. Available online: https://dhsprogram.com/pubs/pdf/FR344/FR344.pdf (accessed on 4 February 2023).
20. WHO. Low Birth Weight. Available online: https://www.who.int/data/nutrition/nlis/info/low-birth-weight (accessed on 4 February 2023).
21. Lee, A.C.; Mullany, L.C.; Tielsch, J.M.; Katz, J.; Khatry, S.K.; LeClerq, S.C.; Adhikari, R.K.; Darmstadt, G.L. Incidence of and Risk Factors for Neonatal Respiratory Depression and Encephalopathy in Rural Sarlahi, Nepal. *Pediatrics* **2011**, *128*, e915–e924. [CrossRef]
22. Rosenbaum, P.L.; Palisano, R.J.; Bartlett, D.J.; Galuppi, B.E.; Russell, D.J. Development of the gross motor function clas-sification system for cerebral palsy. *Dev. Med. Child Neurol.* **2008**, *50*, 249–253. [CrossRef]

23. Eliasson, A.C.; Krumlinde-Sundholm, L.; Rösblad, B.; Beckung, E.; Arner, M.; Öhrvall, A.M.; Rosenbaum, P. The Manu-al Ability Classification System (MACS) for children with cerebral palsy: Scale development and evidence of valid-ity and reliability. *Dev. Med. Child Neurol.* **2006**, *48*, 549–554. [CrossRef]
24. Pirozzo, S.; Papinczak, T.; Glasziou, P. Whispered voice test for screening for hearing impairment in adults and children: Systematic review. *BMJ* **2003**, *327*, 967. [CrossRef]
25. World Health Organization. Hearing Screening: Considerations for Implementation. 2021. Available online: https://www.who.int/publications/i/item/9789240032767 (accessed on 4 February 2023).
26. National Academies of Sciences, Engineering, and Medicine. *Mental Disorders and Disabilities among Low-Income Children*; The National Academies Press: Washington, DC, USA, 2015.
27. Kakooza-Mwesige, A.; Forssberg, H.; Eliasson, A.-C.; Tumwine, J.K. Cerebral palsy in children in Kampala, Uganda: Clinical subtypes, motor function and co-morbidities. *BMC Res. Notes* **2015**, *8*, 166. [CrossRef]
28. Bufteac, E.G.; Andersen, G.L.; Torstein, V.; Jahnsen, R. Cerebral palsy in Moldova: Subtypes, severity and associated impairments. *BMC Pediatr.* **2018**, *18*, 332. [CrossRef]
29. Tsige, S.; Moges, A.; Mekasha, A.; Abebe, W.; Forssberg, H. Cerebral palsy in children: Subtypes, motor function and associated impairments in Addis Ababa, Ethiopia. *BMC Pediatr.* **2021**, *21*, 544. [CrossRef]
30. Jonsson, U.; Eek, M.N.; Sunnerhagen, K.S.; Himmelmann, K. Cerebral palsy prevalence, subtypes, and associated impairments: A population-based comparison study of adults and children. *Dev. Med. Child Neurol.* **2019**, *61*, 1162–1167. [CrossRef]
31. Andersen, G.L.; Irgens, L.M.; Haagaas, I.; Skranes, J.S.; Meberg, A.E.; Vik, T. Cerebral palsy in Norway: Prevalence, sub-types and severity. *Eur. J. Paediatr. Neurol.* **2007**, *12*, 4–13. [CrossRef]
32. Shevell, M.I.; Dagenais, L.; Hall, N.; On behalf of the REPACQ Consortium. Comorbidities in cerebral palsy and their relationship to neurologic subtype and GMFCS level. *Neurology* **2009**, *72*, 2090–2096. [CrossRef]
33. Himmelmann, K.; Beckung, E.; Hagberg, G.; Uvebrant, P. Gross and fine motor function and accompanying im-pairments in cerebral palsy. *Dev. Med. Child Neurol.* **2006**, *48*, 417–423. [CrossRef]
34. Imamura, T.; Ariga, H.; Kaneko, M.; Watanabe, M.; Shibukawa, Y.; Fukuda, Y.; Nagasawa, K.; Goto, A.; Fujiki, T. Neurodevelop-mental Outcomes of Children with Periventricular Leukomalacia. *Pediatr. Neonatol.* **2013**, *54*, 367–372. [CrossRef]
35. Borg, E. Perinatal Asphyxia, Hypoxia, Ischemia and Hearing Loss: An Overview. *Scand. Audiol.* **1997**, *26*, 77–91. [CrossRef]

Disclaimer/Publisher's Note: The statements, opinions and data contained in all publications are solely those of the individual author(s) and contributor(s) and not of MDPI and/or the editor(s). MDPI and/or the editor(s) disclaim responsibility for any injury to people or property resulting from any ideas, methods, instructions or products referred to in the content.

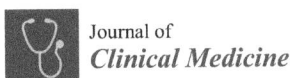

Journal of
Clinical Medicine

Article

Emotion Regulation Is Associated with Anxiety, Depression and Stress in Adults with Cerebral Palsy

Ingrid Honan [1,2,*], Emma Waight [1], Joan Bratel [1], Fiona Given [1], Nadia Badawi [1,3], Sarah McIntyre [1] and Hayley Smithers-Sheedy [1]

1. Cerebral Palsy Alliance Research Institute, Specialty of Child & Adolescent Health, The University of Sydney, Camperdown, NSW 2050, Australia
2. Australian Centre for Health, Independence, Economic Participation and Value Enhanced Care for Adolescents and Young Adults with Cerebral Palsy (CP-Achieve), Melbourne, VIC 3052, Australia
3. Grace Centre for Newborn Care, The Children's Hospital at Westmead, Specialty of Child & Adolescent Health, The University of Sydney, Westmead, NSW 2145, Australia
* Correspondence: ingrid.honan@cerebralpalsy.org.au; Tel.: +61-437617581

Abstract: Emotion regulation difficulties are associated with many neurological conditions and negatively impact daily function. Yet little is known about emotion regulation in adults with cerebral palsy (CP). Our aim was to investigate emotion regulation in adults with CP and its relationship with condition-related and/or socio-demographic factors. In a cross-sectional study of adults with CP, participants completed a survey containing the Difficulties in Emotion Regulation Scale (DERS), Depression Anxiety and Stress Scale-21 (DASS-21), and socio-demographic and condition-related questions. Descriptive statistics, chi-squared and Mann–Whitney tests were performed. Of the 42 adults with CP (x31.5 years, SD13.5) that were tested, 38 had within normal limits DERS total scores; however, a significantly higher proportion of participants experienced elevated scores (i.e., more difficulties with emotion regulation) than would be expected in the general population across five of the six DERs subdomains. Moderate–extremely severe depression and anxiety symptoms were reported by 33% and 60% of participants, respectively. The DERS total scores for participants with elevated depression, anxiety, and stress scores were significantly higher than the DERS totals score for those without elevated depression, anxiety, and stress scores. DERS and DASS-21 scores did not differ significantly by condition-related nor socio-demographic characteristics. In conclusion, emotion regulation difficulties were associated with elevated symptoms of depression and anxiety, which were overrepresented in the adults with CP participating in this study.

Keywords: cerebral palsy; disability; emotion regulation; depression; anxiety

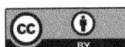

1. Introduction

Cerebral palsy (CP) is an umbrella term for a group of non-progressive motor disorders resulting from damage to or maldevelopment of the immature brain [1]. These disorders are permanent but not unchanging and are frequently accompanied by other conditions, including emotional and behavioural difficulties [1]. Preschool children with CP have been shown to experience more emotional/behavioural difficulties than their peers [2]. Similarly, a large European study of primary school aged children with CP found almost one third had emotion difficulties and 40% had significant social impairments as a result of their emotional or behavioural problems [3]. Other studies of school aged children with CP from Australia and Canada have also identified higher rates of emotional, behavioural, and social difficulties compared with typically developing children [4,5]. A recent study comparing associations between emotion knowledge and emotion regulation abilities of 36 children with CP with 45 typically developing children demonstrated that children with CP exhibited poorer emotion knowledge and poorer emotion regulation skills than their typically developing peers, and that there was an association between emotion regulation abilities and emotion knowledge [6]. However, less is known about how emotional difficulties manifest and impact people with CP in adulthood.

Emotion regulation (ER) refers to how we 'influence which emotions we have, when we have them, and how we experience and express them' [7]. It involves a series of processes, including: a situation, cognitively attending both to the situation and our emotions, appraising our emotions in the situation, and developing a response. Being able to intrinsically experience and regulate our emotions provides us with a feeling of control and allows us to respond to the demands of daily life in a socially acceptable manner [8]. This is useful in education, employment, and in building and maintaining relationships across a lifespan [9–11].

ER difficulties are associated with a range of conditions. More than half of all psychological diagnostic categories (e.g., anxiety and mood disorders) and all personality disorders include ER difficulties as part of the symptomatology required to meet diagnostic criteria [7,12]. ER difficulties are also associated with executive functions and attention deficit hyperactive disorder (ADHD). Given people with CP are more likely to have co-occurring ADHD than the general population, and people with ADHD are at increased risk of experiencing psychological symptoms in adulthood such as anxiety and depression, examining the occurrence of ER difficulties in adults with CP is warranted.

The neural underpinning of ER is also important to examine when considering the likelihood of associations between ER difficulties and CP in adulthood. A model proposed by Etkin et al. (2015) describes how predictions, prediction errors, and valuations contribute towards two forms of ER: model-free regulation and model-based regulation [13]. However, the way in which the neural systems and associated brain regions involved in ER are affected in many conditions is still unclear. It is acknowledged that the dorsal anterior cingulate, insula, amygdala, and periaqueductal grey are all associated with emotional reactivity. Similarly, ER evidence from fields such as Tourette Syndrome, depression, anxiety, traumatic brain injury, and Parkinson's disease suggest that components of the basal ganglia, the amygdala, and/or the connections between these regions play a key role in emotion regulation [14,15]. However, little is known about CP and ER. Some forms of CP, particularly dyskinetic CP, are caused by damage to the basal ganglia [16]. Moreover, brain pathology for people with CP occurs in early development [17], likely impacting plasticity and experiential learning pathways. A recent study examining neural circuitry in adults with CP demonstrated associations between level of functional connectivity in brain regions associated with ER and social skills, and participant well-being scores [18]. As regions of the brain known to control ER have been associated with CP, it is reasonable to hypothesise that adults with CP may experience an increased incidence of ER difficulties than expected in the general population.

Research is required to better understand ER and the relationship between ER and clinical and socio-demographic factors in adults with CP. This is necessary to determine whether there is a need for services and screening to support adults with CP and to assist in managing these challenges. In this study, we aimed to (1) investigate self-reported ER difficulties in adults with CP, and (2) to determine whether ER was associated with other demographic and condition-related factors, including symptoms of mood difficulties (depression, anxiety, and stress), ambulatory status, communication level, living arrangements, employment status, etc. It was hypothesised that (1) adults with CP are more likely to experience ER difficulties than the general population, and (2) that ER difficulties are associated with mood and condition-related factors and socio-demographic factors such as ambulatory status and employment status, respectively.

2. Materials and Methods

2.1. Study Design

This was a cross-sectional study design. The research question was initiated by co-author FG who has a lived experience of CP. Key stages of study design and interpretation of results were informed by lived experience and current best research practice. Methodology and data are reported according to the CHERRIES (Checklist for Reporting Results of Internet E-Surveys) statement [19].

2.2. Ethics

Ethical approval was granted by the Cerebral Palsy Alliance Human Research Ethics Committee (3 November 2018), Victorian Cerebral Palsy Register Governance, and Queensland Cerebral Palsy Register Steering Committee, with data collected throughout 2019. All participants were provided a participant information sheet outlining study protocol and informed consent was obtained.

2.3. Participants, Procedures and Measures

The study was advertised in the NSW/ACT CP Register newsletter and via a study flyer (Appendix A Figure A1). To be eligible, participants were required to have a confirmed diagnosis of CP, be aged $\geq$ 18 years, and have no/mild intellectual impairment as recorded in the CP register. No incentives were offered for participation in the study.

Participants completed a voluntary 15-min paper or online survey. The survey included questions related to socio-demographic and clinical condition, including gender, age, residential postcode, employment status, living arrangements, primary support person, Gross Motor Function Classification System-Expanded and Revised (GMFCS-E&R) [20] level, predominant CP motor type, Communication Function Classification System (CFCS) [21] level, use of Augmentative and Alternative Communication (AAC), receipt of supports/services, and history of any psychological disorder/s, e.g., anxiety/depression. Descriptors were provided alongside classification systems such as the GMFCS and CFCS to allow participants to self-select their level if they did not already know it. Moreover, questions around communication and AAC were asked using branching logic, and participant responses were checked for consistency. See Supplementary Materials for a full copy of the survey.

Other items included the Depression Anxiety and Stress Scale short-form (DASS-21) [22] and the Difficulties of Emotion Regulation Scale-36 (DERS) [23]. The DASS-21 is a validated self-report measure of psychological distress widely used in research and clinical practice. Using a four-point Likert scale 0–3 (never, sometimes, often, almost always) individuals rate their responses to 21 items. Seven items contributed to each of the sub-scales: depression, anxiety, and stress. Cut-off scores have been developed for each sub-scale to indicate mild, moderate, severe, and extremely severe scores. Cut-off scores indicate symptoms relative to the general population, rather than level of severity of a diagnosable disorder, i.e., 'mild' indicates mildly elevated symptoms of depression compared to the general population, not that the individual meets diagnostic criteria for depression in the mild range. The DASS-21 was adapted from the DASS-42 and has demonstrated adequate construct validity and high reliability (0.88 depression, 0.82 anxiety, and 0.90 stress) [22].

DERS is a validated 36-item self-report measure of emotion regulation. Using a five-point Likert scale 1–5 (almost never, sometimes, about half of the time, most of the time, almost always) participants rate responses. Responses were tallied to obtain a total score and six sub-scale scores: non-acceptance of emotional responses (nonaccept), difficulties engaging in goal directed behaviour (goals), impulse control difficulties (impulse), lack of emotional awareness (awareness), limited access to ER strategies (strategies), and lack of emotional clarity (clarity) [23]. Higher scores indicate greater difficulties with ER. Total and sub-scale scores can be converted into age and gender adjusted T-scores, with a mean of 50 and a standard deviation (SD) of 10 [24]. Validity and reliability of DERS is well established, with good internal consistency (Cronbach's α ranging from 0.80 to 0.89) and test–retest reliability for total DERS scores being 0.88 [23].

Online open survey data were collected using REDCap electronic data capture tool, hosted by The University of Sydney. A response was required for all items on the DASS-21 and DERS and participants were able to progress through the survey and review their previous responses at their own pace. The survey was completed by five individuals prior to study commencement to review functionality and acceptability. A copy of the survey is available in Supplementary Materials. In line with ethical requirements, participants who endorsed items suggesting that they were a safety risk to themselves or others were contacted by a registered psychologist and offered support and/or links to services.

2.4. Statistical Analyses

Employment was collapsed into two categories based on participant responses: 'Employed' = full-time, part-time, casual, volunteer, student; 'Unemployed' = unemployed, retired. Similarly, living situation was collapsed into four categories: 'Alone'; 'Share house' = share house or supported accommodation; 'With spouse' = with or without children; 'Other family' = living with parents, living with other children alone or living with other family. GMFCS was collapsed into two categories: 'Ambulant' = GMFCS level I or II; 'Supported mobility' = GMFCS levels III, IV and V. DASS-21 scores were categorised into normal, mild, moderate, severe, and extremely severe groups [22]. Scores were then further collapsed into two groups: "Low" = normal and mild scores and "Elevated" = moderate, severe, extremely severe, based on normative data. "Elevated" scores therefore indicate that an individual endorses feelings of depression equal to or more often/severe than 88 percent of the normative sample, feelings of anxiety equal to or more often/severe than 92 percent of the normative sample, and feelings of stress equal to or more often/severe than 89 percent of the normative sample [22]. These cut-offs were selected as they are considered clinically significant. DERS-36 total scores and sub-scale scores were converted to age and gender adjusted T-scores [24]. DERS T-scores were categorised into two groups; "WNL" (within normal limits) = those who scored ≤ 1.5 SD above the mean (a T-score of ≤ 65), and "Elevated" = those who scored more than 1.5 SD above the mean (a T-score of >65).

Data were analysed using SPSS (Version 24). Descriptive and frequency statistics were run for all variables. Means and proportions were calculated for DASS-21 and DERS sub-scales, and chi-squared tests were performed on DERS scores to compare whether the current sample proportions differed from expected population proportions, based on normative data. Mann–Whitney tests were conducted to examine the relationship between Total DERS scores and DASS-21 sub-scales, with significance set to $p = 0.05$. Mean total DERS T-scores by DASS-21 sub-scale category were calculated and plotted onto a bar graph. Where sample sizes allowed ($n \geq 5$), Mann–Whitney tests were performed to examine relationships between clinical and socio-demographic factors and DASS-21 and DERS scores.

3. Results

After eliminating any duplicate responses, there were 48 respondents who participated in the survey; two were ineligible, two declined consent, and two were incomplete. There were $n = 42$ participants with complete data which were included in the analyses. Table 1 outlines the participant characteristics.

The mean age of participants was 31.5 years (SD 13.48) and 43 percent were males. The majority of participants had spastic hemiplegia and were ambulant (Table 1). Most participants reported that they were effective communicators with no intellectual impairment. When examining socio-demographic factors, $n = 24/42$ (58%) of participants were living with other family members, with the majority of this group living with their parents. Seventy percent of participants were engaged in some form of employment (including volunteer work or study); however, only 22.5 percent of participants were working full-time. Just over 40 percent of participants had received a formal diagnosis of a psychological disorder.

Table 1. Participant characteristics.

Characteristics	Total n = 42
Females; n (%)	24 (57.1)
Age; Mean (SD); Range	31.50 (13.48); (18–72)
CP Type/topography [++] n (%)	
Spastic	30 (73.2)
Hemiplegia	15 (50.0)
Diplegia	8 (26.7)
Quadriplegia	7 (23.3)
Dyskinesia	4 (9.7)
Ataxia	1 (2.4)
Mixed	5 (12.2)
Unknown	1 (2.4)
Intellectual Ability n (%)	
No impairment	37 (88.1)
Mild impairment	5 (11.9)
Functional Communication Level [++] n (%)	
Effective communicator	33 (80.5)
Slow but effective communicator	6 (14.6)
Effective communicator with familiar people	2 (4.9)
Inconsistent communicator	0
Seldom effective communicator	0
AAC; N (%)	
Use AAC	6 (14.3)
GMFCS level; n (%)	
I	14 (33.3)
II	13 (31)
III	4 (9.5)
IV	6 (14.3)
V	5 (11.9)
Gross Motor Function; n (%)	
Ambulant	27 (64.3)
Supported mobility	15 (35.7)
Employment Status [+] n (%)	
Employed	28 (70.0)
Unemployed	12 (30)
Living Arrangement [++] n (%)	
Alone	7 (17.1)
Share house	5 (12.2)
With spouse	5 (12.2)
Other family	24 (58.5)
Primary Support Person; n (%)	
Parent	22 (52.4)
I do not have a primary support person	13 (31.0)
Partner/spouse	2 (4.8)
Sibling	1 (2.4)
Caseworker/advocate/other	4 (9.6)
Psychological Disorder; n (%)	
Diagnosed psychological disorder	17 (40.5)
Routine Services; n (%)	
Receiving routine services	18 (42.9)

[+] N = 40; [++] N = 41.

Examination of self-reported ER using the DERS found that only four participants reported experiencing total elevated DERS scores. Due to small sample size in the elevated group, it was not possible to examine statistical significance. However, when examining sub-scale scores, a higher proportion of participants experienced elevated scores across all sub-scale areas, except lack of emotional clarity, than would be expected in the general population (Table 2).

Table 2. Means and proportions of depression, anxiety, stress and emotion regulation scores.

	Raw DERS	DERS Scores	T-Scores		
	Mean (SD)	Mean (SD)	WNL [1] N (%)	Elevated [2] N (%)	p-Value
Total	81.93 (30.30)	50.95 (14.87)	38 (90.5)	4 (9.5)	Not able to compute
Nonaccept	14.69 (6.99)	55.52 (14.64)	32 (76.2)	10 (23.8)	<0.001
Goals	13.45 (5.29)	49.67 (12.32)	36 (85.7)	6 (14.3)	0.048
Impulse	12.50 (6.31)	51.28 (13.26)	36 (85.7)	6 (14.3)	0.048
Awareness	13.45 (5.53)	51.52 (13.51)	36 (85.7)	6 (14.3)	0.048
Strategies	17.86 (8.26)	52.25 (12.76)	35 (83.3)	7 (16.7)	0.010
Clarity	9.98 (4.41)	49.04 (11.36)	37 (88.1)	5 (11.9)	0.175

	DASS-21 Scores							
	Mean	SD	Range	n (%) Scoring in Ranges				
				Normal	Mild	Moderate	Severe	Extremely Severe
Depression	5.71	3.897	0–18	19 (45.2)	9 (21.4)	8 (19.0)	5 (11.9)	1 (2.4)
Anxiety	7.10	4.143	2–19	10 (23.8)	7 (16.7)	9 (21.4)	6 (14.3)	10 (23.8)
Stress	5.62	4.654	0–20	29 (69.0)	8 (19.0)	0 (0.0)	4 (9.5)	1 (2.4)

[1] WNL = "within normal limits"; [2] Elevated => 1.5 SD from normative mean, 6.68 percent of the normative population would be expected to experience emotion regulation scores 1.5 SD above the mean. Chi-squared goodness-of-fit test performed on DERS scores compared whether sample proportion differed from expected population proportion, based on normative data.

When examining results from the DASS-21 (Table 2) the data for symptoms of depression indicated that 67% percent of participants reported symptoms in the 'normal–mild' range with 33% above this range (moderate–extremely severe). In terms of anxiety, 40% reported symptoms of anxiety in the 'normal–mild' range with the remaining 60% with reported symptoms in the 'moderate–extremely severe' range. The majority (88%) of participants reported symptoms of stress in the 'normal–mild' range.

There was a significant positive relationship between depression, anxiety, and stress, and total DERS scores. DERS total scores for participants with elevated depression, anxiety, and stress scores was significantly higher than the DERS totals score for those without elevated depression, anxiety, and stress scores (Table 3, Figure 1).

Table 3. Non-parametric relationship between depression, anxiety, and stress and total emotion regulation T-scores.

	DASS Low Group			DASS Elevated Group			Change Statistic
	DERS Total T-Score			DERS Total T-Score			
	N	Median	IQR	N	Median	IQR	p-Value
Anxiety	17	42.85	16.64	25	56.82	16.86	0.001
Depression	28	43.16	15.94	14	62.18	16.29	<0.001
Stress	37	49.74	17.65	5	71.64	29.27	0.002

Note: 'Low Group' refers to scores on the DASS that are ≤mild range; 'Elevated Group' refers to scores on the DASS that are ≥moderate range. Mann–Whitney tests were conducted to examine the relationship between Total DERS scores and DASS-21 sub-scales, with significance set to $p = 0.05$.

When examining DERS total T-scores, depression, anxiety, and stress scores by gender and employment status, there were no significant differences across groups (Table 4). Similarly, when examining factors relating to motor condition, there was no significant difference in scores across groups for gross motor function, communication level, or whether or not participants were receiving routine services. Those who had a history of a diagnosed psychological disorder obtained significantly higher DERS total T-scores, anxiety, and stress scores than those who had no history of a diagnosed psychological disorder. There was no difference between groups for depression scores.

Table 4. Non-parametric examination of depression, anxiety, stress, and emotion regulation difficulties by socio-demographic factors.

	DERs Total			Depression			Anxiety			Stress		
	Median	IQR	p-Value	Median	IQR	p-Value	Median	IQR	p-Value	Median	IQR	p-Value
Gross Motor Function												
Ambulant	52.90	10.65	0.232	6.00	5.00	0.225	7.00	5.00	0.117	4.00	5.00	0.518
Supported mobility	43.46	19.08		4.00	3.00		5.00	5.00		4.00	6.00	
Gender												
Male	46.30	26.94	0.416	6.50	6.25	0.289	7.00	7.50	0.574	5.50	7.00	0.898
Female	52.81	19.91		4.00	3.00		6.50	3.75		4.00	3.75	
CFCS												
Effective communicator	49.97	20.75	0.224	5.00	6.25	0.393	6.00	6.00	0.368	4.00	5.25	0.519
Reduced communication	54.36	24.26		6.50	5.75		8.00	8.25		7.00	6.25	
Employment Status [+]												
Employed	52.81	21.18	0.859	5.00	6.75	0.711	6.50	4.75	0.859	4.00	4.75	0.801
Unemployed	48.26	18.81		5.00	4.75		7.00	6.50		5.00	6.50	
Diagnosed psychological disorder												
yes	54.92	9.93	0.018	6.00	5.00	0.091	7.00	6.00	0.033	6.00	4.50	0.008
no	42.85	21.67		4.00	6.50		5.00	5.50		3.00	6.00	
Receiving routine services												
yes	51.46	21.84	0.722	4.50	5.50	0.498	6.00	6.25	0.601	4.00	4.75	0.344
no	51.97	20.84		5.00	5.75		7.00	5.25		6.00	5.00	

Note: Elevated DASS scores are scores ≥ Moderate range; Elevated DERs total scores are T-scores ≥ 1.5 SD above the mean; [+] N = 40; Mann–Whitney nonparametric tests performed.

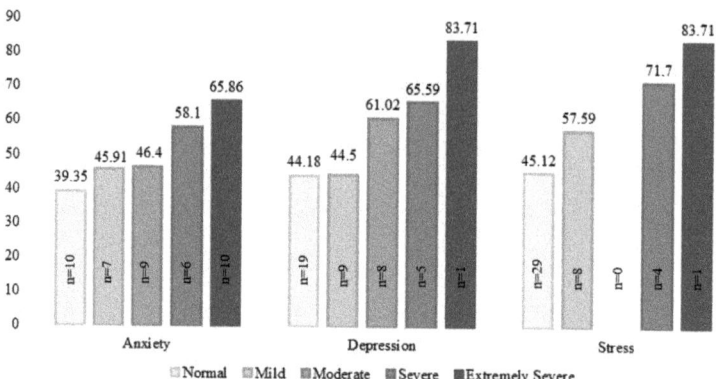

Figure 1. Mean total emotion regulation scores by level of depression, anxiety, and stress.

4. Discussion

To date, there has been little research investigating ER in adults with CP. To begin to explore these factors we conducted a cross-sectional survey of adults with CP with no/mild intellectual impairment. Self-reported ER scores varied widely, with 90% of participant total scores falling within normal limits. However, when examining ER sub-scale scores, a higher proportion of participants scored in the elevated range across all sub-scales, except emotional clarity, than would be expected in the general population. Worryingly, moderate-extremely severe symptoms of depression and anxiety were common; however, most participants' stress scores fell within normal limits. A clear positive relationship was observed between mood and ER scores, whereby people with elevated depression, anxiety, and stress scores experienced more ER difficulties than those without elevated depression, anxiety, and stress scores. Apart from having a diagnosed psychological disorder, no other clinical or socioeconomic factors were associated with the DERS or DASS-21 scores in this sample.

A statistically significant proportion of the total group had elevated sub-scale scores for nonacceptance of emotional responses ($n = 10$, 24%), difficulties engaging in goal-directed behaviour ($n = 6$, 14%), impulse control difficulties ($n = 6$, 14%), lack of emotional awareness ($n = 6$, 14%), and limited access to ER strategies ($n = 7$, 17%). Lower acceptance of emotions, not having strategies, or using less effective ER strategies have been associated with higher depressive symptoms [25,26]. This relationship between ER and mood disorders has been observed in other diagnostic groups, including individuals with traumatic brain injury and eating disorders, [27,28] and suggests that use of effective ER strategies (e.g., mindfulness practices and meditation) may have a role to play in the management of mood disorders [29].

It is understood that adults with CP experience higher rates of mood disorders than the general population [30–32]. Here we found that one third of participants had depression scores falling in the moderate to extremely severe range and more than half had anxiety scores in the moderate to extremely severe range. Whilst data are not diagnostic in nature and therefore not directly comparable, this is considerably higher than what might be expected from population estimates of 10% percent of Australians with depression and 13% percent with anxiety disorder [33]. Interestingly, adults with CP in this study were no more likely to experience stress than the general population. Whilst stress of caregivers of people with CP has been well researched, evidence examining stress in adults with CP is scarce.

The multi-factorial mechanisms responsible for high rates of depression and anxiety in CP are not well understood. In some instances, the brain injury or maldevelopment responsible for an individual's CP may also predispose them to mood disorders and emotion dysregulation [30]. Brain injuries or maldevelopments common in CP can impact the frontal cortex, cerebellum, and limbic system, all of which have important roles in how we regulate emotions, mood, and behaviour [30,34]. Moreover, given that the underlying brain injury or maldevelopment responsible for a person's CP occurs in or before infancy, and ER development occurs across childhood, adolescence, and young adulthood, early injury may have downstream developmental effects. Beyond a biological predisposition, there are a number of other environmental factors that may contribute to mood disorders and associated emotion dysregulation in CP such as pain, social isolation, and marginalisation.

Pain and mood disorders such as depression often co-occur in the general population, with the relationship between pain and mood being bidirectional [35,36]. Chronic pain is reported in both adults and children with CP at a higher rate than the general population, with studies across the world reporting that 33–84% of participants with CP experience pain [30,37–39]. Whilst there is little research describing the contribution of pain to depression in CP, management of pain is essential to support both a good quality of life and to promote mental well-being.

Social isolation and loneliness are also risk factors for mood disorders [40,41]. Whilst not investigated in this study, there is research to suggest that adults with CP experience more social isolation and loneliness than adults without disability [42]. It is hypothesised that this relates to barriers faced in regards to social integration, forming relationships, finding employment, communication, accessing transport for activities outside the home, and having limited accommodation options/choice, all of which can contribute to social isolation [41–43]. In addition to improving quality of life, strategies to support social connectedness may reduce the risk of mood disorders and associated emotion dysregulation in CP.

Strengths and Limitations

To the best of our knowledge, this is the first study to investigate the relationship between ER, mood, and socio-demographic and condition related factors in adults with CP. The research question for this study was originally initiated by author FG who has a lived experience of CP. We found that adults with CP in this study had increased experiences of emotional dysregulation than the general population, had elevated symptoms of depression and anxiety, and that increasing symptoms of depression, anxiety, and stress were associated with poorer emotion regulation. In terms of limitations, this was a preliminary study which aimed to examine ER across adults with CP, and no matched comparison group was included in the design. We did not specifically target any CP motor subgroups for recruitment. The small number of respondents meant it was not statistically viable to investigate ER or mood in some subgroups of interest. Future studies could specifically recruit a sample of adults with dyskinetic CP to investigate emotion dysregulation and mood disorders amongst adults with dyskinetic CP, given dyskinetic CP frequently involves damage to the basal ganglia [44]. As data for this study were collected by a self-report survey, eligibility criteria were limited to individuals with no/mild intellectual impairment, excluding participation for people with CP who had moderate and severe intellectual impairments. Understanding ER and mood in adults with CP and intellectual impairment is also important and should be considered in future research. There was a high proportion of participants ($n = 17$, 40%) who reported having a diagnosed psychological disorder. This highlights a possible self-selection bias with participants who are aware of, or who are experiencing difficulties in this area of their lives potentially being more likely to respond to the study invitation. Conversely, there may have been an underrepresentation of participants with psychological and emotion regulation difficulties who may have chosen not to participate. Finally, the survey was sent to everyone within the eligible age range on the CP registers. The response rate of 42, although expected for a survey study with no immediate benefit for participants, is low. Results, therefore, may not be representative of the broader CP in adulthood population. Finally, data were collected in 2019 before the COVID-19 pandemic. Marginalised groups, including people with disability, have been disproportionately negatively affected by the COVID-19 pandemic and associated societal and policy changes [45]. Similarly, mental health difficulties have increased as a result of the COVID-19 pandemic; therefore, these rates may now be higher than when the data were collected.

5. Conclusions

This is the first study investigating ER amongst adults with CP. Here we observed that the majority of participants had total ER scores within normal limits. However, more participants than expected based on the general population had elevated sub-scale scores, indicating difficulties accepting emotional responses, engaging in goal-directed behaviour, controlling impulses, a lack of emotional awareness, and low belief in and knowledge of strategies to help regulate emotions. Worryingly, a higher proportion of participants reported symptoms of depression than the general population and a relatively high proportion reported symptoms of anxiety. In this study, we found a clear positive relationship between mood and ER scores, whereby participants with elevated depression, anxiety, and stress symptoms reported more ER difficulties than those who did not have elevated depression, anxiety, or stress symptoms. Considering the relationship between mood and ER, use of ER strategies (e.g., mindfulness) may be helpful tools for people with CP and mood difficulties. In the absence of known prevention strategies, screening of emotion regulation and mood difficulties as part of routine health reviews with appropriate onward referral and support should be evaluated.

Supplementary Materials: The following supporting information can be downloaded at: https://www.mdpi.com/article/10.3390/jcm12072527/s1. File S1: Study REDCap Survey.

Author Contributions: Conceptualisation, F.G., H.S.-S., I.H. and E.W.; methodology, I.H., H.S.-S., E.W. and S.M.; data collection, H.S.-S., E.W., S.M. and J.B.; formal analysis, I.H., H.S.-S., E.W. and F.G.; writing—original draft preparation, I.H., H.S.-S. and E.W.; writing—review and editing, I.H., H.S.-S., E.W., S.M., F.G., N.B. and J.B. All authors have read and agreed to the published version of the manuscript.

Funding: This research received no external project funding. HSS received salary support through a National Health and Medical Research Council of Australia Early Career Fellowship (1144566) and Australasian Cerebral Palsy Clinical Trials Network.

Institutional Review Board Statement: The study was conducted in accordance with the Declaration of Helsinki, and approved by Cerebral Palsy Alliance Human Research Ethics Committee (3 November 2018), Victorian Cerebral Palsy Register Governance and Queensland Cerebral Palsy Register Steering Committee.

Informed Consent Statement: Informed consent was obtained from all subjects involved in the study.

Data Availability Statement: The data presented in this study are available on request from the corresponding author. The data are not publicly available due to ethical restrictions.

Acknowledgments: We would like to acknowledge and thank all the individuals with CP who participated in this research. We would also like to acknowledge the support of researchers from the CP registers in the Australian Capital Territory, New South Wales, Queensland CP Register and Victorian CP Register for their assistance with recruitment.

Conflicts of Interest: The authors declare no conflict of interest.

Appendix A

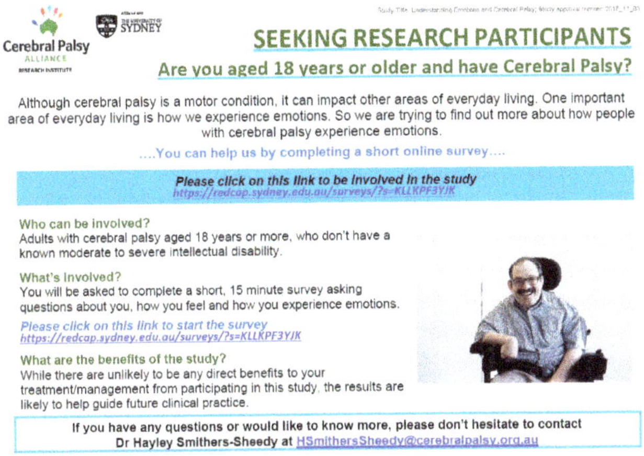

Figure A1. Study invitation flyer.

References

1. Rosenbaum, P.; Paneth, N.; Leviton, A.; Goldstein, M.; Bax, M.; Damiano, D.; Dan, B.; Jacobsson, B. A report: The definition and classification of cerebral palsy April 2006. *Dev. Med. Child Neurol. Suppl.* **2007**, *109* (Suppl. S109), 8–14. [PubMed]
2. Sigurdardottir, S.; Indredavik, M.S.; Eiriksdottir, A.; Einarsdottir, K.; Guðmundsson, H.S.; Vik, T. Behavioural and emotional symptoms of preschool children with cerebral palsy: A population-based study. *Dev. Med. Child Neurol.* **2010**, *52*, 1056–1061. [CrossRef] [PubMed]
3. Parkes, J.; White-Koning, M.; O Dickinson, H.; Thyen, U.; Arnaud, C.; Beckung, E.; Fauconnier, J.; Marcelli, M.; McManus, V.; Michelsen, S.I.; et al. Psychological problems in children with cerebral palsy: A cross-sectional European study. *J. Child Psychol. Psychiatry* **2008**, *49*, 405–413. [CrossRef] [PubMed]
4. Whittingham, K.; Bodimeade, H.L.; Lloyd, O.; Boyd, R.N. Everyday psychological functioning in children with unilateral cerebral palsy: Does executive functioning play a role? *Dev. Med. Child Neurol.* **2014**, *56*, 572–579. [CrossRef] [PubMed]
5. Brossard-Racine, M.; Hall, N.; Majnemer, A.; Shevell, M.I.; Law, M.; Poulin, C.; Rosenbaum, P. Behavioural problems in school age children with cerebral palsy. *Eur. J. Paediatr. Neurol.* **2012**, *16*, 35–41. [CrossRef]
6. Belmonte-Darraz, S.; Montoro, C.I.; Andrade, N.C.; Montoya, P.; Riquelme, I. Alteration of Emotion Knowledge and Its Relationship with Emotion Regulation and Psychopathological Behavior in Children with Cerebral Palsy. *J. Autism Dev. Disord.* **2021**, *51*, 1238–1248. [CrossRef]
7. Gross, J.J. *Emotion Regulation: Conceptual and Empirical Foundations*; The Guilford Press: New York, NY, USA, 2014.
8. John, O.P.; Gross, J.J. Healthy and Unhealthy Emotion Regulation: Personality Processes, Individual Differences, and Life Span Development. *J. Pers.* **2004**, *72*, 1301–1334. [CrossRef]
9. Fried, L. Teaching teachers about emotion regulation in the classroom. *Aust. J. Teach. Educ.* **2011**, *36*, 117–127. [CrossRef]
10. Grandey, A.A. Emotion regulation in the workplace: A new way to conceptualize emotional labor. *J. Occup. Health Psychol.* **2000**, *5*, 95. [CrossRef]
11. Gross, J.J.; John, O.P. Individual differences in two emotion regulation processes: Implications for affect, relationships, and well-being. *J. Pers. Soc. Psychol.* **2003**, *85*, 348–362. [CrossRef]
12. American Psychiatric Association. *Diagnostic and Statistical Manual of Mental Disorders (DSM-5®)*; American Psychiatric Publication: Washington, DC, USA, 2013.
13. Etkin, A.; Büchel, C.; Gross, J.J. The neural bases of emotion regulation. *Nat. Rev. Neurosci.* **2015**, *16*, 693–700. [CrossRef] [PubMed]
14. Ring, H.; Serra-Mestres, J. Neuropsychiatry of the basal ganglia. *J. Neurol. Neurosurg. Psychiatry* **2002**, *72*, 12–21. [CrossRef] [PubMed]
15. Felling, R.J.; Singer, H.S. Neurobiology of Tourette syndrome: Current status and need for further investigation. *J. Neurosci.* **2011**, *31*, 12387–12395. [CrossRef] [PubMed]
16. Monbaliu, E.; Himmelmann, K.; Lin, J.-P.; Ortibus, E.; Bonouvrié, L.; Feys, H.; Vermeulen, R.J.; Dan, B. Clinical presentation and management of dyskinetic cerebral palsy. *Lancet Neurol.* **2017**, *16*, 741–749. [CrossRef]
17. Smithers-Sheedy, H.; Badawi, N.; Blair, E.; Himmelmann, K.; Krägeloh-Mann, I.; McIntyre, S.; Slee, J.; Uldall, P.; Watson, L.; Wilson, M. What constitutes cerebral palsy in the twenty-first century? *Dev. Med. Child Neurol.* **2014**, *56*, 323–328. [CrossRef]
18. Tajik-Parvinchi, D.; MyStory Study Group; Davis, A.; Roth, S.; Rosenbaum, P.; Hopmans, S.N.; Dudin, A.; Hall, G.; Gorter, J.W. Functional connectivity and quality of life in young adults with cerebral palsy: A feasibility study. *BMC Neurol.* **2020**, *20*, 388. [CrossRef]

19. Eysenbach, G. Improving the quality of Web surveys: The Checklist for Reporting Results of Internet E-Surveys (CHERRIES). *J. Med. Internet Res.* **2004**, *6*, e34. [CrossRef]
20. Palisano, R.; Rosenbaum, P.; Bartlett, D.; Livingston, M.; Walter, S.; Russell, D. *GMFCS-E&R*; CanChild Centre for Childhood Disability Research, McMaster University: Hamilton, ON, Canada, 2007; p. 200.
21. Hidecker, M.J.C.; Paneth, N.; Rosenbaum, P.L.; Kent, R.D.; Lillie, J.; Eulenberg, J.B.; Chester, K., Jr.; Johnson, B.; Michalsen, L.; Evatt, M.; et al. Developing and validating the Communication Function Classification System for individuals with cerebral palsy. *Dev. Med. Child Neurol.* **2011**, *53*, 704–710. [CrossRef]
22. Henry, J.; Crawford, J. The short-form version of the Depression Anxiety Stress Scales (DASS-21): Construct validity and normative data in a large non-clinical sample. *Br. J. Clin. Psychol.* **2005**, *44*, 227–239. [CrossRef]
23. Gratz, K.; Roemer, L. Multidimensional Assessment of Emotion Regulation and Dysregulation: Development, Factor Structure, and Initial Validation of the Difficulties in Emotion Regulation Scale. *J. Psychopathol. Behav. Assess.* **2004**, *26*, 41–54. [CrossRef]
24. Giromini, L.; Ales, F.; De Campora, G.; Zennaro, A.; Pignolo, C. Developing age and gender adjusted normative reference values for the difficulties in emotion regulation scale (DERS). *J. Psychopathol. Behav. Assess.* **2017**, *39*, 705–714. [CrossRef]
25. Flynn, J.J.; Hollenstein, T.; Mackey, A. The effect of suppressing and not accepting emotions on depressive symptoms: Is suppression different for men and women? *Pers. Individ. Differ.* **2010**, *49*, 582–586. [CrossRef]
26. Joormann, J.; Stanton, C.H. Examining emotion regulation in depression: A review and future directions. *Behav. Res. Ther.* **2016**, *86*, 35–49. [CrossRef]
27. Shields, C.; Ownsworth, T.; O'Donovan, A.; Fleming, J. A transdiagnostic investigation of emotional distress after traumatic brain injury. *Neuropsychol. Rehabil.* **2016**, *26*, 410–445. [CrossRef]
28. Harrison, A.; Sullivan, S.; Tchanturia, K.; Treasure, J. Emotional functioning in eating disorders: Attentional bias, emotion recognition and emotion regulation. *Psychol. Med.* **2010**, *40*, 1887. [CrossRef] [PubMed]
29. Roemer, L.; Williston, S.K.; Rollins, L.G. Mindfulness and emotion regulation. *Curr. Opin. Psychol.* **2015**, *3*, 52–57. [CrossRef]
30. Peterson, M.D.; Lin, P.; Kamdar, N.; Mahmoudi, E.; Marsack-Topolewski, C.N.; Haapala, H.; Muraszko, K.; Hurvitz, E.A. Psychological morbidity among adults with cerebral palsy and spina bifida. *Psychol. Med.* **2020**, *51*, 1–8. [CrossRef]
31. Whitney, D.G.; Warschausky, S.A.; Ng, S.; Hurvitz, E.A.; Kamdar, N.S.; Peterson, M.D. Prevalence of mental health disorders among adults with cerebral palsy: A cross-sectional analysis. *Ann. Intern. Med.* **2019**, *171*, 328–333. [CrossRef]
32. Smith, K.J.; Peterson, M.; O'Connell, N.E.; Victor, C.; Liverani, S.; Anokye, N.; Ryan, J. Risk of depression and anxiety in adults with cerebral palsy. *JAMA Neurol.* **2019**, *76*, 294–300. [CrossRef]
33. Australia Bureau of Statistics. *National Health Survey: First Results, Australia, 2017–2018*; Australia Bureau of Statistics: Canberra, Australia, 2018.
34. Lanciego, J.L.; Luquin, N.; Obeso, J.A. Functional neuroanatomy of the basal ganglia. *Cold Spring Harb. Perspect. Med.* **2012**, *2*, a009621. [CrossRef]
35. Miller, L.R.; Cano, A. Comorbid chronic pain and depression: Who is at risk? *J. Pain* **2009**, *10*, 619–627. [CrossRef] [PubMed]
36. Goesling, J.; Clauw, D.J.; Hassett, A.L. Pain and depression: An integrative review of neurobiological and psychological factors. *Curr. Psychiatry Rep.* **2013**, *15*, 421. [CrossRef] [PubMed]
37. Van Der Slot, W.M.; Nieuwenhuijsen, C.; Van Den Berg-Emons, R.J.; Bergen, M.P.; Hilberink, S.R.; Stam, H.J.; Roebroeck, M.E. Chronic pain, fatigue, and depressive symptoms in adults with spastic bilateral cerebral palsy. *Dev. Med. Child Neurol.* **2012**, *54*, 836–842. [CrossRef] [PubMed]
38. Whitney, D.G.; A Hurvitz, E.; Ryan, J.M.; Devlin, M.J.; Caird, M.S.; French, Z.P.; Ellenberg, E.C.; Peterson, M.D. Noncommunicable disease and multimorbidity in young adults with cerebral palsy. *Clin. Epidemiol.* **2018**, *10*, 511. [CrossRef] [PubMed]
39. Jahnsen, R.; Villien, L.; Aamodt, G.; Stanghelle, J.; Holm, I. Musculoskeletal pain in adults with cerebral palsy compared with the general population. *J. Rehabil. Med.* **2004**, *36*, 78–84. [CrossRef]
40. Matthews, T.; Danese, A.; Wertz, J.; Odgers, C.L.; Ambler, A.; Moffitt, T.E.; Arseneault, L. Social isolation, loneliness and depression in young adulthood: A behavioural genetic analysis. *Soc. Psychiatry Psychiatr. Epidemiol.* **2016**, *51*, 339–348. [CrossRef]
41. Wang, J.; Mann, F.; Lloyd-Evans, B.; Ma, R.; Johnson, S. Associations between loneliness and perceived social support and outcomes of mental health problems: A systematic review. *BMC Psychiatry* **2018**, *18*, 156. [CrossRef]
42. Balandin, S.; Berg, N.; Waller, A. Assessing the loneliness of older people with cerebral palsy. *Disabil. Rehabil.* **2006**, *28*, 469–479. [CrossRef]
43. Michelsen, S.I.; Uldall, P.; Hansen, T.; Madsen, M. Social integration of adults with cerebral palsy. *Dev. Med. Child Neurol.* **2006**, *48*, 643–649. [CrossRef]
44. Krägeloh-Mann, I.; Helber, A.; Mader, I.; Staudt, M.; Wolff, M.; Groenendaal, F.; DeVries, L. Bilateral lesions of thalamus and basal ganglia: Origin and outcome. *Dev. Med. Child Neurol.* **2002**, *44*, 477–484. [CrossRef]
45. Cho, M.; Kim, K.M. Effect of digital divide on people with disabilities during the COVID-19 pandemic. *Disabil. Health J.* **2022**, *15*, 101214. [CrossRef] [PubMed]

Disclaimer/Publisher's Note: The statements, opinions and data contained in all publications are solely those of the individual author(s) and contributor(s) and not of MDPI and/or the editor(s). MDPI and/or the editor(s) disclaim responsibility for any injury to people or property resulting from any ideas, methods, instructions or products referred to in the content.

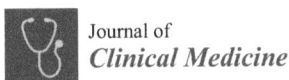

Perspective

Hip Surveillance and Management of Hip Displacement in Children with Cerebral Palsy: Clinical and Ethical Dilemmas

Jason J. Howard [1], Kate Willoughby [2], Pam Thomason [3], Benjamin J. Shore [4], Kerr Graham [2] and Erich Rutz [2,*]

1. Nemours Children's Hospital, Wilmington, DE 19803, USA
2. Department of Orthopaedics, The Royal Children's Hospital, Parkville 3052, Australia
3. The Hugh Williamson Gait Laboratory, The Royal Children's Hospital, Parkville 3052, Australia
4. Boston Children's Hospital, Boston, MA 02115, USA
* Correspondence: erich_rutz@hotmail.com; Tel.: +61-3-9345-7645

Abstract: Hip displacement is the second most common musculoskeletal deformity in children with cerebral palsy. Hip surveillance programs have been implemented in many countries to detect hip displacement early when it is usually asymptomatic. The aim of hip surveillance is to monitor hip development to offer management options to slow or reverse hip displacement, and to provide the best opportunity for good hip health at skeletal maturity. The long-term goal is to avoid the sequelae of late hip dislocation which may include pain, fixed deformity, loss of function and impaired quality of life. The focus of this review is on areas of disagreement, areas where evidence is lacking, ethical dilemmas and areas for future research. There is already broad agreement on how to conduct hip surveillance, using a combination of standardised physical examination measures and radiographic examination of the hips. The frequency is dictated by the risk of hip displacement according to the child's ambulatory status. Management of both early and late hip displacement is more controversial and the evidence base in key areas is relatively weak. In this review, we summarise the recent literature on hip surveillance and highlight the management dilemmas and controversies. Better understanding of the causes of hip displacement may lead to interventions which target the pathophysiology of hip displacement and the pathological anatomy of the hip in children with cerebral palsy. We have identified the need for more effective and integrated management from early childhood to skeletal maturity. Areas for future research are highlighted and a range of ethical and management dilemmas are discussed.

Keywords: cerebral palsy; hip displacement; hip surveillance; GMFCS; adductor-psoas release; hip reconstruction; guided growth; salvage surgery

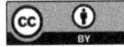

1. Introduction

Hip displacement (HD) is common in non-ambulatory children with cerebral palsy (CP) and may result in pain, limitations in sitting ability and impaired Health Related Quality of Life (HRQoL) [1,2]. In a large, population-based study, the prevalence of HD, defined as migration percentage (MP) > 30%, was 35% for the whole CP population, rising to 90% for children at Gross Motor Function Classification System (GMFCS) Level V [3]. Prevalence was related in a linear fashion to GMFCS Level but not to motor type [1,3]. In recent years, there has been an increasing interest in hip surveillance (HS) and preventive and reconstructive surgery [4,5]. Reports from single-site studies, state-wide studies, national studies and systematic reviews are largely positive about the benefits of HS in detecting HD in CP [5–10]. However, questions remain pertaining to the HS process, the efficacy of non-operative treatments, the efficacy of soft tissue releases in younger children, the timing and dose of reconstructive osteotomies and the need for salvage procedures (i.e., joint resection). The common association of multiple co-morbidities, leading to a higher risk of post-operative medical complications, further impacts clinical decision-making [1]. The frailty of some children with severe CP raises clinical and ethical questions about surgical management. The purpose of this review is to identify areas where knowledge is lacking and where future research efforts might be focused to help answer these questions (Figure 1).

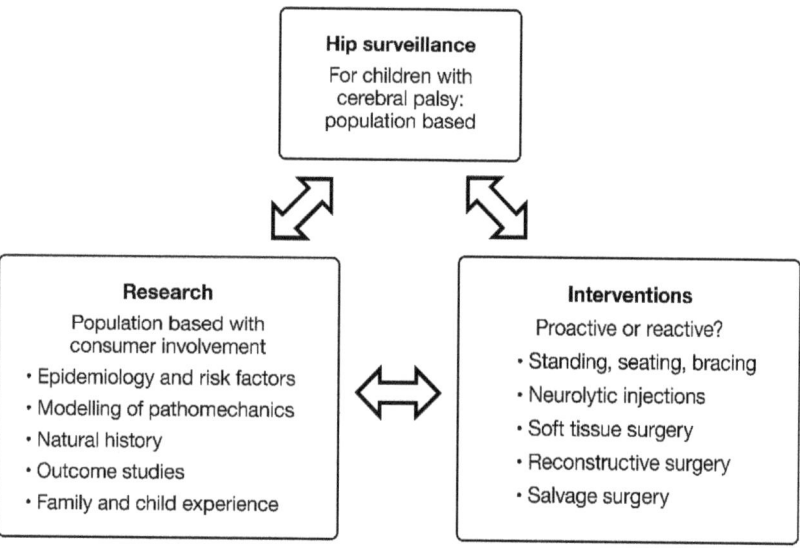

Figure 1. Hip surveillance, research and interventions. Copyright Bill Reid, Pam Thomason and Kerr Graham, RCH Melbourne. Hip surveillance for children with CP improves the knowledge and research base. It can help us understand why hips dislocate and effects of intervention on the natural history of hip migration. Hip surveillance usually leads to interventions, which can be proactive or reactive and include both non-operative and operative approaches. Hip surveillance, research and outcome studies are inextricably linked. Each informs the other.

2. Hip Surveillance for Children with Cerebral Palsy

Detecting a disease early—when it may be easier to treat—is intuitively attractive, but the benefits and potential harms require careful evaluation. Screening and surveillance programs can be successful, but there may be unintended consequences. It has been stated that: 'all screening programs do harm . . . some do good as well' [1,11,12].

HS for children with CP involves both clinical and radiographic examinations based on a risk assessment linked to gross motor function, rather than the development of symptoms, to help subvert a natural history typified by painful osteoarthritis and impairment [1,5–11]. This may prevent some children from developing symptomatic dislocation if HS detects HD early enough for treatment to make a difference in outcome (Figure 2). Although the reported prevalence of pain in children with CP and dislocated hips is variable, it reached >80% in some studies [13,14]. However, given that some with HD may never develop pain, children may be subjected to physical, emotional and financial harms from interventions that may have little clinical impact [11]. As with many screening programs, the trade-offs between potential benefits and harms relating to HS is complex and not fully understood [11,12] (Figure 2).

Clinicians who have embraced hip surveillance may have been influenced historically by the miseries of neglected hip dislocation in teenagers and young adults with severe CP. On top of marked restrictions in gross motor function and the inability to walk, the development of HD can be a source of pain, impair the ability to sit comfortably and significantly reduce quality of life [2,6].

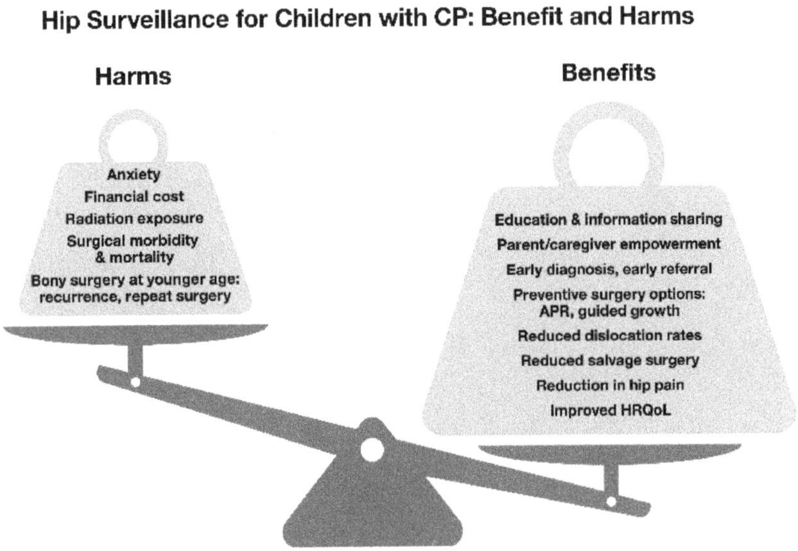

Hip Surveillance for Children with CP: Benefit and Harms

Harms
- Anxiety
- Financial cost
- Radiation exposure
- Surgical morbidity & mortality
- Bony surgery at younger age: recurrence, repeat surgery

Benefits
- Education & information sharing
- Parent/caregiver empowerment
- Early diagnosis, early referral
- Preventive surgery options: APR, guided growth
- Reduced dislocation rates
- Reduced salvage surgery
- Reduction in hip pain
- Improved HRQoL

Figure 2. The benefits and harms of hip surveillance. Copyright Bill Reid, Kate Willoughby and Kerr Graham, RCH Melbourne. Some of the potential benefits and harms of hip surveillance are shown as a 'see-saw' or 'teeter-totter'. Through hip surveillance, early identification of hip displacement and referral to orthopaedics provide options for surgical management. This, in turn, introduces additional potential harms and benefits. There is strong evidence that the benefits outweigh the harms for children with cerebral palsy as a population. The benefit to harm experience however is not just for study cohorts or populations, but is experienced by individual children and their families. While early bony surgery is safe and effective in the short term, the associated harm is a high recurrence and surgery revision rate. This could be reduced, perhaps, through 'temporising' surgical options such as adductor-psoas muscle release (APR) and/or guided growth. As noted elsewhere, surgery is safer and more successful when conducted in the context of an experienced, multidisciplinary team which includes high volume, experienced surgeons.

3. Lessons from the History of Hip Surveillance

The first studies on the aetiology and prevention of hip dislocations in children with CP were published more than 70 years ago. Dr. Mercer Rang was one of the first clinicians to advocate for hip surveillance for children with CP and to develop educational materials to promote the concept. He educated clinicians and parents about HD, advocating for yearly clinical and radiographic examinations for children with CP and severe limitations in walking [15]. This remains the core of contemporary hip surveillance [6–10].

Dr Rang produced instructive posters to remind all staff of their responsibility to check children for silent hip dysplasia on a regular basis. He called this approach 'The Art of Preventive Orthopaedics'. He wryly observed that 'he had not met a child with CP who had been helped by having a dislocated hip' [15]. In 1985, he published a study of adductor release surgery in children with CP [16]. This is one of the many studies on the treatment of HD prior to the introduction and widespread use of the GMFCS, a valid and reliable classification of functional severity [1,17]. This makes the data harder to interpret by contemporary standards, given the less reliable classification used at the time emphasizing motor type and topographical patterns [1,18]. At a mean follow-up of approximately 4 years, Dr Rang and his colleagues reported good outcomes in 80% of children and identified predictive factors for success or failure following adductor surgery [16]. Implicit in Dr. Rang's publications was the principle that dislocation could be prevented in the majority of children with CP by a single, well-timed soft tissue surgery, adductor-psoas release (APR). Unfortunately, a large recent population-based study incorporating the

GMFCS does not support this optimistic view of APR surgery, which in turn changes the benefit-to-harm calculation with respect to the application of HS to determine the need and timing of surgery for HD [19] (Figure 2).

HS programs were introduced and refined in Southern Sweden (CPUP) and in Australia over the past 20–30 years [6–9]. HS has also been endorsed and supported by numerous professional bodies including the Australian Academy of Cerebral Palsy and Developmental Medicine (AusACPDM), the American Academy of Cerebral Palsy and Developmental Medicine (AACPDM) and the Paediatric Orthopaedic Society of North America (POSNA) [7,9,20]. HS programs have been introduced in many other countries as well, including the United Kingdom, Canada and India [5,19,21,22].

Children with developmental dysplasia of the hip (DDH) are screened most intensively in the neonatal period because the majority of hips are unstable at birth. Children with CP usually have normal hips at birth, and surveillance rather than screening is applied for children who are considered to be at high risk of HD, especially those who are non-ambulant (GMFCS IV and V) [3,23]. Clinical examination—involving the assessment of hip adductor and flexor contractures—is important in the overall assessment of the child, but it is unreliable in detecting hip displacement and incomplete without radiology [15,23]. HS programs are based on regular high-quality radiographs of the hips with the timing and frequency determined by studies which have identified the relative risk according to GMFCS level [3,23]. The extent that the femoral head is uncovered by the acetabular roof is measured from pelvic radiographs using the migration percentage (MP), a quantitative measure of HD with face validity and acceptable reliability [20,22–25]. The predictors and associations of HD in CP have been studied and reported but there is no universally agreed threshold for MP to define significant HD, to indicate referral to orthopaedic surgeons, or to determine the need for preventive, reconstructive or salvage surgery [24–26].

Within a MP threshold range of 30–40%, referral to an orthopaedic service is usually advised [20–23]. Unlike DDH, non-operative treatments for cerebral palsy hip displacement (CPHD) are relatively ineffective [27]. That said, operative treatments are invasive and have substantial failure rates and risks of medical and surgical complications [1,28,29]. The preventive APR surgery, initially advocated by Dr. Rang, has a high failure rate in recent, longer-term studies [16,19,30–32]. It is now apparent that a substantial percentage of children with severe CP (GMFCS IV and V) will require bony reconstructive surgery to maintain good 'hip health' [32]. Some may require revision or repeated episodes of bony reconstructive surgery to achieve acceptable hip morphology at skeletal maturity [30–32] (Figure 3). This knowledge contributes to the ethical and clinical dilemmas surrounding HS and the management of asymptomatic HD in young people with CP. How many operations are acceptable to children, parents and surgeons for a condition which, at the time of first diagnosis, is often asymptomatic [1,3]?

Figure 3 illustrates the journey of a child with CP, from birth towards skeletal maturity as a road travelled with various exits and destinations. There is an interaction between hip surveillance and options for preventive and reconstructive surgery, with the goal of avoiding salvage surgery and reaching skeletal maturity with good hip health, defined in broad terms a pain-free, mobile hip with morphology at Melbourne Cerebral Palsy Hip Classification Scale (MCPHCS) Grades 1–3 (Supplementary Materials S1).

At birth, the hip is normal. In early childhood, hip displacement is usually silent and the rate of increase in MP can be between 6% and 12% per annum, for children functioning at GMFCS V.

The option for children of BoNT-A and bracing of the hip has been shown to be ineffective: 'wrong way, go back!'

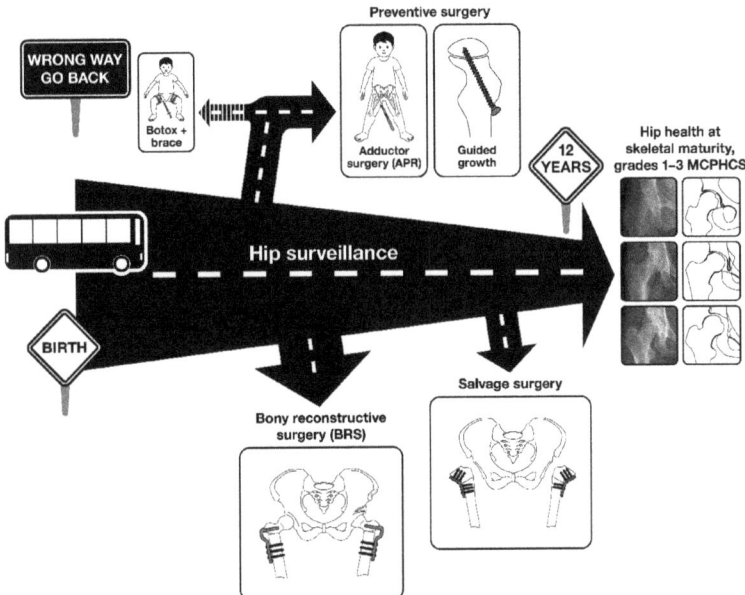

Figure 3. The hip surveillance journey. Copyright Bill Reid, Pam Thomason and Kerr Graham, RCH Melbourne.

The second preventive option is adductor psoas release (APR) surgery. In some children, APR surgery can stop the progression of MP and in others the rate of progression is reduced. After APR surgery, the number of hips which will stabilise for the long-term is not clearly known. APR surgery has been used for approximately 80 years and the results in the literature are mixed. In contrast, the third preventive option, 'guided growth' is a minimally invasive, relatively new intervention which may have a major impact on the femoral deformity, in younger children who are growing rapidly. Studies to date are short-term and many questions remain unanswered. This technology requires both long-term studies and controlled studies to define its role.

As indicated in the figure, hip surveillance should continue and if there is a continued progression in MP after APR or guided growth, the next exit is for bony reconstructive surgery. This is most often between the ages of 6 and 12 years, before irreversible femoral head damage occurs. Severe femoral head damage may leave salvage surgery as the only option. The road in the diagram is shown to narrow, indicating that in the second decade the hip and the child may run out of time and out of options. By the time of the adolescent growth spurt, some hips will have dislocated and have irreversible damage leaving salvage surgery as the only option for the hip, the child and the family.

4. How Do We Judge the Success of Hip Surveillance?

The goal of HS can be defined narrowly as: the detection of significant HD in children with CP within a given population. This can facilitate timely referral to an orthopaedic surgeon and the option for early intervention. Using such criteria, Kentish and colleagues demonstrated that this goal could be achieved in a large state with low population density and maintained over a 5-year period, despite the many geographical and health care delivery challenges [7]. However, it may not be logical to separate the process of HS from the outcome of management of HD. The purpose of HS is not referral alone, but instead is to facilitate the maintenance of 'hip health' in the most vulnerable children with CP [13]. Good 'hip health' describes a hip which is pain-free and mobile, without significant fixed deformity. Good 'hip health' facilitates comfortable sitting, standing and walking in some children. It also facilitates activities of daily living (ADLs) such as dressing, bathing and perineal hygiene. The hip morphology required to meet these demands varies by GMFCS level and has not yet been precisely defined. Hips with MP < 40% and which are Grades 1–3 according to the Melbourne Cerebral Palsy Hip Classification Scale (MCPHCS E&R, Supplementary Materials S1) have a combination of good or acceptable hip morphology and low pain scores. These children and youth are typically able to sit comfortably with few restrictions [13,33] (Figure 3).

There are several population-based studies which show that HS improves the outcome of CPHD, favouring preventive and reconstructive procedures over salvage surgery [6,8,34]. Prior to HS, children with CP in one tertiary centre were presenting for salvage surgery at a rate of 4–8 per annum. After the introduction of HS, the rates for preventive and reconstructive surgeries increased while salvage surgery was temporarily eliminated [6]. In Southern Sweden, the 20-year results of hip surveillance, combined with a responsive surgical program, resulted in very low rates of dislocated hips and salvage surgery [8]. A contrary view was expressed by Larsen et al. who reported that HS had failed to reduce hip pain in adolescents at long-term follow-up [35]. Perhaps it was the surgical program that failed to reduce hip pain rather than the HS [35].

5. Net Zero Is Neither Possible Nor Desirable

A reasonable goal of HS would be detection of all hips with MP > 30% and referral for assessment and consideration of orthopaedic surgery [6–10]. This should result in a reduction in late dislocations and the need for salvage surgery to its lowest possible level [6,8,32,34]. Achieving a zero rate of late hip dislocation—and the associated salvage surgery—is probably not attainable. Children with advanced hip disease may move from a country or state without HS to one with state-wide HS [8]. The parents of some children with CP are willing to have their children enrolled in a HS program but decline the option of invasive surgery, especially when their children are asymptomatic. A number of children at GMFCS V have limited life expectancy and may be too frail for bony reconstructive surgery [1,36]. There is a danger that frail children detected by HS as having progressive increase in MP might be offered invasive surgery and suffer premature mortality. Every child with CP is a candidate for HS but some may not be candidates for hip surgery [28,29,35] (Figure 2). Approximately 20% of children with severe CP suffer premature mortality by the age of 4 years, without prior surgical intervention [1,36]. Withholding surgical intervention for children with severe CP and HD presents an ethical dilemma, as it is difficult to determine which children would be at higher risk of mortality after hip surgery. The complication rate after hip surgery in non-ambulant children is high and when 'failure to cure' is included, the complication rate rose to 54% in one study [28].

6. Knowledge Gaps with Respect to Hip Surveillance

Given the high prevalence of CPHD in non-ambulant children, those functioning at GMFCS IV and V have been the focus of research in this area [3]. Although the prevalence is lower in ambulant children, the sequelae of late dislocation are magnified by higher functional demands and communication ability [1,3,17,18]. The majority of children with hemiplegia function at GMFCS level I or II, rarely, if ever, suffer hip dislocation [1,3,18]. Late-onset, symptomatic hip subluxation in the second decade, however, can be a problem in children with Type IV hemiplegia, according to the Winters Gage Hicks Classification (WGH) [37]. These children have flexion, adduction and internal rotation alignment of the hip and may present de novo with hip pain if not under regular HS. Although the prevalence is low, we are not aware of population-based studies which identify the precise rate of HD in Type IV hemiplegia. Smaller studies of surgical outcomes of symptomatic HD in Type IV hemiplegia suggest that this can be a difficult management problem, often requiring major reconstructive surgery [37]. A better understanding of the natural history of HD in hemiplegia would be very useful to guide the practice of HS for these children, the largest subgroup of children with CP [3,38]. Although the Type IV hemiplegia phenotype can be recognised by a combination of clinical examinations and three-dimensional gait analysis, the WGH Types are overlapping, not discrete and there are problems with the reliability of the classification [1,38].

Ambulant children with diplegia (GMFCS I-III) have lower rates of HD but natural history, optimum HS guidelines and clinical management have not been well studied [3]. Miller and colleagues recently reported four children with asymmetric diplegic CP functioning at GMFCS levels II and III, with the more involved hip showing rapid, progressive displacement at a later age [39]. They noted the current HS guidelines may not adequately identify HD in children with asymmetric diplegia and pelvic obliquity. Modifications to current HS guidelines may be warranted [39].

It has been assumed that the risk of progressive HD is negligible after triradiate cartilage (TRC) closure—a proxy for the onset of skeletal maturity—and thus HS could safely be discontinued after that point [9]. A recent large study, however, has demonstrated that there is a risk of further hip displacement in children with CP after closure of the TRC especially for those with risk factors including male gender, pelvic obliquity, high MP and no prior surgery [40]. For those youth at risk, the authors suggested that HS be continued up until age 18 years, with at least an x-ray every 2 years [40].

7. Hip Surveillance Leads to Bony Reconstructive Surgery When Children Are Younger

The treatment effects of all interventions are weak in comparison to the biomechanical forces which predispose the hip to primary or recurrent displacement [3]. Most operative interventions lead to an improvement in MP or a reduced rate of progression in MP [16,19,30–32] (Figure 3). Despite the release of adductors, flexors and proximal hamstrings, there is a tendency to progressive HD and, if HS is neglected, dislocation [19,28,32,33]. Recent thinking points to abnormalities in proximal femoral growth secondary to a lack of functional ambulation, rather than muscle imbalance due to spastic contractures alone, as being causative for CPHD [41]. Management must include strategies which ensure stable, pain-free hips with good morphology, after skeletal maturity [13]. Outcome studies with follow-up to an age younger than skeletal maturity are provisional, at best (Figure 3).

Early detection of HD by HS leads to early referral to orthopaedic surgery. When APR is the first-choice preventive option, early failure will often lead to consideration of bony reconstructive surgery (BRS) at an earlier age [13,19] (Figure 3). This might seem to be a good thing, with early bony correction of proximal femur and acetabular deformities intuitively leading to better outcomes. However, the success of bony reconstructive surgery is inversely related to the age at surgery [28,30,32]. Younger children have more years of growth ahead of them during which re-displacement may occur [33,40]. This is logical when it is remembered that the factors which contribute to hip displacement—such as adductor spasticity, weakness of the hip abductors and limited weight-bearing—remain present and largely unchanged after orthopaedic surgery [1,3,17]. The risk period for recurrence is mainly, but not exclusively, related to the interval between bony reconstructive surgery and skeletal maturity [40].

8. The Cause of Hip Displacement in Children with Cerebral Palsy: Spasticity or Weakness?

Hip displacement and dislocation have historically been linked to muscle imbalance across the hip joint and spasticity in the hip adductors and flexors [15,16,42]. There is evidence from musculoskeletal modelling to support the role of muscle imbalance and increased contact forces [42]. However, modelling depends on forces measured during gait, and extrapolation of these data to the non-ambulant child are problematic. In recent years the emphasis has shifted to include the role of abnormal proximal femoral geometry. In population-based studies of CPHD, the prevalence of displacement (MP > 30%) was directly related to GMFCS level, but not to motor type [3]. Mean femoral neck anteversion (FNA) and neck shaft angle (NSA) increased stepwise from GMFCS I to V [43,44]. In children with hypotonia, the prevalence of CPHD was the same as for children with hypertonia [3,41].

These data suggest that activity limitations may make a stronger contribution to HD than adductor spasticity [1,3,17,41–43]. A fundamental question is whether abnormal femoral geometry is a primary response to activity limitations and hip abductor weakness, or a secondary response to spastic contractures of the hip adductors and flexors [3,39,42]. Ulusaloglu and colleagues compared proximal femoral and acetabular geometry in non-ambulatory children with spastic CP (GMFCS IV, V) to non-ambulatory children with spinal muscular atrophy (SMA, Types I and II). They reported an earlier onset of HD in SMA, with similar radiographic features in the two groups, despite CP being characterised by spasticity and SMA by hypotonia [41]. A recent study identified laxity of the capsule and ligaments as the primary pathology in HD in children with CP, but offered no supporting evidence [45]. Whilst joint laxity is a fundamental factor in DDH there is no clinical or experimental evidence to suggest that it plays a primary role in CPHD [3,39,41,42,45]. Understanding pathological anatomy and pathophysiology of CPHD is important as it may have a major role in the design, planning and selection of management strategies (Figures 3 and 4).

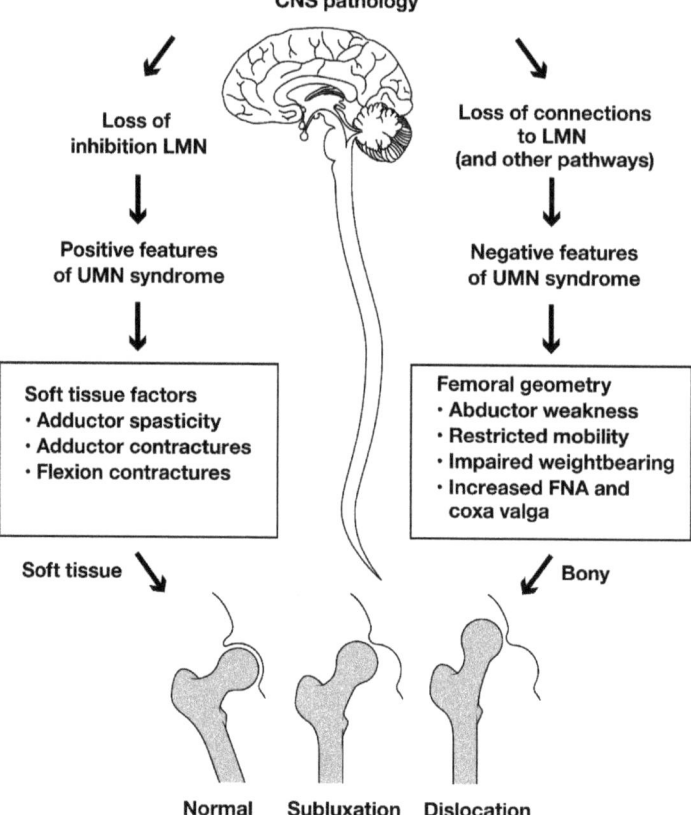

Figure 4. The pathophysiology of hip displacement in children with cerebral palsy. Copyright Bill Reid, Jason Howard and Kerr Graham, RCH Melbourne.

The cause of hip displacement in children with severe CP has been considered to be secondary to the positive features of the UMN Syndrome, which include adductor spasticity and contractures of the hip adductors and flexors. This leads to muscle imbalance across the hip joint. More recently, the negative features of the UMN Syndrome have also been considered and these include profound alterations in proximal femoral geometry. It is hypothesised that abductor weakness and limitations in weight-bearing lead to persistence of femoral neck anteversion (FNA), progressive lateral tilting of the proximal femoral epiphysis leading to increasing head shaft angle (HSA) and coxa valga or increased neck shaft angle (NSA). Probably it is a combination of both the positive and negative features of the UMN Syndrome which have such a strong deleterious effect on the growing hip in children with severe CP. Guided growth may be a logical intervention to directly address abnormal proximal femoral geometry.

The emphasis on adductor spasticity and contracture has led to an emphasis on abduction bracing, spasticity reduction by injections of Botulinum Neurotoxin A (BoNT-A) and APR surgery [45–47]. The outcomes of these interventions, in comparison to bony reconstructive surgery which addresses the abnormal proximal femoral geometry, are unpredictable and often disappointing [48]. The identification of persistent or recurrent coxa valga and secondary acetabular dysplasia in non-ambulant children with CP, suggests a possible role for guided growth of the proximal femur [49,50]. We suggest that muscle imbalance *and* abnormal proximal femoral geometry acting together may contribute to CPHD which we suggest is a more accurate term than 'spastic hip disease' [1,3,41,44].

9. The Natural History of Hip Displacement in Children with Cerebral Palsy

There are few studies of the natural history of hip displacement in children with CP since children who are receiving HS are usually offered early intervention, while those not receiving HS tend to present late, often with an established, painful dislocation [51]. What is known is that most hips in children with CP are normal at birth, although a very small number have congenital dislocations, such as in DDH [51]. In a large study of untreated children with CP, dislocation occurred in 10% of children by progressive lateral displacement of the femoral head from the acetabulum [51]. This resulted in secondary acetabular dysplasia, femoral head deformity and frank arthrosis [6]. The prevalence of painful degenerative arthritis in this cohort was very high, with the majority presenting around the time of the pubertal growth spurt requiring salvage surgery [6]. More recently, Terjersen reported a cohort of 76 children with CP who were followed for five years before treatment [52]. Age and ambulatory ability were the main predictors of the speed of HD. Children who could not walk had a 12% increase in MP per annum compared to 2% in children who could walk, with or without support [52]. In CPHD, abductor weakness and ambulatory ability may be more important than adductor spasticity [1,43].

For children functioning at GMFCS Level V, the annual increase in MP in one study was 6.2%. The annual increase in femoral neck shaft angle was 3.4 degrees. This confirms the contributions of progressive coxa valga to lateral displacement of the femoral head from the acetabulum and secondary acetabular dysplasia. [53]. Fortunately, in a comprehensive review, Lins and colleagues have demonstrated that this bleak natural history can be favourably improved by appropriate HS and timely intervention [54].

10. Non-Operative Treatment for Early CPHD

Specialised seating and orthotic systems have been trialled for children with severe CP with varying outcomes with respect to managing HD. The majority of studies were uncontrolled and had short-term follow-up [25]. There is limited evidence that specialised seating and orthotic devices can prevent progressive HD in non-ambulant children with CP [25]. Given the strong natural history leading to hip dislocation, it would be surprising if these forces could be negated by an orthotic device. It would also seem improbable, from first principles, that the progressive coxa valga seen in non-ambulatory children with CP could be reversed by non-operative means [43–45].

Despite this, a recent study of a novel hip brace reported slowing of HD by daily wear of at least 12 h [45]. Unfortunately, participants were not matched in terms of baseline MP. The authors suggest that a primary aetiological factor in CPHD is laxity of the joint capsule and surrounding ligaments. It was claimed that the brace was designed to reduce coxa valga but no evidence was offered in support of this improbable claim [45]. Given the failure of other non-operative modalities over the long-term, despite short-term success, longitudinal follow-up of this cohort is awaited with interest [13,45,46].

11. Injections of Botulinum Neurotoxin A Combined with Bracing

Injection of botulinum toxin A (BoNT-A) to the hip adductors, hip flexors and hamstrings has been practiced for many years for the reduction of focal spasticity in children with CP [46,47]. However, the evidence that repeated injections of BoNT-A can prevent or even slow HD is mixed. Repeated injections of BoNT-A combined with an abduction brace did not prevent progressive HD in a large, randomised clinical trial of three years duration [46]. There was a delay in progression to surgery but no difference in long-term outcomes. The outcomes reported were: the amount of surgery required, final hip morphology and pain levels [13]. There are several short-term studies which reported more favourable outcomes but without a control group and long-term follow-up, so the evidence is not compelling [47]. At the population level, injections of BoNT-A had no impact on the prevalence of CPHD or scoliosis [55].

12. Adductor-Psoas Releases for CPHD: 80% Success or 80% Failure?

Both Silver et al. and Presedo et al. reported high success rates from early adductor surgery in non-ambulant children with CP [16,56]. However, these early studies pre-date the use of the GMFCS to stratify patient risk, and both studies had relatively short-term follow-up. With a combination of risk stratification by GMFCS and long-term follow-up, the 60–80% success rate of soft tissue surgery is replaced by a 60–80% failure rate in children functioning at GMFCS IV and V [17,28]. This led Shore and colleagues to the conclusion that 'adductor surgery works least for those children who need it most' [17].

When hip surveillance leads to the identification of early hip displacement in children with no symptoms, it would be ideal to offer a minimally invasive soft tissue surgical approach with good long-term outcomes [11,15]. Adductor surgery seems to work best for younger children with MP between 30% and 50% and abduction <30 degrees [15,30,31] (Figure 5). For many children, a temporary improvement or decreased progression rate in MP can be anticipated after APR. With long-term follow-up, the improvement in MP may continue in ambulant children but a relapse is common after 3–10 years, with continued progression of hip displacement in non-ambulant children [17].

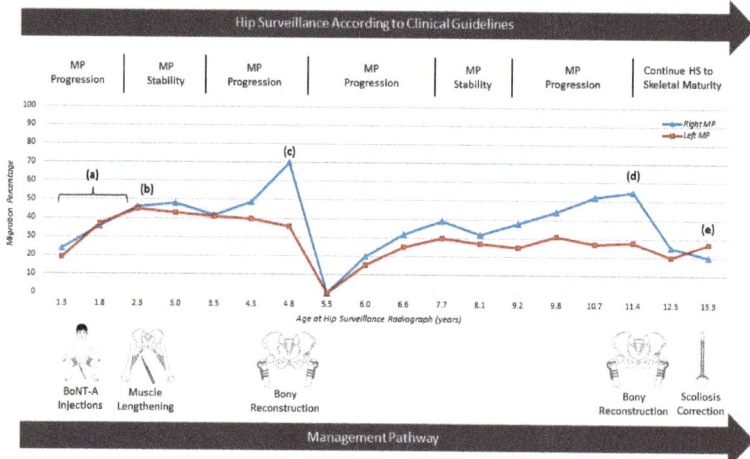

Figure 5. Hip surveillance and response to interventions for hip displacement for a child from age 1–13 years. Copyright Kate Willoughby, RCH Melbourne. The red line shows serial MP for the left hip; the blue line shows serial MP for the right hip, over time. This figure shows the interplay between the hip surveillance and management pathways of a girl who functioned at GMFCS IV and had regular HS and multiple interventions over a 13-year period.

Hip surveillance commenced according to national guidelines with the first radiograph soon after her first birthday. No benefit was gained from repeated injections of BoNT-A and bracing, with progression in MP recorded (a). The treatment with BoNT-A was during the era when the efficacy of this intervention for hip displacement was undecided. APR surgery at 2 years of age (b) resulted in a stable MP for only 2 years. Rapid progression in MP led to bilateral VDROs at age 4 years (c) and the MPs returned to zero. Guided growth may have been a better option at such a young age. MPs gradually increased over the next 6 years and a second episode of bony reconstructive surgery was performed at age 11 years (d), followed by posterior spinal fusion at age 13 years (e). Approaching skeletal maturity, the patient has a level pelvis, mobile pain-free hips which are MCPHCS Grade 3. This has been achieved at significant cost to the child, family and the health care service. More durable interventions and fewer episodes of major intervention are required.

The contemporary view of APR surgery as a primary intervention for HD is that it is a useful intervention, but more often to delay the need for bony reconstructive surgery than a means to achieve long-term hip stability in non-ambulant children [43] (Figures 3 and 5). More prospective studies are required to see if there are sub-groups of non-ambulant children who by virtue of age, low MP or other factors might respond more favourably to APR surgery [11,16,30,31]. Chemo-denervation of the obturator nerve at the time of APR surgery may reduce post-operative pain and spasm, and might prolong the effect on hip stability [43]. However, no comparative studies or clinical trials have been conducted.

13. Guided Growth and Proximal Femoral Geometry in CPHD

Given the limited efficacy for APR in non-ambulant children, and the relatively high recurrence rate after reconstructive osteotomies for younger children (<6 years old), the most optimal treatment of early detected CPHD has yet to be determined [28,32,56,57]. To avoid major, invasive bony reconstructive surgery, there has been an increased interest in recent years in using guided growth in the proximal femur to correct some of the bony deformities that develop in non-ambulant children [44]. These include coxa valga, a horizontal tilt to the proximal femoral epiphysis and increased neck-shaft-angle (NSA). Increased head-shaft angle (HSA) is another useful radiological index to describe the abnormal proximal femoral geometry in children with CP, defined as the angle between the proximal femoral growth plate and the femoral shaft [58]. In typically developing children, HSA starts high and decreases over time, consistent with the acquisition of weight-bearing and ambulation [59]. Concurrently, femoral NSA also decreases, likely related to this medialisation of the proximal femoral physis. By contrast, in children with CP, the HSA starts high and remains high, associated with increased coxa valga, progressive increase in MP and secondary acetabular dysplasia [41,59]. These changes have been theorised to be linked to abnormal joint forces and result in these changes in proximal femoral growth, and thus geometry [41,44,59].

If abnormal growth is the primary driver, then interventions which modulate the growth of the proximal femur—by reversal of coxa valga—would seem logical. In addition, guided growth has the potential to provide dynamic correction of proximal femoral deformity during growth in contrast to the acute but static correction offered by hip reconstruction [43,48]. Hsieh and colleagues reported the use of inferomedial screw epiphysiodesis of the proximal femur to reduce the lateral physeal tilt, in the proximal femoral physis [60]. In their study, they reported significant decreases in HSA, MP and AI following guided growth, with longer duration of follow-up and smaller index MP having better outcomes. Further, in their comparative study of adductor surgery, Sheu and colleagues reported significant reductions in MP and a lower rate of MP > 40% in the group augmented with proximal femoral guided growth [61]. The reduction in MP, though significant, was relatively modest in this study, perhaps related to the older age at index procedure (mean 8.1 years). A recent systematic review investigating the role of guided growth in children with CP (178 hips) also reported significant reductions in MP (35% to 26%), HSA (162° to 149°) and AI (22° to 18°), but the mean age at surgery was quite high at 7.2 years. The studies also included many ambulant children who are known to be at low risk of progressive hip displacement, and the mean follow-up was too short for strong recommendations [40,50].

Given these promising outcomes, coupled with limited efficacy for APR alone for non-ambulant children with early HD, two of our authors' (JJH, BJS) institutions have maintained typical indications for APR surgery (MP > 40% or MP > 30% and progressive) but have augmented this treatment with the use of guided growth. This is achieved with the percutaneous placement of a cannulated screw across the inferomedial proximal femoral physis (Figure 6). For children under 5 years of age, substantial improvements in MP have been realised with this additional treatment, along with a low complication rate. Future comparative studies are planned to substantiate these favourable early results and to determine the longer-term outcomes of this minimally invasive treatment. Whether it will offer a convincing role as an index surgery for hip displacement remains to be seen. Inserting a screw across the proximal femoral physis every 12 to 24 months carries some risks of general anaesthesia, but much less than what would be expected from early reconstructive osteotomies [50].

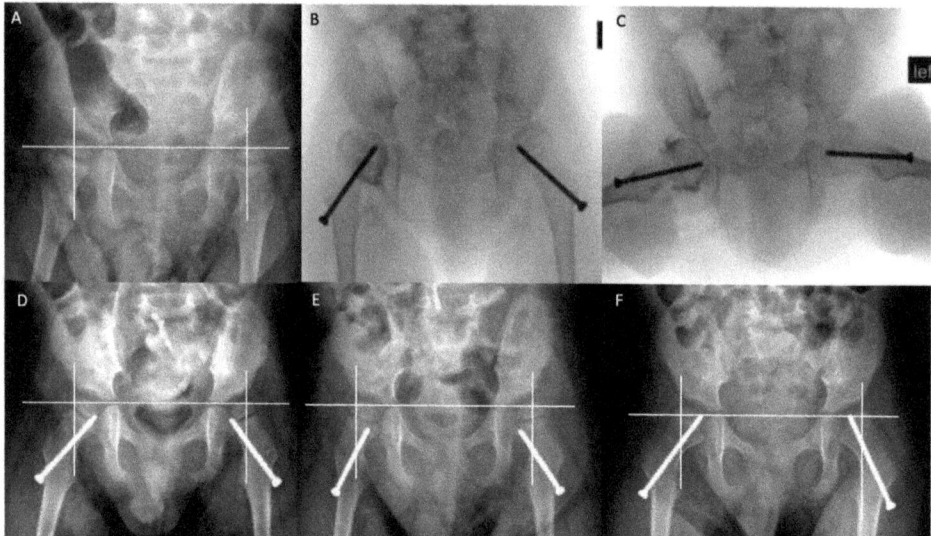

Figure 6. Guided growth in the management of the younger child with early, severe hip displacement. Copyright Jason J Howard, Nemours Children's Hospital. Serial radiographs of a 3-year-old boy with severe cerebral palsy, functioning at GMFCS V, with progressive hip displacement, left greater than right. (**A**) Pre-operative AP radiograph, MP: right 34%, left 67%. (**B,C**) Intra-operative fluoroscopic images showing bilateral hip arthrograms and inferomedial proximal femoral screw epiphysiodesis also known as 'guided growth'. (**D**) Five-month post-operative follow-up radiograph. (**E**) Twelve-month post-operative follow-up radiograph. Note that the epiphysis has 'grown off' the screw bilaterally due to high growth velocity at this early age. (**F**) Sixteen-month post-operative follow-up radiograph, post screw exchange. MP: right 25%, left 27%. Images courtesy Jason J. Howard.

14. Bony Reconstructive Surgery for CPHD

At present, the gold standard intervention for the prevention of progressive hip displacement and for the correction of hip dislocation is a one-stage hip reconstruction [43,48]. This consists of a bilateral adductor lengthening, bilateral varus derotation osteotomies of the proximal femur (VDRO) and pelvic osteotomy or acetabuloplasty, when indicated. There are many cohort studies which report a high success rate in terms of improved hip morphology at medium- to long-term follow-up. However, many studies report high rates of complications including mortality [28,29,62–66]. In one study, the mortality rate was 4% and the overall complication rate was 25%, rising to 68% in children with gastrostomies or tracheostomies [62]. These rates may not be acceptable to the parents of children with CP who have asymptomatic hip dysplasia detected by routine HS.

Recurrent hip displacement and avascular necrosis are two of the most disappointing late outcomes after reconstructive surgery [28,62–66]. Earlier studies of AVN after hip reconstruction in children with CP used or adapted the classifications for AVN in DDH [64,65]. In contrast, Park and colleagues devised a new classification and reported a prevalence of 43% [66]. They reported both risk factors and outcomes.

Despite the significant morbidity and mortality which is associated with bony reconstructive surgery, this surgery has been reported to have good short-term and long-term outcomes [43,48]. Bony reconstructive surgery may be preferable to the uncertain results of salvage hip surgery [1,6,43]. For parents and carers to make an informed choice, the treating team must be aware of their teams' success rate, failure rate and complication rate [48,57].

The components of a full hip reconstruction are typically adductor lengthening, VDRO and acetabuloplasty. The indications for open reduction and capsulorraphy are not well-defined and there is little published evidence to guide decision-making. Rates for capsulotomy and capsulorraphy vary in the literature and may be related to the utilisation of hip surveillance and the severity and duration of hip dislocation for the specific patient and for the population of children with CP [43,48,57]. Dynamic arthrography is a promising tool to guide intra-operative decision-making as to when acetabuloplasty may be required in BRS, after VDRO. Arthrographic assessment of the labrum after VDRO provides objective information to help surgeons standardise decision-making regarding the indications for acetabuloplasty [43].

15. Bilateral Surgery for Unilateral Hip Displacement?

In children who are functioning at GMFCS IV and V HD may, on MP alone, appear to be unilateral or asymmetric (Figure 7). Some children may present with MP > 40% in only one hip but both hips have similar degrees of increased femoral neck anteversion and coxa valga. Increased MP may be related to the severity of adductor spasticity and contracture, but abnormalities in proximal femoral geometry seem to be more related to the biomechanical environment of the growing hip. Specific factors include GMFCS level, hip abductor weakness and limitations in weight bearing [3,17,44]. Unilateral APR or bony reconstructive surgery are associated with a high rate of displacement in the contralateral hip in long-term follow-up [1,43]. Most surgeons recommend bilateral APR and bilateral reconstructive surgery [43,48,67–69]. Bilateral surgery is more durable, maintains symmetry and has only marginal increased risks of morbidity [68,69] (Figure 7).

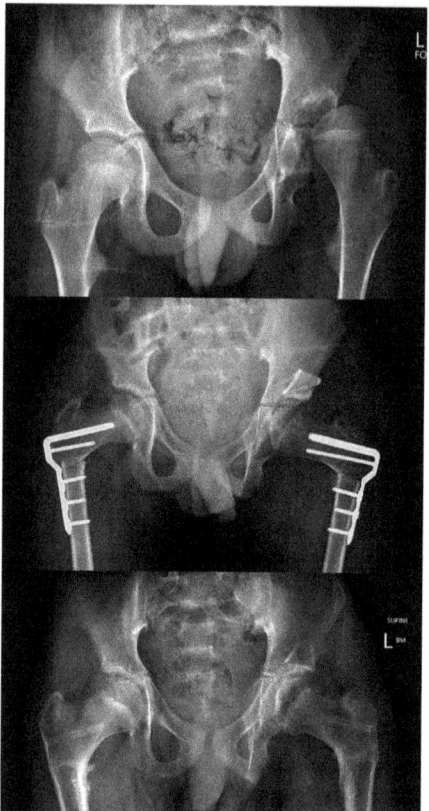

Figure 7. Bilateral surgery for unilateral CPHD. Copyright Kerr Graham, RCH Melbourne. These are the radiographs of a boy aged 10 years, GMFCS IV with clinical and radiographic unilateral (left) CPHD. The top image is immediately pre-operative. The middle image is 7 days after bilateral APR, bilateral VDRO and left San Diego Acetabuloplasty. The bottom image is at 2-year follow-up, after removal of implants. Bilateral surgery gives the best opportunity for symmetry and durability of outcome with marginal increases in surgical adverse events and morbidity.

16. Reconstructive Surgical Outcomes and Surgeon Volume

An additional clinical and ethical dilemma is posed by the observation by Shore and colleagues that the outcomes of reconstructive surgery in children with CP are influenced by surgeon volume [57]. In a large study from a specialist tertiary centre, surgeon volume was an independent predictor of the need for surgical revision [57]. The importance of surgeon volume has been identified in many areas of surgical practice. The importance of surgeon volume to outcomes requires further study in CPHD. For the present, we suggest that when children with CPHD require surgery, it should ideally be by a high-volume surgeon, working in a specialised tertiary centre, well-supported by a multidisciplinary medical, anaesthetic and pain management team [43,57,63].

17. Scoliosis and Pelvic Obliquity

The group of children with CP who are most at risk of developing hip displacement/dislocation in the first decade of life are also the children who are most at risk of developing scoliosis in the second decade of life [70,71]. The careful work done through hip surveillance and by the hip reconstruction surgeon can be undone by the sudden development of scoliosis and pelvic obliquity [70–74]. Surgery to correct scoliosis usually involves instrumentation and arthrodesis of the spine from T2 to the pelvis [70]. Hips which have previously been managed by 'successful' reconstructive surgery can become symptomatic all over again, following loss of motion in spinal segments after surgery for scoliosis [72]. Despite this, a recent study has reported that scoliosis surgery did not influence a change in MP postoperatively—neither positively nor negatively—regardless of the extent of pelvic obliquity correction [75]. The ideal alignment of the spine–pelvic–femoral axis requires further elucidation [74].

18. Femoral Head Deformity: Salvage or Reconstruction?

With respect to bony reconstructive surgery, one of the unknowns is the degree of femoral head deformity which is amenable to reconstruction versus progressing to salvage surgery. Prior to the long-term outcome study by Rutz and colleagues, many surgeons lacked confidence in the ability of the femoral head to remodel following reconstructive surgery [45]. Probably, too many femoral heads have been excised and this may have led to too many children being subjected to salvage surgery [40,43].

A recent study of non-ambulant children with CP investigated the status of femoral head deformity at skeletal maturity, finding an MP > 30% at triradiate cartilage closure was associated with a 'more severe' outcome at final follow-up [76]. This more severe head shape was also associated with a higher risk of worse osteoarthritis by Tönnis grading. Interestingly, the authors found that prior reconstructive surgery had no impact on head shape at skeletal maturity which they felt was likely due to a lack of complete containment of the femoral epiphysis. Additional work is required to precisely define the degree of femoral head deformity which is amenable to reconstructive surgery versus the degree of deformity which would be better managed by a salvage surgical option [45,76].

19. Palliation of CPHD and the Role of Salvage Surgery

Some clinicians are not convinced by the value of hip surveillance and the need for bony reconstructive surgery in the management of CPHD in the non-ambulant child. This is supported by the observation that not all dislocated hips will be symptomatic and therefore some adopt a reactive approach, meaning to offer intervention only when hips become symptomatic [5]. The only hips in our centre which did not become symptomatic at long-term follow-up were a minority of children with early, complete, bilateral dislocations [6,13]. It might be appropriate to consider a reactive approach for asymptomatic, bilateral dislocations, especially in frail children functioning at GMFCS V with limited life expectancy [36].

The range of surgical procedures described for salvage of a painful dislocated hip in children with CP include at least eight widely used and radically different procedures, from arthrodesis, excision arthroplasty, osteotomy, to total joint replacement [43]. When multiple surgical procedures are offered to treat a single condition, it is often an indication that no one procedure is very effective or acceptable to the target population. The majority of outcome studies from salvage surgery are relatively small case series. There are few comparative studies and follow-up has generally been short- to medium-term. The majority of studies lack adequate documentation of pain before and after surgery as well as valid patient reported outcome measures (PROMS) [43,77–80]. A notable exception was the study by Koch et al. [79]. They compared the outcomes of three surgical groups to injection of the painful hip with local anaesthetic and corticosteroid. The study was strengthened by a standardised approach to surgery and routine use of visual analogue scales (VAS) to assess pain. The disadvantage of injecting the hip was the need for repeated injections which became less effective over time. Both resection arthroplasty and interposition arthroplasty were effective in reducing pain scores and were supported by parental satisfaction scores [79].

The recent publication of a study which reported racial disparities in both the risk of requiring a salvage procedure and the rate of post-operative complications points to yet another clinical and ethical dilemma in the management of CPHD which, to date, has gone unrecognised and unreported [80]. As this is the first report of this important ethical issue, further studies are required.

20. Summary, Conclusions and Future Directions

The purpose of this review is not to undermine confidence in HS, which we think offers the only realistic opportunity to learn about natural history and risk factors for hip displacement in children with CP. This information gives clinicians and parents the ability to have a conversation regarding management options which are not available once a hip dislocates and has reached the 'point of no return' in terms of femoral head deformity. However, there are many unanswered questions regarding hip surveillance and the surgical management of hip displacement which require further study.

There is a remarkable level of agreement and congruence in HS guidelines from many countries around the world for children with bilateral, severe CP, GMFCS IV and V. In contrast HS protocols for ambulant children are lacking in strong evidence and this is reflected in uncertainty and variation in HS protocols. This is the key area for future research.

We do not question the need to refer children with hip displacement to orthopaedic surgeons for surgery for the prevention of progressive hip displacement or the reconstruction of displaced hips. It is rather a plea for controlled studies, long-term outcome studies, patient reported outcome measures and family centred studies.

Key areas for future studies include identifying better preventive strategies to avoid BRS, or at least to delay BRS until older age when outcomes are more predictable. The long-term results of APR surgery require further study. The potential role for guided growth as a preventive strategy requires urgent investigation. This would ideally be in the form of comparative surgical studies and clinical trials which include patient-reported outcomes and long-term follow-up.

Supplementary Materials: The following supporting information can be downloaded at: https://www.mdpi.com/article/10.3390/jcm12041651/s1, Supplementary Materials S1: The Melbourne Cerebral Palsy Hip Classification System (MCPHCS) Expanded and Revised.

Author Contributions: Conceptualisation, J.J.H., P.T., K.W., B.J.S., K.G. and E.R.; data curation and contributions/publications to the original literature on which this study is based: J.J.H., P.T., K.W., B.J.S., K.G. and E.R.; writing—original draft preparation, K.G.; writing—review and editing, J.J.H., P.T., K.W., B.J.S., K.G. and E.R.: All authors have read and agreed to the published version of the manuscript.

Funding: This research received no external funding. KG acknowledges support from NHMRC, CP-Achieve.

Institutional Review Board Statement: Not applicable.

Informed Consent Statement: Not applicable.

Data Availability Statement: Not applicable.

Acknowledgments: The authors acknowledge illustrations prepared by Bill Reid and secretarial support from Josephine Skelton.

Conflicts of Interest: The authors declare no conflict of interest.

References

1. Graham, H.K.; Rosenbaum, P.; Paneth, N.; Dan, B.; Lin, J.P.; Damiano, D.L.; Becher, J.G.; Gaebler-Spira, D.; Colver, A.; Reddihough, D.S.; et al. Cerebral palsy. *Nat. Rev. Dis. Prim.* **2016**, *2*, 15082. [CrossRef]
2. Ramstad, K.; Jahnsen, R.B.; Terjesen, T. Severe hip displacement reduces health-related quality of life in children with cerebral palsy. *Acta Orthop.* **2017**, *88*, 205–210. [CrossRef]
3. Soo, B.; Howard, J.J.; Boyd, R.N.; Reid, S.M.; Lanigan, A.; Wolfe, R.; Reddihough, D.; Graham, H.K. Hip displacement in cerebral palsy. *J. Bone Joint Surg. Am.* **2006**, *88*, 121–129. [CrossRef]
4. Shore, B.; Spence, D.; Graham, H. The role for hip surveillance in children with cerebral palsy. *Curr. Rev. Musculoskelet. Med.* **2012**, *5*, 126–134. [CrossRef]

5. Aroojis, A.; Mantri, N.; Johari, A.N. Hip displacement in cerebral palsy: The role of surveillance. *Indian J. Orthop.* **2021**, *55*, 5–19. [CrossRef]
6. Dobson, F.; Boyd, R.N.; Parrott, J.; Nattrass, G.R.; Graham, H.K. Hip surveillance in children with cerebral palsy. Impact on the surgical management of spastic hip disease. *J. Bone Joint Surg. Br.* **2002**, *84*, 720–726. [CrossRef]
7. Kentish, M.; Wynter, M.; Snape, N.; Boyd, R. Five-year outcome of state-wide hip surveillance of children and adolescents with cerebral palsy. *J. Pediatr. Rehabil. Med.* **2011**, *4*, 205–217. [CrossRef]
8. Hägglund, G.; Alriksson-Schmidt, A.; Lauge-Pedersen, H.; Rodby-Bousquet, E.; Wagner, P.; Westbom, L. Prevention of dislocation of the hip in children with cerebral palsy: 20-year results of a population-based prevention programme. *Bone Joint J.* **2014**, *96-b*, 1546–1552. [CrossRef]
9. Wynter, M.; Gibson, N.; Willoughby, K.L.; Love, S.; Kentish, M.; Thomason, P.; Graham, H.K. Australian hip surveillance guidelines for children with cerebral palsy: 5-year review. *Dev. Med. Child Neurol.* **2015**, *57*, 808–820. [CrossRef]
10. Gordon, G.S.; Simkiss, D.E. A systematic review of the evidence for hip surveillance in children with cerebral palsy. *J. Bone Joint Surg Br.* **2006**, *88*, 1492–1496. [CrossRef]
11. Gray, J.A.; Patnick, J.; Blanks, R.G. Maximising benefit and minimising harm of screening. *BMJ* **2008**, *336*, 480–483. [CrossRef]
12. Toovey, R.; Willoughby, K.L.; Hodgson, J.M.; Graham, H.K.; Reddihough, D.S. More than an X-ray: Experiences and perspectives of parents of children with cerebral palsy when engaging in hip surveillance. *J. Paediatr. Child Health* **2020**, *56*, 130–135. [CrossRef]
13. Wawrzuta, J.; Willoughby, K.L.; Molesworth, C.; Ang, S.G.; Shore, B.J.; Thomason, P.; Graham, H.K. Hip health at skeletal maturity: A population-based study of young adults with cerebral palsy. *Dev. Med. Child Neurol.* **2016**, *58*, 1273–1280. [CrossRef]
14. Ramstad, K.; Terjesen, T. Hip pain is more frequent in severe hip displacement: A population-based study of 77 children with cerebral palsy. *J. Pediatr. Orthop. B* **2016**, *25*, 217–221. [CrossRef]
15. Rang, M. Cerebral palsy. In *Lovell and Winter's Paediatric Orthopaedics*, 3rd ed.; Morrissey, R., Ed.; JB Lippincott: Philadelphia, PA, USA, 1990; Volume 1, pp. 465–506.
16. Silver, R.L.; Rang, M.; Chan, J.; de la Garza, J. Adductor release in nonambulant children with cerebral palsy. *J. Pediatr. Orthop.* **1985**, *5*, 672–677. [CrossRef]
17. Palisano, R.; Rosenbaum, P.; Walter, S.; Russell, D.; Wood, E.; Galuppi, B. Development and reliability of a system to classify gross motor function in children with cerebral palsy. *Dev. Med. Child Neurol.* **1997**, *39*, 214–223. [CrossRef]
18. Howard, J.; Soo, B.; Graham, H.K.; Boyd, R.N.; Reid, S.; Lanigan, A.; Wolfe, R.; Reddihough, D.S. Cerebral palsy in Victoria: Motor types, topography and gross motor function. *J. Paediatr. Child Health* **2005**, *41*, 479–483. [CrossRef]
19. Shore, B.J.; Yu, X.; Desai, S.; Selber, P.; Wolfe, R.; Graham, H.K. Adductor surgery to prevent hip displacement in children with cerebral palsy: The predictive role of the Gross Motor Function Classification System. *J. Bone Joint Surg. Am.* **2012**, *94*, 326–334. [CrossRef]
20. Shore, B.J.; Shrader, M.W.; Narayanan, U.; Miller, F.; Graham, H.K.; Mulpuri, K. Hip surveillance for children with cerebral palsy: A survey of the POSNA Membership. *J. Pediatr. Orthop.* **2017**, *37*, e409–e414. [CrossRef]
21. Miller, S.D.; Mayson, T.A.; Mulpuri, K.; O'Donnell, M.E. Developing a province-wide hip surveillance program for children with cerebral palsy: From evidence to consensus to program implementation: A mini-review. *J. Pediatr. Orthop. B* **2020**, *29*, 517–522. [CrossRef]
22. Protocol for Hip Surveillance in Cerebral Palsy. Available online: http://www.nice.org.uk (accessed on 27 November 2022).
23. Gibson, N.; Wynter, M.; Thomason, P.; Baker, F.; Burnett, H.; Graham, H.K.; Kentish, M.; Love, S.C.; Maloney, E.; Stannage, K.; et al. Australian hip surveillance guidelines at 10 years: New evidence and implementation. *J. Pediatr. Rehabil. Med.* **2022**, *15*, 31–37. [CrossRef]
24. Parrott, J.; Boyd, R.N.; Dobson, F.; Lancaster, A.; Love, S.; Oates, J.; Wolfe, R.; Nattrass, G.R.; Graham, H.K. Hip displacement in spastic cerebral palsy: Repeatability of radiologic measurement. *J. Pediatr. Orthop.* **2002**, *22*, 660–667. [CrossRef]
25. Kulkarni, V.A.; Davids, J.R.; Boyles, A.D.; Cung, N.Q.; Bagley, A. Reliability and efficiency of three methods of calculating migration percentage on radiographs for hip surveillance in children with cerebral palsy. *J. Child Orthop.* **2018**, *12*, 145–151. [CrossRef]
26. Hermanson, M.; Hägglund, G.; Riad, J.; Rodby-Bousquet, E.; Wagner, P. Prediction of hip displacement in children with cerebral palsy: Development of the CPUP hip score. *Bone Joint J.* **2015**, *97-b*, 1441–1444. [CrossRef]
27. Miller, S.D.; Juricic, M.; Hesketh, K.; Mclean, L.; Magnuson, S.; Gasior, S.; Schaeffer, E.; O'donnell, M.; Mulpuri, K. Prevention of hip displacement in children with cerebral palsy: A systematic review. *Dev. Med. Child Neurol.* **2017**, *59*, 1130–1138. [CrossRef]
28. Ruzbarsky, J.J.; Beck, N.A.; Baldwin, K.D.; Sankar, W.N.; Flynn, J.M.; Spiegel, D.A. Risk factors and complications in hip reconstruction for nonambulatory patients with cerebral palsy. *J. Child Orthop.* **2013**, *7*, 487–500. [CrossRef]
29. Shea, J.; Nunally, K.D.; Miller, P.E.; Difazio, R.; Matheney, T.H.; Snyder, B.; Shore, B.J. Hip reconstruction in nonambulatory children with cerebral palsy: Identifying risk factors associated with postoperative complications and prolonged length of stay. *J. Pediatr. Orthop.* **2020**, *40*, e972–e977. [CrossRef]
30. Kiapekos, N.; Broström, E.; Hägglund, G.; Åstrand, P. Primary surgery to prevent hip dislocation in children with cerebral palsy in Sweden: A minimum 5-year follow-up by the national surveillance program (CPUP). *Acta Orthop.* **2019**, *90*, 495–500. [CrossRef]
31. Wagner, P.; Hägglund, G. Hip development after surgery to prevent hip dislocation in cerebral palsy: A longitudinal register study of 252 children. *Acta Orthop.* **2022**, *93*, 45–50. [CrossRef]

32. Hosseinzadeh, P.; Baldwin, K.; Minaie, A.; Miller, F. Management of hip disorders in patients with cerebral palsy. *JBJS Rev.* **2020**, *8*, e0148. [CrossRef]
33. Burns, F.; Stewart, R.; Reddihough, D.; Scheinberg, A.; Ooi, K.; Graham, H.K. The cerebral palsy transition clinic: Administrative chore, clinical responsibility, or opportunity for audit and clinical research? *J. Child Orthop.* **2014**, *8*, 203–213. [CrossRef]
34. Wordie, S.J.; Robb, J.E.; Hägglund, G.; Bugler, K.E.; Gaston, M.S. Hip displacement and dislocation in a total population of children with cerebral palsy in Scotland. *Bone Joint J.* **2020**, *102-b*, 383–387. [CrossRef]
35. Larsen, S.M.; Ramstad, K.; Terjesen, T. Hip pain in adolescents with cerebral palsy: A population-based longitudinal study. *Dev. Med. Child Neurol.* **2021**, *63*, 601–607. [CrossRef]
36. Blair, E.; Langdon, K.; McIntyre, S.; Lawrence, D.; Watson, L. Survival and mortality in cerebral palsy: Observations to the sixth decade from a data linkage study of a total population register and National Death Index. *BMC Neurol.* **2019**, *19*, 111. [CrossRef]
37. Rutz, E.; Passmore, E.; Baker, R.; Graham, H.K. Multilevel surgery improves gait in spastic hemiplegia but does not resolve hip dysplasia. *Clin. Orthop. Relat. Res.* **2012**, *470*, 1294–1302. [CrossRef]
38. Tsitlakidis, S.; Horsch, A.; Schaefer, F.; Westhauser, F.; Goetze, M.; Hagmann, S.; Klotz, M.C.M. Gait classification in unilateral cerebral palsy. *J. Clin. Med.* **2019**, *8*, 1652. [CrossRef]
39. Miller, S.; Leveille, L.; Juricic, M.; Mulpuri, K. Late hip displacement identified in children at Gross Motor Function Classification System II and III with asymmetric diplegia and fixed pelvic obliquity. *J. Am. Acad. Orthop. Surg. Glob. Res. Rev.* **2022**, *6*, e20.00094. [CrossRef]
40. Asma, A.; Ulusaloglu, A.; Shrader, M.W.; Miller, F.; Rogers, K.J.; Howard, J.J. Hip displacement after triradiate cartilage closure in nonambulatory cerebral palsy: Who needs continued radiographic surveillance? *J. Bone Joint Surg. Am.* **2022**, *105*, 27–34. [CrossRef]
41. Ulusaloglu, A.C.; Asma, A.; Rogers, K.J.; Shrader, M.W.; Graham, H.K.; Howard, J.J. The influence of tone on proximal femoral and acetabular geometry in neuromuscular hip displacement: A comparison of cerebral palsy and spinal muscular atrophy. *J. Child Orthop.* **2022**, *16*, 121–127. [CrossRef]
42. Miller, F.; Slomczykowski, M.; Cope, R.; Lipton, G.E. Computer modeling of the pathomechanics of spastic hip dislocation in children. *J. Pediatr. Orthop.* **1999**, *19*, 486–492. [CrossRef]
43. Howard, J.J.; Khot, A.; Graham, H.K. The hip in cerebral palsy. Part VIII Neuromuscular conditions. In *The Pediatric and Adolescent Hip*; Alshryda, S., Howard, J.J., Huntley, J.S., Schoenecker, J.G., Eds.; Springer: Cham, Switzerland, 2019; Chapter 18; pp. 467–530.
44. Robin, J.; Graham, H.K.; Selber, P.; Dobson, F.; Smith, K.; Baker, R. Proximal femoral geometry in cerebral palsy: A population-based cross-sectional study. *J. Bone Joint Surg. Br.* **2008**, *90*, 1372–1379. [CrossRef]
45. Kim, B.R.; Yoon, J.A.; Han, H.J.; Yoon, Y.I.; Lim, J.; Lee, S.; Cho, S.; Shin, Y.B.; Lee, H.J.; Suh, J.H.; et al. Efficacy of a hip brace for hip displacement in children with cerebral palsy: A randomized clinical trial. *JAMA Netw. Open* **2022**, *5*, e2240383. [CrossRef]
46. Graham, H.K.; Boyd, R.; Carlin, J.B.; Dobson, F.; Lowe, K.; Nattrass, G.; Thomason, P.; Wolfe, R.; Reddihough, D. Does botulinum toxin a combined with bracing prevent hip displacement in children with cerebral palsy and "hips at risk"? A randomized, controlled trial. *J. Bone Joint Surg. Am.* **2008**, *90*, 23–33. [CrossRef]
47. Lee, Y.; Lee, S.; Jang, J.; Lim, J.; Ryu, J.S. Effect of botulinum toxin injection on the progression of hip dislocation in patients with spastic cerebral palsy: A pilot study. *Toxins* **2021**, *13*, 872. [CrossRef]
48. Rutz, E.; Vavken, P.; Camathias, C.; Haase, C.; Jünemann, S.; Brunner, R. Long-term results and outcome predictors in one-stage hip reconstruction in children with cerebral palsy. *J. Bone Joint Surg. Am.* **2015**, *97*, 500–506. [CrossRef]
49. McCarthy, J.J.; Noonan, K.J.; Nemke, B.; Markel, M. Guided growth of the proximal femur: A pilot study in the lamb model. *J. Pediatr. Orthop.* **2010**, *30*, 690–694. [CrossRef]
50. Lebe, M.; van Stralen, R.A.; Buddhdev, P. Guided growth of the proximal femur for the management of the Hip at Risk' in children with cerebral palsy—A systematic review. *Children* **2022**, *9*, 609. [CrossRef]
51. Cooke, P.H.; Cole, W.G.; Carey, R.P. Dislocation of the hip in cerebral palsy. Natural history and predictability. *J. Bone Joint Surg. Br.* **1989**, *71*, 441–446. [CrossRef]
52. Terjesen, T. Development of the hip joints in unoperated children with cerebral palsy: A radiographic study of 76 patients. *Acta Orthop.* **2006**, *77*, 125–131. [CrossRef]
53. Park, J.Y.; Choi, Y.; Cho, B.C.; Moon, S.Y.; Chung, C.Y.; Lee, K.M.; Sung, K.H.; Kwon, S.S.; Park, M.S. Progression of hip displacement during radiographic surveillance in patients with cerebral palsy. *J. Korean Med. Sci.* **2016**, *31*, 1143–1149. [CrossRef]
54. Lins, L.A.B.; Watkins, C.J.; Shore, B.J. Natural history of spastic hip disease. *J. Pediatr. Orthop.* **2019**, *39* (Suppl. S1), s33–s37. [CrossRef]
55. Lin, C.Y.; Chung, C.H.; Matthews, D.J.; Chu, H.Y.; Chen, L.C.; Yang, S.S.; Chien, W.C. Long-term effect of botulinum toxin A on the hip and spine in cerebral palsy: A national retrospective cohort study in Taiwan. *PLoS ONE* **2021**, *16*, e0255143. [CrossRef]
56. Presedo, A.; Oh, C.W.; Dabney, K.W.; Miller, F. Soft-tissue releases to treat spastic hip subluxation in children with cerebral palsy. *J. Bone Joint Surg. Am.* **2005**, *87*, 832–841. [CrossRef]
57. Shore, B.J.; Zurakowski, D.; Dufreny, C.; Powell, D.; Matheney, T.H.; Snyder, B.D. Proximal Femoral Varus Derotation Osteotomy in children with cerebral palsy: The effect of age, Gross Motor Function Classification System Level, and surgeon volume on surgical success. *J. Bone Joint Surg. Am.* **2015**, *97*, 2024–2031. [CrossRef]
58. Hermanson, M.; Hägglund, G.; Riad, J.; Wagner, P. Head-shaft angle is a risk factor for hip displacement in children with cerebral palsy. *Acta Orthop.* **2015**, *86*, 229–232. [CrossRef]

59. Van der List, J.P.; Witbreuk, M.M.; Buizer, A.I.; van der Sluijs, J.A. The head-shaft angle of the hip in early childhood: A comparison of reference values for children with cerebral palsy and normally developing hips. *Bone Joint J.* **2015**, *97-b*, 1291–1295. [CrossRef]
60. Hsieh, H.C.; Wang, T.M.; Kuo, K.N.; Huang, S.C.; Wu, K.W. Guided growth improves coxa valga and hip subluxation in children with cerebral palsy. *Clin. Orthop. Relat. Res.* **2019**, *477*, 2568–2576. [CrossRef]
61. Sheu, H.; Lee, W.C.; Kao, H.K.; Yang, W.E.; Chang, C.H. The effectiveness of adding guided growth to soft tissue release in treating spastic hip displacement. *J. Orthop. Sci.* **2022**, *27*, 1082–1088. [CrossRef]
62. Stasikelis, P.J.; Lee, D.D.; Sullivan, C.M. Complications of osteotomies in severe cerebral palsy. *J. Pediatr. Orthop.* **1999**, *19*, 207–210. [CrossRef]
63. DiFazio, R.; Vessey, J.A.; Miller, P.; Van Nostrand, K.; Snyder, B. Postoperative complications after hip surgery in patients with cerebral palsy: A retrospective matched cohort study. *J. Pediatr. Orthop.* **2016**, *36*, 56–62. [CrossRef]
64. Koch, A.; Jozwiak, M.; Idzior, M.; Molinska-Glura, M.; Szulc, A. Avascular necrosis as a complication of the treatment of dislocation of the hip in children with cerebral palsy. *Bone Joint J.* **2015**, *97-b*, 270–276. [CrossRef]
65. Phillips, L.; Hesketh, K.; Schaeffer, E.K.; Andrade, J.; Farr, J.; Mulpuri, K. Avascular necrosis in children with cerebral palsy after reconstructive hip surgery. *J. Child Orthop.* **2017**, *11*, 326–333. [CrossRef]
66. Park, B.K.; Park, H.; Park, K.B.; Rhee, I.; Kim, S.; Kim, H.W. Fate of hips complicated by avascular necrosis of the femoral head following reconstructive surgery in nonambulatory patients with cerebral palsy. *Sci. Rep.* **2022**, *12*, 11767. [CrossRef]
67. Kamisan, N.; Thamkunanon, V. Outcome of bilateral hip reconstruction in unilateral hip subluxation in cerebral palsy: Comparison to unilateral hip reconstruction. *J. Orthop.* **2020**, *20*, 367–373. [CrossRef]
68. Sung, K.H.; Kwon, S.-S.; Chung, C.Y.; Lee, K.M.; Kim, J.; Lee, S.Y.; Park, M.S. Fate of stable hips after prophylactic femoral varization osteotomy in patients with cerebral palsy. *BMC Musculoskelet. Disord.* **2018**, *19*, 130. [CrossRef]
69. Miller, S.D.; Juricic, M.; Baraza, N.; Fajardo, N.; So, J.; Schaeffer, E.K.; Shore, B.J.; Narayanan, U.; Mulpuri, K. Unilateral versus bilateral reconstructive hip surgery in children with cerebral palsy: A survey of pediatric orthopedic surgery practice and decision-making. *J. Child Orthop.* **2022**, *16*, 325–332. [CrossRef]
70. McCarthy, J.J.; D'Andrea, L.P.; Betz, R.R.; Clements, D.H. Scoliosis in the child with cerebral palsy. *J. Am. Acad. Orthop. Surg.* **2006**, *14*, 367–375. [CrossRef]
71. Willoughby, K.L.; Ang, S.G.; Thomason, P.; Rutz, E.; Shore, B.; Buckland, A.J.; Johnson, M.B.; Graham, H.K. Epidemiology of scoliosis in cerebral palsy: A population-based study at skeletal maturity. *J. Paediatr. Child Health* **2022**, *58*, 295–301. [CrossRef]
72. Crawford, L.; Herrera-Soto, J.; Ruder, J.A.; Phillips, J.; Knapp, R. The fate of the neuromuscular hip after Spinal Fusion. *J. Pediatr. Orthop.* **2017**, *37*, 403–408. [CrossRef]
73. Cobanoglu, M.; Chen, B.P.; Perotti, L.; Rogers, K.; Miller, F. The impact of spinal fusion on hip displacement in cerebral palsy. *Indian J. Orthop.* **2021**, *55*, 176–182. [CrossRef]
74. Buckland, A.J.; Woo, D.; Kerr Graham, H.; Vasquez-Montes, D.; Cahill, P.; Errico, T.J.; Sponseller, P.D. Residual lumbar hyperlordosis is associated with worsened hip status 5 years after scoliosis correction in non-ambulant patients with cerebral palsy. *Spine Deform.* **2021**, *9*, 1125–1136. [CrossRef]
75. Asma, A.; Cobanoglu, M.; Ulusaloglu, A.C.; Rogers, K.J.; Miller, F.; Howard, J.J.; Shah, S.A.; Shrader, M.W. Hip Displacement Does Not Change After Pelvic Obliquity Correction During Spinal Fusion in Children With Cerebral Palsy. *J. Pediatr. Orthop.* **2023**, *43*, e127–e131. [CrossRef]
76. Ulusaloglu, A.C.; Asma, A.; Rogers, K.J.; Shrader, M.W.; Miller, F.; Howard, J.J. Femoral head deformity associated with hip displacement in cerebral palsy: Results at skeletal maturity. *J. Pediatr. Orthop.* **2022**, *accepted, in press*. [CrossRef]
77. De Souza, R.C.; Mansano, M.V.; Bovo, M.; Yamada, H.H.; Rancan, D.R.; Fucs, P.M.; Svartman, C.; de Assumpcao, R.M. Hip salvage surgery in cerebral palsy cases: A systematic review. *Rev. Bras. Ortop.* **2015**, *50*, 254–259. [CrossRef]
78. Hwang, L.; Varte, L.; Kim, H.W.; Lee, D.H.; Park, H. Salvage procedures for the painful chronically dislocated hip in cerebral palsy. *Bone Joint J.* **2016**, *98-B*, 137–143. [CrossRef]
79. Koch, A.; Krasny, J.; Dziurda, M.; Ratajczyk, M.; Jozwiak, M. Parents and caregivers satisfaction after palliative treatment of spastic hip dislocation in cerebral palsy. *Front Neurol.* **2021**, *12*, 635894. [CrossRef]
80. Brown, L.; Cho, K.M.; Tarawneh, O.H.; Quan, T.; Malyavko, A.; Tabaie, S.A. Race Is associated with risk of salvage procedures and postoperative complications after hip procedures in children with cerebral palsy. *J. Pediatr. Orthop.* **2022**, *42*, e925–e931. [CrossRef]

Disclaimer/Publisher's Note: The statements, opinions and data contained in all publications are solely those of the individual author(s) and contributor(s) and not of MDPI and/or the editor(s). MDPI and/or the editor(s) disclaim responsibility for any injury to people or property resulting from any ideas, methods, instructions or products referred to in the content.

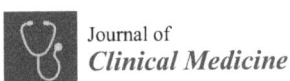

Protocol

Co-Design of an Intervention to Increase the Participation in Leisure Activities Including Adolescents with Cerebral Palsy with GMFCS Levels IV and V: A Study Protocol

Rocío Palomo-Carrión [1,2], Caline Cristine De Araújo Ferreira Jesus [3,*], Camila Araújo Santos Santana [4], Raquel Lindquist [5], Roselene Alencar [5], Helena Romay-Barrero [1,2], Elena Contell-Gonzalo [6], Karolinne Souza Monteiro [3], Elena Pinero-Pinto [7] and Egmar Longo [3]

1 Faculty of Physiotherapy, University of Castilla-La Mancha, 45071 Toledo, Spain
2 Hemi Child-Research Unit, University of Castilla-La Mancha, 45071 Toledo, Spain
3 Rehabilitation Sciences Graduate Program, Faculty of Health Science of Trairi, Federal University of Rio Grande do Norte, Santa Cruz 59078-900, Brazil
4 Department of Physical Therapy, Federal University of São Carlos, São Carlos 13565-905, Brazil
5 Department of Physical Therapy, Faculty of Health Science, Federal University of Rio Grande do Norte, Campus Universitário Lagoa Nova, Natal 59076-740, Brazil
6 Corseford School, Capability Scotland, Renfrewshire PA10 2NT, UK
7 Department of Physical Therapy, Faculty of Nursery, Physiotherapy and Podiatry, University of Seville, 41004 Seville, Spain
* Correspondence: calinefisio@gmail.com

Abstract: The participation of adolescents with cerebral palsy (CP) within the community is reduced compared to their peers and is a barrier to their socialization, self-determination and quality of life. Patient and Public Involvement (PPI) is a key strategy for successful interventions, especially when involvement of the stakeholders takes place at all stages of the research. Co-design can be crucial for success as researchers, patients with CP and their families work together to bring the necessary elements to the interventions to be designed. The objectives will be: (1) To co-design an intervention aimed at improving the participation of adolescents with significant motor disabilities within the community in partnership with adolescents with CP, families and rehabilitation professionals. (2) To assess the feasibility of the co-design process in partnership with interested parties. The study will be based on Participatory Action Research (PAR) and will be held in Spain and Brazil. In both countries, the study will be carried out remotely with nine adolescents aged 12 to 17 years with CP, Gross Motor Function Classification System (GMFCS) levels IV–V, their families and six health professionals (physiotherapists and occupational therapists). Different dialogue groups will be created to involve adolescents, families and health professionals to the research's project. To manage their involvement in the co-design process, the Involvement Matrix (IM) will be used, and according to the IM phases, four steps will be included in the research: (1) Preparation; (2) Co-design; (3) Analysis: results of the intervention protocol and the study's feasibility and (4) Dissemination of results. Partnering with the public to design an intervention to improve participation can bring better results compared to protocols designed only by health professionals. In addition, it will allow for knowing the needs of adolescents with CP in terms of participation within the community. The study will also explore which roles were chosen by all participants and how they felt while actively participating in the process of co-designing an intervention protocol and their own perspectives on the use of the involvement matrix.

Keywords: cerebral palsy; co-design; intervention; participation; involvement matrix; public and patient involvement; adolescents

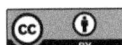

1. Introduction

Cerebral palsy (CP) is one of the most common physical disabilities, affecting approximately 2–3/1000 children [1]. It describes a group of permanent disorders that affect the development of movement and posture and contribute to activity limitations [1,2]. CP is a chronic health condition, which can increase the risk of developing problems related to mental health, chronic pain, fatigue and stress. These are highly comorbid in these patients, reducing their possibilities of interacting in the community [3]. Adolescents with CP experience limitations in their performance of day-to-day activities and restrictions on their participation in home, school and community life [4].

The International Classification of Functioning, Disability, and Health (ICF) by the World Health Organization (WHO) defines participation as a person's involvement in life situations (WHO, 2001) [5]. Recently, participation has been understood from a Family of Participation-related Constructs (fPRC) perspective, which describes participation in terms of attendance (being there) and involvement (level of engagement) [6]. Participation is context-dependent and may predominantly be influenced by characteristics of the environment over characteristics of the individual, focuses on the societal level and is related to quality of life [7,8]. The participation of young people with CP within the community is reduced compared to their peers and is an impediment to socialization, self-determination and quality of life of the individual [8,9]. Participation depends on different factors such as children's gross motor function and adaptive behavior for participation. Children's ability to communicate and family support are important considerations for improving children's social skills in life situations [10]. Thus, understanding the needs for participation within the community of adolescents with CP who have severe motor disabilities, giving them a voice through a collaborative process, can contribute to the success of the intervention.

A participative methodology facilitates democratic dialogue in the development and implementation of interventions and service improvement directed to that specific public, as they can share their real needs. Patient and public involvement (PPI) comprises the active involvement of patients and members of the public in the design and research process [11]. It aims to ensure that research is relevant to the intended audience and that their views are taken into account. PPI in research is currently being defined as "research being carried out 'with' or 'by' members of the public rather than 'to', 'about' or 'for' them" [12]. End-users are most often involved only in the early stages and/or in the final stages of research [13]. However, PPI can take place at any stage of the research process, from the development of the initial research questions through to specific aspects of study design, including data analysis and dissemination [11–13].

According to Bailey et al. (2015) [13], involving children and young people with disabilities in research is of vital importance as they are in an ideal position to opine on what works for them and their families. When dealing with young people with chronic diseases, researchers argue that the PPI improves the relevance and quality of projects and contributes to the personal development of this public. In addition, there seems to be a consensus that the involvement of young people with chronic diseases should become an integral and standard element of the projects that affect them. Van Schelven et al. (2020) [14] stated that these young people have always had a passive role in health and social assistance projects, as research subjects, recipients of an intervention and users of an instrument and that nowadays there is a growing consensus that they should be actively involved in matters that concern them.

In this sense, the Involvement Matrix (IM) [15] was developed to support conversation and discussion about roles and expectations, aiming for sustainable partnerships in research. This tool was jointly built by researchers and patients in the Netherlands to promote the collaboration of patients (from the age of 12) in projects and research. Using the IM ensures that the public is included in all phases of the research project and in an orderly manner, according to their preferences and interests [16]. The IM includes five roles for involvement (Listener, Co-thinker, Advisor, Partner, and Decision-maker) over three main phases of research projects (Preparation, Execution, and Implementation) [16,17]. This tool aims to support PPI in research projects, allowing different levels of involvement, which is useful to clarify the expectations during the process. It can be used prospectively to discuss strategies to be developed with the patients in different phases of projects, and retrospectively to discuss if the strategies were carried out satisfactorily [16,17].

Involving patients, caregivers and health professionals in the early stages of intervention development and evaluation is widely recognized as a good practice to elicit the opinions of users and professionals in order to create a credible and motivating program [17–22]. McDermott et al. (2010) [23] further state that the views of users and professionals are integral in the development of an intervention, which can help to clarify the mechanisms by which the intervention works, identify potential barriers to change, provide information about individual needs to users, and explore questions that can be used to develop and refine the intervention model.

Few studies [14,24] using a participative methodology have involved children and adolescents with more severe disabilities such as CP GMFCS level IV–V as active participants in research. In addition, it is known that interventions for children and adolescents with CP, especially at levels with greater dependence such as GMFCS levels IV and V, are strongly focused on components of the ICF such as function and structure, rather than activity, participation and contextual factors (physical environment, social environment, attitudinal environment, and personal factors unrelated to a child's health condition). Thus, our objective will be to co-design an intervention to promote participation of young people with CP levels IV and V in partnership with the public and to assess the feasibility of the co-designing process in partnership with interested parties.

2. Materials and Methods

2.1. Study Design

The study will be based on the Participatory Action Research (PAR) [25], a term that encompasses numerous approaches to research in which researchers work collaboratively with stakeholders through an iterative cycle of fieldwork or practice, reflection, planning, research and action [12]. It is supported by a recommendation to execute research "with" people rather than "about" people. PAR is a qualitative research approach that seeks to maximize the participation of the people whose lives are researched about. It includes people affected by the research topic as researchers themselves [26]. To achieve this, young people with chronic conditions (cerebral palsy GMFCS levels IV–V), their families and health professionals will be involved. In this way, it is intended to be able to allow the public to whom the intervention is directed to decide on its execution based on their needs and expectations, obtaining results according to their perspectives and actually based on their own experiences [27]. Being able to involve the participants themselves in the initial stage of the research allows it to be targeted to their objectives and not those of the researcher. It gives validity and objectivity to the intervention by focusing on the user. In addition, involving families and health professionals allows for a greater awareness of the youth's own reality. Thus, researchers and the public have a shared role and this allows the co-design of a viable intervention, whose objective is to make it possible to improve participation within the community [19].

2.2. Setting and Participants

This study was approved by the Ethics Committee of FIDMAG in Brazil (CAEE: 51319321.1.0000.5568) and Hermanas Hospitalarias (FIDMAG hospitable sisters Research Foundation) in Spain (PR-2022-07) according to the World Medical Association's Declaration of Helsinki. Before the study began, the written informed consent of all participants: adolescents, families and pediatric physiotherapist and occupational therapist will be requested.

This research will be carried out remotely (online) in Brazil and Spain, with nine adolescents aged 12 to 17 years, diagnosed with CP, GMFCS level IV and V, their families and six health professionals (physiotherapists and occupational therapists) in each country.

The sample size is based on research by Brooks et al. [28]. This study is also a co-design study involving youth with neuro-disability, parents and physicians. The sample they recruited has characteristics similar to those of this project. In this protocol, the sample will be recruited from different centers in Brazil and Spain.

Selection Criteria

Inclusion Criteria

Adolescents with CP from 12 to 17 years old, levels IV–V within the Gross Motor Function Classification System (GMFCS). They must have sufficient communication skills with support as needed, for example from using augmentative and alternative communication (AAC), help from another person or sign language translator. Other inclusion criteria are: participation of their family members, physiotherapists and occupational therapists who agree to participate in the study.

Exclusion Criteria

Adolescents who do not have the possibility of communicating with any AAC because there is no communicative interaction or functional communication, a problem answering questions and collaborating, other health conditions such as spina bifida or muscular dystrophy, and families, physiotherapists and occupational therapists who do not have time to participate in the meetings. Any participant who does not agree to sign the informed consent form will be excluded.

2.3. Recruitment

Recruitment will be intentional, as it is understood that the selection of participants in qualitative research often involves objective sampling, prioritizing the inclusion of information-rich cases from which much can be learned about issues of central importance. Importantly, purposeful sampling is highly adaptable and therefore applicable to many of the varied goals of engaging patients and the public as research partners.

Adolescents and their families will be recruited through known support networks, associations, philanthropic institutions and social networks. Rehabilitation professionals will be recruited for having previous experience working with the ICF participation constructs (the consultation of this information will be through publications, clinical background, ICF-attended courses or congress presentations by the professional).

2.4. Setting

The research will be carried out in Brazil and Spain, online, to facilitate the execution of the meetings. In this way, it will be possible to compare the participation of the same population in different countries, the influencing factors and how the approach works according to the perspectives of the parties involved in the research.

2.5. Assessment Tools

To manage the involvement of the public in this research we will use the "Involvement Matrix" (IM) (Figure 1) with the adolescents, their families and the rehabilitation professionals [16].

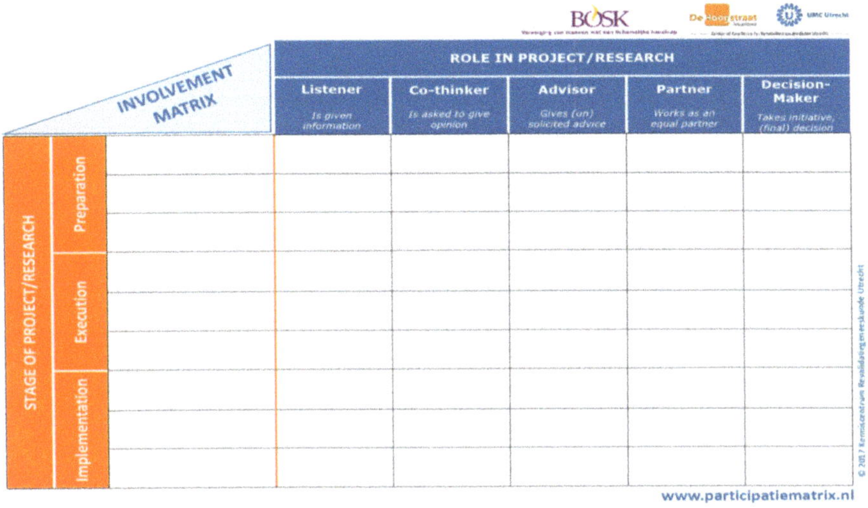

Figure 1. Involvement Matrix; Accessed on 1 March 2019, www.kcrutrecht.nl/involvement-matrix. © Center of Excellence for Rehabilitation Medicine Utrecht, used with permission.

Initially, the tool will be translated into Spanish and Portuguese simultaneously and cross-culturally adapted for its proper use, as recommended by the Dutch team that developed the IM. This includes the five roles for involvement represented in Figure 2. When using the IM, all participants involved in the research project will fit into one of these roles, according to their preferences on each study phase [17]:

- Listener is a less active role but certainly not less important in the project;
- Co-thinker can also involve asking questions and giving feedback, as well as giving an opinion when asked;
- Advisor gives feedback from project leaders to patients on whether or not advice has been followed at any time;
- Partner is valuable not only at the start of a project but also at the intermediate and final phases. The partner has the same function as the main researcher;
- Decision-maker requires project leaders to have a 'hands off' attitude.

Figure 2. Illustration of the five roles for involvement in the Involvement Matrix. Accessed on 1 March 2019, www.kcrutrecht.nl/involvement-matrix. © Center of Excellence for Rehabilitation Medicine Utrecht, used with permission.

To evaluate the participation and the environmental barriers of adolescents in the community, we will use the Participation and Environment Measure for Children and Youth (PEM-CY) [29,30]. The PEM-CY is a parent-report instrument that examines participation and environment across three settings: home, school and community. It can be used to improve our understanding of the participation of children and young people with and without disabilities aged from 5 to 17 years and the environmental factors that support or hinder their participation in the home, school and community. It provides an overall environmental supportiveness score, as well as sub-scores that summarize the impact of particular features of the environment on participation in a given setting and the adequacy of available resources. For this research, only the community section of the PEM-CY will be used, considering the Spanish and Portuguese versions of the scale for the respective countries. A previously trained research assistant will pass the questionnaire to the adolescent and his/her caregiver so that the answers reflect the thinking of both, and not just the caregiver, as the scale recommends. The use of PEM-CY helps adolescents and their families to understand what it means to participate in the community, in addition to what can help or hinder participation.

2.5.1. Qualitative Tools

Semi-structured interviews will be conducted with adolescents, families and health professionals, in order to identify their opinions on the intervention proposal, as well as on the design of the study aimed at the PPI in research. The interview guide for adolescents, families and health professionals is presented in Figure S1 (Supplementary Materials).

Research Phases

This research will be conducted based on the phases suggested by the IM, having the following steps: preparation, co-design, analysis and dissemination of results (Figure 3) [17]. The objectives are related to the different phases included in the IM (phase 1 to phase 3). The main objective "To co-design an intervention aimed at improving the participation of adolescents with significant motor disabilities within the community in alliance with adolescents with CP, families and rehabilitation professionals" will be achieved from phase 1 to phase 2 of the IM, according to the Preparation and Execution parts in the IM.

To reach this objective we will answer the following research questions:

- What are the needs of adolescents with CP within the community?
- What barriers do you find in enhancing your participation in leisure activities?
- What are your perspectives on how to improve your participation?
- Do families and health professionals have the same perspectives on participation in the community as adolescents with CP?

The secondary objective "To assess the feasibility of the co-design process in partnership with interested parties" will be obtained in the last phase of IM, related to Implementation in IM. To reach this objective, we will answer the next research questions: Is it feasible to involve young people with CP, their families and professionals in the research? Is it possible to carry out their involvement in all phases of the study? Would the role in which they choose to become involved in the investigation be the right one?

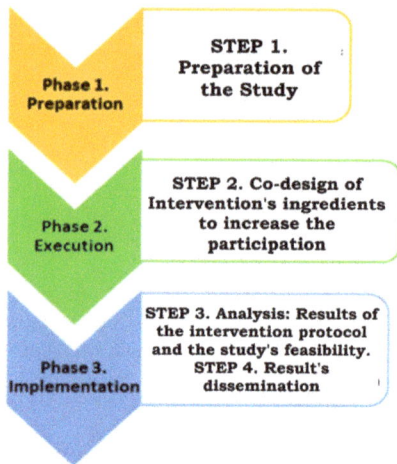

Figure 3. Research steps in the different phases of the Involvement Matrix.

2.5.2. Phase (1) Preparation Phase-Step 1

(1.1) Involvement Matrix Translation

The preparation phase corresponds with Step 1 in the research project, PREPARATION. Phase 1 begins with the translation of the IM into Portuguese and Spanish and, later, its back-translation being later sent to the original authors to release the use of the tool in the research. The process will be similar and concomitant in both countries. The translations into Portuguese and Spanish will be performed by two pediatric physiotherapists independently. When all documents are ready, two versions will be analyzed by five pediatric physiotherapists and three online meetings will be performed to discuss the versions and consider changes to include in the final version to be understood in Spanish and Portuguese. When the meetings are over and we have the best and correct version for both countries, the final version will be back-translated into English by a pediatric physiotherapist. Finally, the back-translated version will be sent to the authors for checking and permission to use in both countries.

(1.2) Participants' Recruitment

The recruitment of participants will be carried out intentionally, as explained in Section 2.1. Table 1 illustrates the details of this process in both countries and Table 2 shows the content and number of meetings that will be held with the different participants in the research project.

Table 1. Recruitment process that will be addressed in both countries.

Country	Spain	Brazil
Places of recruitment	Fundació Aspace Catalunya em Barcelona (Aspace Foundation-Catalonia)	Associations, support networks and social networks
Type of meetings	Remote	Remote
Number of Adolescents with CP	9	9
Number of families of adolescents with CP	9	9
Health professionals: PTs	3	3
Health professionals: OTs	3	3

Table 2. Duration and content of the meetings that will be held in the research project in both countries.

Country	Spain	Brazil	Description	Duration of Each Group (min)
Presentation meeting	1	1	Presentation of the project and the IM to all stakeholders	60
Discussion groups-Participation	2	2	Presentation of the concept of participation based on the ICF and its meaning in practice	60–90
PEMCY questionnaire	9	9	Application of the PEM-CY community session	60–90
Discussion groups-Participation + PEMCY results	2	2	Discussion of the concept of participation now based on the results of the application of PEM-CY	60–90

Table 2. Cont.

Country	Spain	Brazil	Description	Duration of Each Group (min)
Discussion Group-*What is a community participation intervention?*	1	1	Discussion about what is an intervention aimed to improve the participation of young people with disabilities in the community	60–90
Discussion Group-intervention draft	2	2	Co-design of an intervention draft aimed at the participation of young people with CP GMFCS IV-V in leisure activities	60–90
Meetings with the external public	1	1	Presentation of protocol results so far and capture criticism and suggestions from an external group made up of adolescents with CP GMFCS IV and V	60
Discussion Group-final version	3	3	Co-design of final version with all ingredients that should be present in the intervention for CP to increase the community participation	60–90
Semi-structured interviews and open-ended questions	24	24	A guide with questions will be used	60–90

(1.3). Discussion/Development/Group Meetings (Shown in Figure 4)

A first meeting will be held for the presentation by the responsible researcher of the research project to all the participants, where we will use the *IM* in order to facilitate the discussion about what roles and responsibilities the participants would like to have within the project and how to achieve this in practice.

Subsequently, focus groups will be organized to discuss the concept of participation focused on the ICF with the project participants, divided into three groups: adolescents, their families and health professionals. To support the participation of adolescents with CP in remote meetings, open questions will be established, asking them who wants to participate first so as not to generate rejection. If participation is not forthcoming, direct and more specific questions will be asked so that they can participate. In addition, if the adolescent wishes, the presence of a caregiver will always be allowed so that they can have the security and calm of being able of becoming involved in the meeting. They will be given enough time to communicate and their word will be respected.

A health professionals' discussion group 1 will be created with all the health professionals to discuss the concept of PARTICIPATION. At first, they will be asked for their thoughts, and their understanding of the construct of participation (what they understand by "participation" according to their knowledge? What do they think about it? What do they know about it?). Afterwards, a dialogue will be opened between the attendees, using games and activities to create the understood concept of participation and building its definition. The Adolescents and Families (discussion group 2) will be created by adolescents and their families to reflect deeply and according to their own experiences on PARTICIPATION: What are their perspectives? How do they think it influences their condition? What barriers are present? As in the previous discussion group (health professionals), a dialogue will be performed to create the concept of participation and building its definition according to adolescents' and families' perspectives. In order to assess the participation and environment of the participating adolescents, the "community" session of the PEM-CY will be used [29,30]. This instrument considers the perception of parents and/or guardians to obtain information about involvement, frequency and desire for change in participation, as well as barriers and facilitators of the environment. To encourage the involvement of adolescents, researchers will be present online with families and adolescents when the questionnaire is answered by parents, to facilitate the inclusion of the adolescents' voices if they have a desire for change.

After that, a meeting with health professionals (discussion group 1) will be held in order to present the result of the application of the PEM-CY questionnaire (community section). In addition, a meeting will be held to present these results with the adolescents and their families with the same purpose (discussion group 2). The presentation of the results of the PEM-CY (community section) will allow an understanding of what the restrictions of adolescents are in that context to analyze the barriers. Additionally, it could be possible to think of different strategies to favor their execution and how to design interventions to promote participation in the community.

At the end of the preparation phase, a meeting will be held with all participants (discussion group 3) in a focus group format, to think more easily about which ingredients should be part of the intervention protocol in terms of components, people involved and place of performance. It will provide a collaborative discussion about models of intervention to promote participation, taking components of the Pathways and Resources for Engagement and Participation (PREP) as an example [31]. PREP was developed in Canada and has been used as an evidence-based approach to enhance participation through modifying the environment, however, the research of Anaby et al. [32] includes adolescents with moderate motor impairment. Using PREP as an example will help adolescents, families and professionals to think more easily about which ingredients should be part of the intervention protocol in terms of components, people involved and place of performance [32,33].

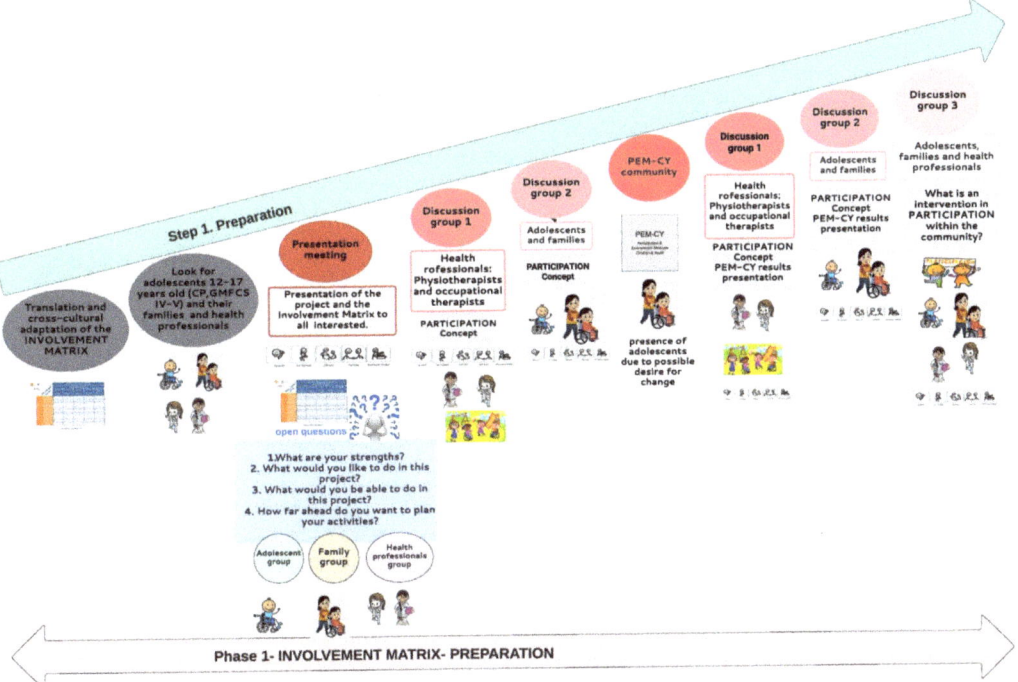

Figure 4. Step 1 of project's research in phase 1 of the Involvement Matrix: PREPARATION.

2.5.3. Phase (2) Execution Phase-Step 2 (Shown in Figure 5)

The Execution phase corresponds with Step 2 in the research project, CO-DESIGN. This phase is characterized by the stage where the participants will co-design an intervention protocol that encourages the participation of adolescents with CP GMFCS IV and V in leisure activities. It will initially consist of two brainstorming meetings (draft versions) where all participants will discuss and build necessary ingredients for an intervention protocol that will promote the participation of adolescents in the selected leisure activities.

(2.1) Intervention Checking

After the draft versions obtained in both meetings, a group external to the project (two adolescents, two family members and four health professionals, two OT and two PT) will be invited to express their opinion on the intervention protocol's preliminary version.

After this stage, the intervention protocol proposal to increase the participation in leisure activities of adolescents with GMFCS IV and V will end with three meetings.

(2.2) Co-Design Evaluation

At the end of this phase 2, Execution in the IM, semi-structured interviews and open questions (Figure S1) for all participants will be carried out to identify the experience in the use of the IM and their roles in the co-design of the intervention protocol. To obtain information (co-design evaluation follow-up) from the intervention protocol application, to identify the strengths and limitations that occurred in its implementation, and to maintain their involvement in research and co-working to collect needs from the same population and other issues, different dialogue groups will be built to continue the discussion. These dialogue groups, constituted of adolescents with CP, families, health professionals and researchers will continue co-designing and co-working in relation to their own needs and to have a voice in the community, increasing the visibility of these young people and their families in society, as well as their engagement in research.

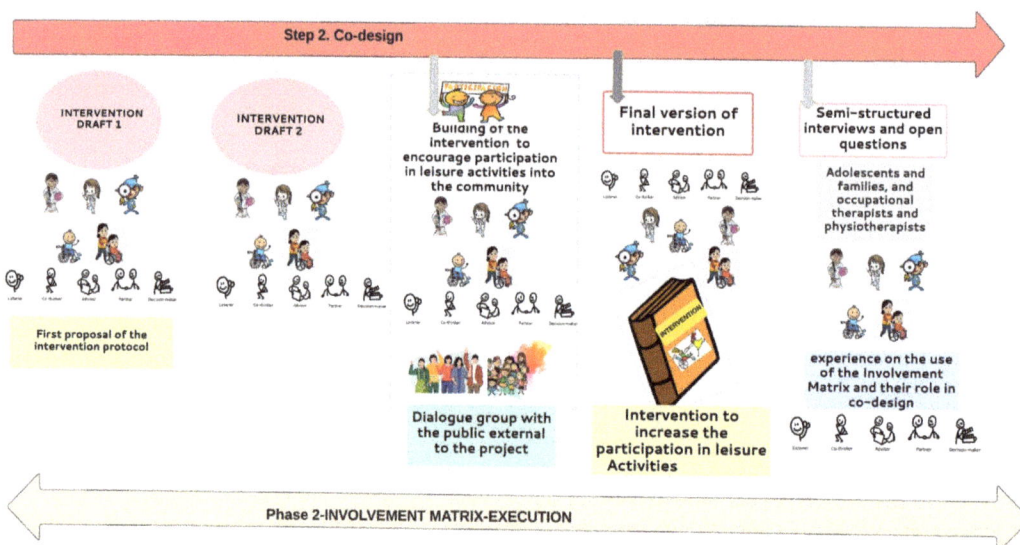

Figure 5. Step 2 of project's research (co-design) in phase 2 of Involvement Matrix: EXECUTION.

3. Analysis Procedure

3.1. Data Analysis of Co-Design Experiences and Role

The sample descriptive analysis will be performed through the SPSS statistical program [34]. For qualitative analysis, we will conduct an inductive thematic analysis of qualitative data collected in verbatim transcripts of audio recordings of meetings, materials used during the meetings and responses to open-ended questions to analyze members' perceptions, barriers and facilitators to patient involvement in the co-design and in the IM use [35]. Analysis will be conducted during the course of the study by H.R.B using the N-Vivo software (QSR International, NVivo Qualitative Data Analysis Software) [36].

The content of the analysis will be shared with the participants of the process, so that they can give their opinion, suggest changes, and validate the results.

3.2. Participation of the Public in the Selection and Dissemination of Results and Analysis of the Feasibility of the Co-Design of the Study and Strategies of Dissemination

Phase (3) Implementation Phase-Step 3 and Step 4

Feasibility and Acceptability Analysis

Finally, the feasibility and acceptability (of PPI) on the participants' involvement in the co-design of the final version of the intervention protocol will be analyzed, in the following aspects: evaluation of data collection ("How appropriate are the data collection procedures and purpose of the study?"). Follow-up questions address the participants' ability to answer and be involved in the phases of the co-design (e.g., comprehension, capacity), the appropriateness of the amount of data collection, whether they are relatively complete and usable and if the use of the Involvement Matrix is appropriate to involve participants in a structured way and to co-design an intervention protocol; evaluation of acceptability and adequacy, of the study's co-design and study's procedures ("Are the study procedures suitable for and acceptable to participants?"). Meetings attendance, and engagement; time, capacity and understanding of the procedures and co-design; acceptability and satisfaction of the co-design to participants; evaluation of resources and the ability to manage and implement the study, adherence to the project (through attendance at meetings depending on the role acquired and execution of the phases and sub-phases corresponding to the IM), evaluation of the preliminary participants' opinions on involvement in the study ("Does the research team have the resources and ability to manage the study and intervention?"). Follow-up questions address whether or not the research team has the space, administrative capacity, expertise, skills and time to conduct the study; ethics in implementing the study; budgetary considerations.

Dissemination Strategies (Shown in Figure 6)

The data analysis and dissemination will be carried out jointly with the research participants. To obtain information about the experience of involvement (strengths and limitations) in the intervention protocol, different dialogue groups will be formed. These dialogue groups, constituted of adolescents with CP, families, health professionals and researchers will continue co-designing and co-working in relation to their own needs and to have a voice in the community, increasing the visibility of these young people and their families in society, as well as their engagement in research.

The advisor, co-thinker and the researcher will select the most relevant results to be disseminated related to their interest and to give more support to adolescents who share the same condition (CP). The information will be analyzed and organized through the partners and decision-makers to be published in different ways: papers, websites, congresses. The results of semi-structured interviews, open questions and experience of the use of the involvement matrix and their role in the co-design will be disseminated according to their roles (partners and decision-makers). Adolescents with CP and their families will create dialogue groups to give support to the public with the same characteristics.

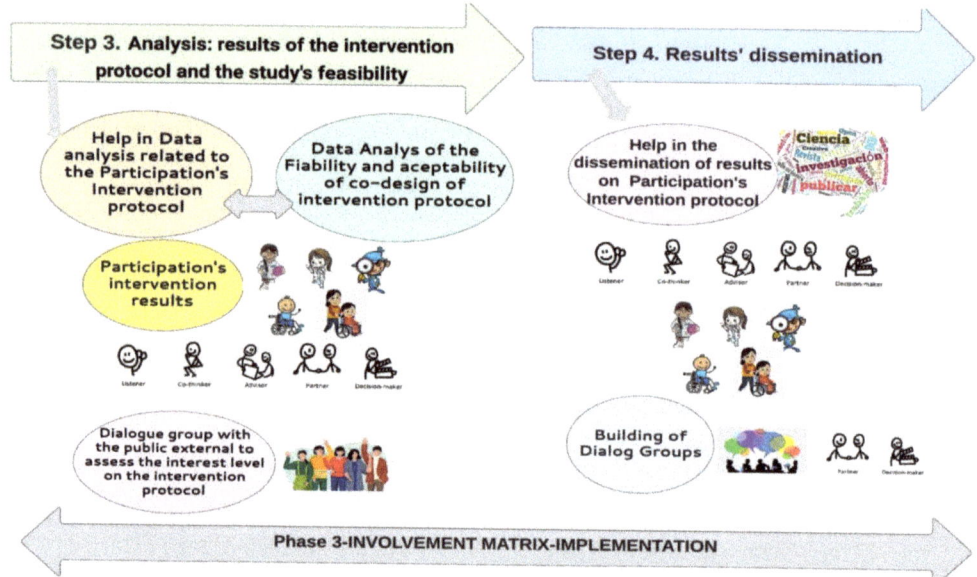

Figure 6. Steps 3 and 4 of project's research in phase 3 of Involvement Matrix: IMPLEMENTATION.

Coordination Brazil–Spain to Analyze the Data and Interpretation of Results from the Research Project

For the execution of both projects in Brazil and Spain, continuous coordination will be carried out between the responsible researchers on a weekly basis. For this, points of reflection will be established on which were the chosen roles, how the participants are involved in the meetings, structuring the meetings so that the same concepts can be addressed and can also be adjusted to the needs of the participants involved in each project. A comparison of the profiles that collaborate in the co-design is created in order to have information when interpreting the data and to see whether, therefore, personal characteristics can influence the planning, adherence and design of the protocol.

At the end of the project, the barriers encountered by the participants from Brazil and those from Spain will be compared. What were ingredients introduced to encourage community participation of adolescents for each country? Were there similarities in the choice? How was the implementation developed in each country.

4. Time Line

The study commenced in October 2022 with the first two tasks included in Figure 4, of Step 1 of Phase 1. An action schedule summarized in Table 3 is planned.

Table 3. Anticipated time line of the project.

		Oct–Dec 2022	Jan–Mar 2023	Apr–Jun 2023	Jul–Sep 2023	Oct–Dec 2023	Jan–Mar 2024
Phase 1. Step 1		X	X				
Phase 2. Step 2				X	X		
Phase 3	Step 3					X	
	Step 4						X

X: Execution time of the phase/step corresponding to the research project.

5. Discussion and Perspectives

The purpose of this paper is to present a protocol involving adolescents with CP, GMFCS levels IV–V, their families and health professionals. The aim is to co-design a preliminary protocol about the ingredients that should be included in the intervention to improve the participation of these adolescents in the community, considering various perspectives. Public and patient perspectives can be sought through their involvement and through participating in interviews or focus groups to provide data for others to analyze, interpret and act on [37].

PPI offers a methodology where researchers are in a continuous and reciprocal relationship with participants and make decisions with them about the research. The research is carried out with them and therefore satisfies their wishes, favoring its implementation in the population that shares the same condition [37,38]. This interaction can better ensure that research incorporates the participants' voices including their priorities and preferences [39].

Researchers should involve the public and patients and to plan potential roles, responsibilities and tasks for their study as early as possible [39]. Therefore, the IM is a very useful tool that allows the participation of the public from an early stage in the design of the research project. In addition, it offers the possibility of choosing the role with which they want to get involved in the different stages of the design, creating learning opportunities for all participants according to their interest. It offers the opportunity to create an orderly and coordinated work together with the researcher and the participants to promote the co-design of the research [17,39].

The design of a preliminary intervention protocol that encourages the participation in leisure activities of adolescents with a chronic condition within the community will allow professionals and families from Brazil and Spain to consider their lived experiences. Using this study, it could be possible to guide the intervention based on their real needs, motivations and interests. The implementation in both countries will allow a comparison of the differences and similarities between both preliminary intervention protocols designed, the needs of some adolescents with CP regarding participation in the community, what were the roles chosen by all the participants, the relationships and dialogues established in the different dialogue groups created and the results obtained regarding the co-design of the intervention protocol and their own perspectives on the use of the IM [14,40,41].

The ultimate goal of an intervention should be to increase patient participation, but based on their own interests, hence the need to give them a voice. Considering that the study population has several factors present (communication problems, mobility, etc.) that limit their ability to be heard, it will allow them to feel motivated by entering the co-design of the research and will encourage their families and the health professionals to consider their needs. In addition, their active participation in disseminating the results will make it possible for the designed intervention protocol to be accepted by other young people with CP GMFCS IV and V and to create dialogue groups that give this group a "voice", making it possible to improve life conditions. In order to increase the participation in most of adolescents with CP levels GMFCS IV–V, with profound intellectual disability (IQ < 25), or with communication impairments, we will facilitate their inclusion in research through different strategies through the results in this preliminary pilot study. The adolescents with severe disabilities will be able to watch images of the ingredients of the leisure activities chosen by the participants in this pilot study and videos of the adolescents performing the activities in the community, and we will record the behavior and reaction to these stimuli: facial and body response of motivation, rejection, etc., which will indicate their satisfaction or not with the activities. In addition, information will be collected with the help of their families in order to know their tastes regarding different leisure activities in the community and, therefore, to be able to co-design a program of ingredients of leisure activities that would increase their participation in the community.

As perspectives that will be obtained after this research project based on the PPI, the following topics could be included:

- What is the current participation of young people of adolescents with CP within the community like?
- Detection of barriers present in the community;
- Facilitators that increase participation: Improvements in access, adaptations and resources for participation according to the needs of young people with CP;
- Places within the community where the participation of young people with CP is encouraged (schools, leisure places, home, etc.);
- Role that the family and health professionals should have in the implementation of leisure activities within the community to encourage the participation of young people;
- Usefulness of the involvement of the PPI in the co-design of the intervention program to encourage the participation of young people with CP (GMFCS IV-V) within the community;
- Feasibility of co-designing the intervention protocol to encourage the participation of young people with CP (GMFCS IV-V) within the community;
- What should an intervention protocol to improve participation for adolescents GMFCS IV–V be like?

Supplementary Materials: The following supporting information can be downloaded at: https://www.mdpi.com/article/10.3390/jcm12010182/s1, Figure S1: Open questions for participants.

Author Contributions: Conceptualization, R.P.-C., C.C.D.A.F.J., C.A.S.S., R.L., R.A., H.R.-B., E.C.-G., K.S.M., E.P.-P. and E.L.; methodology, R.P.-C., C.C.D.A.F.J., C.A.S.S., K.S.M. and E.L.; writing—original draft preparation, R.P.-C., C.C.D.A.F.J. and E.L.; writing—review and editing, R.P.-C., C.C.D.A.F.J., C.A.S.S., R.L., R.A., H.R.-B., E.C.-G., K.S.M., E.P.-P. and E.L. All authors have read and agreed to the published version of the manuscript.

Funding: This research was funded by Coordenação de Aperfeiçoamento de Pessoal de Nível Superior—(CAPES). Graduate Program in Rehabilitation Sciences. Federal University of Rio Grande do Norte—Faculty of Health Sciences of Trairi (UFRN-FACISA), Brazil, grant number 001.

Institutional Review Board Statement: The study was conducted according to the guidelines of the Declaration of Helsinki and approved by the Ethics Committee of FIDMAG in Brazil (CAAE: 51319321.1.0000.5568) and Hermanas Hospitalarias in Spain (PR-2022-07).

Informed Consent Statement: Not applicable.

Acknowledgments: We would like to thank Marjolijn Ketelaar (author and developer of the Involvement Matrix tool (IM)) for her great help, continuous support and guidance in the process of executing the research protocol.

Conflicts of Interest: The authors declare no conflict of interest.

References

1. Sadowska, M.; Sarecka-Hujar, B.; Kopyta, I. Cerebral Palsy: Current Opinions on Definition, Epidemiology, Risk Factors, Classification and Treatment Options. *Neuropsychiatr. Dis. Treat.* **2020**, *16*, 1505–1518. [CrossRef] [PubMed]
2. Rosenbaum, P.; Paneth, N.; Leviton, A.; Goldstein, M.; Bax, M.; Damiano, D.; Dan, B.; Jacobsson, B. A report: The definition and classification of cerebral palsy April 2006. *Dev. Med. Child Neurol. Suppl.* **2007**, *109*, 8–14. [PubMed]
3. Weber, P.; Bolli, P.; Heimgartner, N.; Merlo, P.; Zehnder, T.; Kätterer, C. Behavioral and emotional problems in children and adults with cerebral palsy. *Eur. J. Paediatr. Neurol.* **2016**, *20*, 270–274. [CrossRef] [PubMed]
4. King, G.; Lawm, M.; King, S.; Rosenbaum, P.; Kertoy, M.K.; Young, N.L. A Conceptual Model of the Factors Affecting the Recreation and Leisure Participation of Children with Disabilities. *Phys. Occup. Ther. Pediatr.* **2003**, *23*, 63–90. [CrossRef]
5. World Health Organization (WHO). *International Classification of Functioning, Disability and Health*; World Health Organization (WHO): Genova, Switzerland, 2001; ISBN 9241545429.
6. Imms, C.; Granlund, M.; Wilson, P.H.; Steenbergen, B.; Rosenbaum, P.L.; Gordon, A.M. Participation, both a means and an end: A conceptual analysis of processes and outcomes in childhood disability. *Dev. Med. Child Neurol.* **2017**, *59*, 16–25. [CrossRef] [PubMed]
7. Shields, N.; Synnot, A. Perceived barriers and facilitators to participation in physical activity for children with disability: A qualitative study. *BMC Pediatr.* **2016**, *16*, 9. [CrossRef] [PubMed]

8. Sienko, S. Understanding the factors that impact the participation in physical activity and recreation in young adults with cerebral palsy (CP). *Disabil. Health J.* **2019**, *12*, 467–472. [CrossRef]
9. Engel-Yeger, B.; Jarus, T.; Anaby, D.; Law, M. Differences in Patterns of Participation Between Youths With Cerebral Palsy and Typically Developing Peers. *Am. J. Occup. Ther.* **2009**, *63*, 96–104. [CrossRef] [PubMed]
10. Rožkalne, Z.; Mukāns, M.; Vētra, A. Transition-Age Young Adults with Cerebral Palsy: Level of Participation and the Influencing Factors. *Medicina* **2019**, *55*, 737. [CrossRef] [PubMed]
11. Boyd, H.; McKernon, S.; Mullin, B.; Old, A. Improving healthcare through the use of co-design. *N. Z. Med. J.* **2012**, *125*, 76–87.
12. Harrison, J.D.; Auerbach, A.D.; Anderson, W.; Fagan, M.; Carnie, M.; Hanson, C.; Banta, J.; Symczak, G.; Robinson, E.; Schnipper, J.; et al. Patient stakeholder engagement in research: A narrative review to describe foundational principles and best practice activities. *Health Expect.* **2019**, *22*, 307–316. [CrossRef] [PubMed]
13. Bailey, S.; Boddy, K.; Briscoe, S.; Morris, C. Involving disabled children and young people as partners in research: A systematic review. *Child. Care. Health Dev.* **2015**, *41*, 505–514. [CrossRef] [PubMed]
14. Van Schelven, F.; Van Der Meulen, E.; Kroeze, N.; Ketelaar, M.; Boeije, H. Patient and public involvement of young people with a chronic condition: Lessons learned and practical tips from a large participatory program. *Res. Involv. Engagem.* **2020**, *6*, 59. [CrossRef]
15. Involvement Matrix. Available online: https://www.kcrutrecht.nl/involvement-matrix/ (accessed on 10 November 2022).
16. Hoddinott, P.; Pollock, A.; O'cathain, A.; Boyer, I.; Taylor, J.; Macdonald, C.; Oliver, S.; Donovan, J.L. How to incorporate patient and public perspectives into the design and conduct of research [version 1; peer review: 3 approved, 2 approved with reservations]. *F1000Research* **2018**, *7*, 752. [CrossRef] [PubMed]
17. Smits, D.W.; Van Meeteren, K.; Klem, M.; Alsem, M.; Ketelaar, M. Designing a tool to support patient and public involvement in research projects: The Involvement Matrix. *Res. Involv. Engagem.* **2020**, *6*, 30. [CrossRef] [PubMed]
18. Morris, C.; Shilling, V.; Mchugh, C.; Wyatt, K. Why it is crucial to involve families in all stages of childhood disability research. *Dev. Med. Child Neurol.* **2011**, *53*, 769–771. [CrossRef] [PubMed]
19. Kirwan, J.R.; de Wit, M.; Frank, L.; Haywood, K.L.; Salek, S.; Brace-McDonnell, S.; Lyddiatt, A.; Barbic, S.P.; Alonso, J.; Guillemin, F.; et al. Emerging Guidelines for Patient Engagement in Research. *Value Health* **2017**, *20*, 481–486. [CrossRef] [PubMed]
20. Damschroder, L.J.; Aron, D.C.; Keith, R.E.; Kirsh, S.R.; Alexander, J.A.; Lowery, J.C. Fostering implementation of health services research findings into practice: A consolidated framework for advancing implementation science. *Implement. Sci.* **2009**, *4*, 50. [CrossRef]
21. Greenhalgh, T.; Hinton, L.; Finlay, T.; Macfarlane, A.; Fahy, N.; Clyde, B.; Chant, A. Frameworks for supporting patient and public involvement in research: Systematic review and co-design pilot. *Health Expect.* **2019**, *22*, 785–801. [CrossRef]
22. Smith, E.; Bélisle-Pipon, J.-C.; Resnik, D. Patients as research partners; how to value their perceptions, contribution and labor? *Citiz. Sci. Theory Pract.* **2019**, *4*, 15. [CrossRef] [PubMed]
23. McDermott, L.; Yardley, L.; Little, P.; Ashworth, M.; Gulliford, M. Developing a computer delivered, theory based intervention for guideline implementation in general practice. *BMC Fam. Pract.* **2010**, *11*, 90. [CrossRef] [PubMed]
24. Wintels, S.C.; Smits, D.W.; van Wesel, F.; Verheijden, J.; Ketelaar, M.; van der Leest, A.; de Groot, C.; Snel, D.; van de Water, J.; Sluiter, L.; et al. How do adolescents with cerebral palsy participate? Learning from their personal experiences. *Health Expect.* **2018**, *21*, 1024. [CrossRef] [PubMed]
25. Cusack, C.; Cohen, B.; Mignone, J.; Chartier, M.J.; Lutfiyya, Z. Participatory action as a research method with public health nurses. *J. Adv. Nurs.* **2018**, *74*, 1544–1553. [CrossRef] [PubMed]
26. Baum, F.; MacDougall, C.; Smith, D. Participatory action research. *J. Epidemiol. Community Health* **2006**, *60*, 854. [CrossRef] [PubMed]
27. Tremblay, M.C.; Bradette-Laplante, M.; Bérubé, D.; Brière, É.; Moisan, J.; Niquay, D.; Dogba, M.J.; Légaré, F.; McComber, A.; McGavock, J.; et al. Engaging indigenous patient partners in patient-oriented research: Lessons from a one-year initiative. *Res. Involv. Engagem.* **2020**, *6*, 44. [CrossRef] [PubMed]
28. Brooks, R.; Lambert, C.; Coulthard, L.; Pennington, L.; Kolehmainen, N. Social participation to support good mental health in neurodisability. *Child. Care. Health Dev.* **2021**, *47*, 675–684. [CrossRef]
29. Coster, W.; Law, M.; Bedell, G.; Khetani, M.; Cousins, M.; Teplicky, R. Development of the participation and environment measure for children and youth: Conceptual basis. *Disabil. Rehabil.* **2012**, *34*, 238–246. [CrossRef]
30. Coster, W.; Bedell, G.; Law, M.; Khetani, M.A.; Teplicky, R.; Liljenquist, K.; Gleason, K.; Kao, Y.C. Psychometric evaluation of the Participation and Environment Measure for Children and Youth. *Dev. Med. Child Neurol.* **2011**, *53*, 1030–1037. [CrossRef]
31. Waisman-Nitzan, M.; Ivzori, Y.; Anaby, D. Implementing Pathways and Resources for Engagement and Participation (PREP) for Children with Disabilities in Inclusive Schools: A Knowledge Translation Strategy. *Phys. Occup. Ther. Pediatr.* **2022**, *42*, 526–541. [CrossRef]
32. Anaby, D.R.; Law, M.; Feldman, D.; Majnemer, A.; Avery, L. The effectiveness of the Pathways and Resources for Engagement and Participation (PREP) intervention: Improving participation of adolescents with physical disabilities. *Dev. Med. Child Neurol.* **2018**, *60*, 513–519. [CrossRef]
33. Law, M.; Anaby, D.; Teplicky, R.; Turner, L. *Pathways and Resources for Engagement and Participation, a Practice Model for Occupational Therapists*; CanChild: Hamilton, ON, Canada, 2016.
34. IBM Corp. *Released 2021. IBM SPSS Statistics for Windows*, Version 28.0; IBM Corp: Armonk, NY, USA.
35. Braun, V.; Clarke, V. Using thematic analysis in psychology. *Qual. Res. Psychol.* **2006**, *3*, 77–101. [CrossRef]

36. Zamawe, F.C. The Implication of Using NVivo Software in Qualitative Data Analysis: Evidence-Based Reflections. *Malawi Med. J.* **2015**, *27*, 13–15. [CrossRef] [PubMed]
37. Harrison, J.D.; Anderson, W.G.; Fagan, M.; Robinson, E.; Schnipper, J.; Symczak, G.; Hanson, C.; Carnie, M.B.; Banta, J.; Chen, S.; et al. Patient and Family Advisory Councils (PFACs): Identifying Challenges and Solutions to Support Engagement in Research. *Patient* **2018**, *11*, 413–423. [CrossRef] [PubMed]
38. Frank, L.; Forsythe, L.; Ellis, L.; Schrandt, S.; Sheridan, S.; Gerson, J.; Konopka, K.; Daugherty, S. Conceptual and practical foundations of patient engagement in research at the patient-centered outcomes research institute. *Qual. Life Res.* **2015**, *24*, 1033–1041. [CrossRef] [PubMed]
39. Marlett, N.; Shklarov, S.; Marshall, D.; Santana, M.J.; Wasylak, T. Building new roles and relationships in research: A model of patient engagement research. *Qual. Life Res.* **2015**, *24*, 1057–1067. [CrossRef] [PubMed]
40. Hersh, D.; Israel, M.; Shiggins, C. The ethics of patient and public involvement across the research process: Towards partnership with people with aphasia. *Aphasiology* **2021**, 1–27. [CrossRef]
41. Dada, S.; May, A.; Bastable, K.; Samuels, A.; Tönsing, K.; Wilder, J.; Casey, M.; Ntuli, C.; Reddy, V. The involvement matrix as a framework for involving youth with severe communication disabilities in developing health education materials. *Health Expect.* **2022**, *25*, 1004–1015. [CrossRef]

Disclaimer/Publisher's Note: The statements, opinions and data contained in all publications are solely those of the individual author(s) and contributor(s) and not of MDPI and/or the editor(s). MDPI and/or the editor(s) disclaim responsibility for any injury to people or property resulting from any ideas, methods, instructions or products referred to in the content.

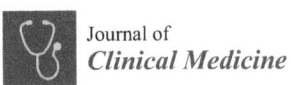

Article

Examining the Role of Sublingual Atropine for the Treatment of Sialorrhea in Patients with Neurodevelopmental Disabilities: A Retrospective Review

Kayla Durkin Petkus [1,2,*], Garey Noritz [1] and Laurie Glader [1]

[1] Division of Complex Care, Nationwide Children's Hospital, Columbus, OH 43205, USA; garey.noritz@nationwidechildrens.org (G.N.); laurie.glader@nationwidechildrens.org (L.G.)
[2] Department of Pharmacy, Nationwide Children's Hospital, Columbus, OH 43205, USA
* Correspondence: kayla.petkus@nationwidechildrens.org

Abstract: Sialorrhea is common in children with neurodevelopmental disabilities (NDD) and is reported in >40% of children with cerebral palsy (CP). It causes a range of complications, including significant respiratory morbidity. This single-center retrospective chart review aims to document sublingual atropine (SLA) utilization to guide further study in establishing its role in secretion management for children with NDD. A chart review was completed for patients with NDD ≤ 22 years of age treated with SLA at a free-standing children's hospital between 1 January 2016 and 1 June 2021. Descriptive statistics were generated to summarize findings. In total, 190 patients were identified, of which 178 met inclusion criteria. The average starting dose for SLA was 1.5 mg/day, or 0.09 mg/kg/day when adjusted for patient weight. Eighty-nine (50%) patients were prescribed SLA first line for secretion management while 85 (48%) patients tried glycopyrrolate prior to SLA. SLA was used after salivary Botox, ablation, and/or surgery in 16 (9%) patients. This study investigates SLA as a potential pharmacologic agent to treat sialorrhea in children with NDD. We identify a range of prescribing patterns regarding dosing, schedule, and place in therapy, highlighting the need for further evidence to support and guide its safe and efficacious use.

Keywords: atropine; cerebral palsy; sialorrhea; pediatric; drooling; sublingual; developmental disorders; neurodevelopmental disorders

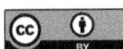

1. Introduction

Sialorrhea, or excessive drooling, is a common problem for children with neurodevelopmental disabilities (NDD), particularly those with motor disabilities. Prevalence among children with cerebral palsy (CP), the most common motor NDD, is over 40% [1]. The term CP describes "a group of permanent disorders of the development of movement and posture, causing activity limitation, that are attributed to nonprogressive disturbances that occurred in the developing fetal or infant brain. The motor disorders of cerebral palsy are often accompanied by disturbances of sensation, perception, cognition, communication, and behavior, by epilepsy, and by secondary musculoskeletal problems [2]." In the US, the prevalence of CP is estimated between 1.5 and 4 per 1000 live births [3]. Other childhood motor disabilities in which sialorrhea is common include the muscular dystrophies, spinal muscular atrophy, sequelae of traumatic brain injury, and neurodegenerative conditions such as Rett syndrome and the leukodystrophies. Children with craniofacial abnormalities, airway abnormalities, or tracheostomies may also have significant sialorrhea. Finally, drooling is a common symptom amongst people with intellectual disability disorder, and it is a reasonably common side effect of medication commonly used in children with neurologic disorders, including benzodiazepines and atypical neuroleptics.

Sialorrhea can manifest anteriorly, as spillage of saliva over the lips, or posteriorly, with pooling of secretions in the oropharynx. Anterior sialorrhea tends to be associated with skin breakdown and irritation, odor, and can impact social relationships and self-esteem. Posterior sialorrhea can have serious medical sequelae, such as difficulty with airway clearance, chronic aspiration, and recurrent pneumonia [4]. Pulmonary issues are a leading cause of morbidity in children with complex medical conditions, accounting for 29% of hospitalizations in the population [5–7]. Respiratory disease is also the most common cause of death for both children and adults with CP, underscoring the importance of providing effective interventions, such as sialorrhea reduction, to curb pulmonary complications [8,9].

Both anterior and posterior sialorrhea affect the health and quality of life of children and their families. As such, numerous strategies were developed in an effort to reduce symptoms. Common approaches to management range from least to most invasive. These typically include behavioral interventions, pharmacologic treatments, targeted salivary gland injections with botulinum toxin, and finally, surgeries, which include salivary duct ligation, re-routing, or gland excision [10]. Ultrasound-guided salivary gland ablation using ethanol is an emerging intervention [11]. Treatment appears to be effective with all agents, but studies are heterogeneous, with generally low-level evidence and inconsistency in outcome measures [10–15].

Behavioral treatments for sialorrhea are based on principles of behavior modification and include reinforcement, prompting, self-management, extinction, overcorrection, instruction, and fading. These are discussed in a recent systematic review, which concluded that "Low-level evidence suggests behavioural interventions may be useful for treatment of drooling in children with neurodisability [15]".

Among pharmacologic agents used to treat sialorrhea, anticholinergics are the most common. Glycopyrrolate, scopolamine, trihexyphenidyl, and benztropine are the most studied agents [10,16–21]. More recently, sublingually administered atropine (SLA) appeared in the literature [22]. As a newer agent to be utilized in this context, atropine's recommended dosing and place in treatment is still being established.

Atropine competitively blocks acetylcholine from binding to muscarinic receptors in the central nervous system, smooth muscle, and secretory glands. Submucosal glands are innervated by parasympathetic neurons and predominantly have M1 and M3 muscarinic receptors. Activation of these receptors by acetyl choline is blocked by atropine, inhibiting secretions from the nose, mouth, pharynx, and bronchi. Ultimately, this leads to drying of the mucus membranes in these areas [23,24].

Injectable forms (intramuscular (IM), intravenous (IV), and subcutaneous (SubQ)) of atropine have an approved indication to inhibit salivation and secretions in the preoperative/intraoperative setting. Recommended dosing for inhibition of salivation in infants, children, and adolescents is 0.02 mg/kg/dose administered IM, IV, or SubQ. Doses may be repeated every 4 to 6 h as needed for secretions. The maximum total dose for infants and children less than 12 years of age is 1 mg per procedure, while the maximum total dose for children greater than or equal to 12 years of age is 2 mg per procedure [25].

A study completed by Volz-Zang and colleagues assessed how oral versus intramuscular administration of atropine affected the heart rate and salivary flow in seven healthy adults. They found that a 0.03 mg/kg dose of atropine administered orally demonstrated an 84.3% maximum reduction in salivary flow. The orally administered dose did not cause a significant increase in heart rate, especially when compared to intramuscular administration of the medication. They attributed their findings to low absorption of the oral dose and to lower vagal tone in the salivary glands compared to the heart [26]. Schwartz et al. additionally demonstrated systemic bioavailability of SLA at 60%, which is achieved via an intravenous route in healthy adults [27]. Whether there is a direct local effect on the salivary glands remains unclear. Available studies suggest a more limited side effect profile for SLA compared to alternative agents, such as glycopyrrolate and scopolamine, which have well-documented potential effects of constipation, urinary retention, and behavioral changes, among others [28–31]. The reduced systemic absorption, the report to date of minimal adverse effects, and the rapidity of a drying effect from the sublingual administration of atropine make it an attractive option for treating children with sialorrhea.

Most reports of using SLA in the literature are in palliative settings for adults, case reports involving pediatric patients, or for the treatment of pharmacologically induced sialorrhea [32–34]. In a pediatric case report, dosing of SLA for sialorrhea was reported as atropine 0.5% ophthalmic drop, given as one drop (0.25 mg) sublingually every six hours as needed. Based on the need for suctioning, it was estimated that the onset of action was between 15 and 30 min and the duration of action was approximately 4 h [33].

Two prospective studies evaluated efficacy in pediatric patients with NDD [30,31]. Dias et al. performed an uncontrolled open clinical trial of 33 children with cerebral palsy, 25 of whom completed the study. Significant reduction in drooling was reported as reflected in the validated parent reported Drooling Impact Scale across all but two variables [30,35]. Norderyd et al. evaluated 19 children in a prospective single system design where participants served as their own controls, 11 of whom completed the study. Significant reduction in drooling was measured using the Visual Analogue Scale, another parent reported instrument [31]. Both studies found tolerable adverse effects [30,31]. Dias' study identified fever and flushing (1), irritability (1), flushing and irritability (1), and flushing and angioedema (1) in 4 of 33 patients [30]. Norderyd reported that excessive dry mouth occurred most frequently (7), followed by difficulty with voiding, constipation, and behavioral changes (3 in each case). All side effects disappeared with cessation of treatment [31]. Azapagasi et al. conducted a retrospective chart review of 25 hospitalized children receiving SLA for 7 days, 20 of whom had outcome data available. Significant reduction in the Teacher Drooling Scale, a 5-point reporting scale, was reported over a two-day period ($p < 0.001$). Side effects were not reported [36].

The literature for SLA is thus sparse and the evidence is generally of a low level. Although it paints an optimistic view of the potential for SLA to be used in the treatment of sialorrhea in children and young adults with NDD, further study is clearly warranted. The current study was undertaken to describe use of SLA, including dosing regimens and place in therapy, in an effort to glean patterns of real-world use and to inform potential dosing regimens for prospective study.

2. Materials and Methods

This study is a retrospective electronic chart review evaluating SLA use for sialorrhea within a free-standing children's hospital. Data were extracted from our electronic health record for patients who received an outpatient prescription order for atropine 1% ophthalmic solution, atropine 0.5% ophthalmic solution, and/or atropine 0.5% oral solution (compounded at our institution once the 0.5% ophthalmic solution was discontinued by manufacturers in 2014) for sublingual administration between 1 January 2016 and 1 June 2021. Patients with NDD of childhood, an umbrella term for conditions associated with neurologic impairment that impacts physical, cognitive, linguistic, and behavioral development and function, were eligible. Inclusion criteria included being 22 years of age or younger at therapy initiation and being treated with SLA either alone or in conjunction with other anti-cholinergic therapies for secretion management. Exclusion criteria included use of SLA for other indications, absence of NDD, age > 22 years at treatment initiation, incomplete data, and/or patients with protected chart information.

Patient information including date of birth, sex, and unifying diagnosis was collected to describe our population. For the first and last SLA prescription listed in the patient's chart, date of prescription, patient dosing weight, medication, dose, and frequency were collected. Doses were calculated based on product concentration and assuming the established criteria that 20 drops is equal to one milliliter of clear solution [37]. For daily dose and weight-based dose calculations, all "as needed" doses were considered to be given as scheduled, and doses were rounded to the maximum dose if a dosing range was given. Additional analysis was completed to assess if dosing differed depending on the patient's age at the start of therapy (<1 year, 1–<3 year, 3–<12 year, and ≥12 year) to incorporate common age cut offs for dosing of another anticholinergic agent, glycopyrrolate, in other studies.

A manual chart review of all medication history was performed to identify whether the patient previously received alternative anticholinergic therapies for the treatment of sialorrhea (i.e., glycopyrrolate, scopolamine, trihexyphenidyl, and/or benztropine). Timing of when these agents were utilized for secretion management in relation to SLA therapy was assessed. A manual chart review was also completed to evaluate prior administration of salivary gland botulinum toxin injection, salivary gland surgery, and/or salivary gland ablation.

Descriptive statistics were generated to summarize our findings. Data are presented as means, ranges, and percentages. A two-tailed paired *t*-test was completed to assess significance of change from starting to final dose. This study was approved by the Institutional Review of Nationwide Children's Hospital and a waiver of consent was granted.

3. Results

On initial chart review, 190 eligible patients were prescribed SLA for the treatment of sialorrhea. Seven patients were excluded due to missing or incomplete chart data, 3 patients were removed due to protected chart information, and 2 were removed due to the absence of a neurodevelopmental diagnosis. The remaining 178 patients were included in the analysis. Patient demographic information is included in Table 1. The average age at initiation of atropine was 7.8 years, and 96 patients were male (54%). Ninety-eight patients (55%) had a confirmed diagnosis of cerebral palsy (CP). It is quite possible that children with some of the diagnoses listed, such as brain injury or genetic disorder, met criteria for a diagnosis of CP but did not carry the diagnosis in their chart, resulting in an underestimate of this subpopulation. Almost half of the initial prescriptions ($n = 88$, 49.4%) were generated through the pulmonary service. Fifty-five prescriptions (30.9%) were written by the complex care division, which cares for children with medical complexity. The remaining prescriptions were written by various subspecialties, including neonatal services, neurology, acute care, physical medicine, aero-digestive, palliative care, and otorhinolaryngology, or at discharge from the general pediatric hospital service.

Table 1. Demographic information.

	Total $n = 178$ n (%)
Age in years at initiation of atropine	
Average (range)	7.8 (2 months–22 years)
<1 year	21 (11.8%)
1–<3 years	26 (14.6%)
3–<12 years	80 (44.9%)
>12 years	51 (28.7%)
Gender	
Male	96 (54%)
Female	82 (46%)
Underlying Diagnosis	
Cerebral Palsy	98 (55.1%)
Genetic/syndromic disorder	35 (19.7%)
Neuromuscular disease	17 (9.6%)
Neurodegenerative condition	11 (6.2%)
Brain injury	5 (2.8%)
Developmental disorder	4 (2.2%)
Multiple congenital anomalies	4 (2.2%)
Unknown/other	4 (2.2%)

Dose and dosing frequency of SLA ranged greatly among patients [Table 2]. Doses ranged from 1 to 3 drops given at a time, and frequency ranged from every 4 to every 24 h, often accompanied by indications of "may increase up to X" for both dosing and scheduling. The most common starting frequency was written as twice daily ($n = 63$, 35.4%)

and approximately one-third of the prescriptions were written for "as needed" (PRN) dosing. Final dosing strategies were also quite varied and open to adjustment.

Table 2. SLA dosing by drop.

	Initial n = 178 n (%)	Final n = 178 n (%)
Drops per dose		
Atropine 0.5%		
1 drop	9 (5%)	0 (0%)
2 drop	6 (3.4%)	1 (0.56%)
Atropine 1%		
1 drop	125 (70.2%)	126 (70.8%)
2 drop	36 (20.2%)	47 (26.4%)
3 drop	2 (1.12%)	3 (1.7%)
4 drop	0 (0%)	1 (0.56%)
Frequency of dosing		
QDay	44 (24.7%)	37 (20.8%)
BID	63 (35.4%)	60 (33.7%)
TID	38 (21.3%)	42 (23.6%)
4 times daily	19 (10.7%)	25 (14%)
6 times daily	14 (7.9%)	14 (7.9%)
Total drops per day		
Atropine 0.5%		
1 drop	2 (1.1%)	0 (0%)
2 drop	3 (1.337%)	0 (0%)
3 drop	1 (0.56%)	0 (0%)
4 drop	1 (0.56%)	1 (0.56%)
6 drop	5 (2.8%)	0 (0%)
12 drop	3 (1.7%)	0 (0%)
Atropine 1%		
1 drop	36 (20.2%)	31 (17.4%)
2 drop	51 (28.7%)	48 (27%)
3 drop	24 (13.5%)	28 (15.7%)
4 drop	25 (14%)	31 (17.4%)
6 drop	17 (9.6%)	21 (11.8%)
8 drop	7 (3.9%)	10 (5.6%)
9 drop	1 (0.56%)	1 (0.56%)
12 drop	2 (1.1%)	7 (3.9%)
Rx written as PRN	66 (37%)	79 (44.4%)

Abbreviations: QDay, once daily; BID, twice daily; TID, three times daily; and Rx, prescription.

The most common starting dose was atropine 1% drops, 2 total drops per day, regardless of age or weight at the start of therapy, and ranged up to 12 drops per day. Dosing by drop was converted to mg/day as well as mg/kg/day to allow for analysis of weight-based treatment strategies and for direct comparison to results of prior studies. It is important to note that prescriptions were not written in a weight-based manner, but rather reflected the practicality of using doses standardized by common concentration and drop volume. The difference between average starting and final mg/day was significantly different (1.5 mg vs. 1.8 mg, $p \leq 0.001$), but when adjusted for patient weight, there was no significant difference based on mg/kg/day ($p = 0.635$). Upon examining the variance in mg/kg dosing between initial and final prescriptions for SLA, 128 patients (72%) had no change in dose, while 40 patients (22%) had an increase in dose. By comparison, mg/kg dosing remained consistent.

Initial and final sublingual atropine dosing, expressed as drops, are presented in this table and resemble the "real life" approach to dosing this medication. Please note that all doses provided as ranges were rounded up for the purpose of analysis.

We found that SLA dosing for sialorrhea management in this population was quite variable. For ease of analysis, a side-by-side table is provided [Table 3] to allow for comparison of prescribing patterns in this study with the three studies previously mentioned [30,31,36].

Table 3. Comparison of available data. "Side-by-side" comparison of patient populations, products used, directions for use, and dosing data found in our study versus that available in the literature. Some calculations were completed to extrapolate directions/doses from their original form to ease comparison.

Study	Our Study	Dias et al. [30]	Norderyd et al. [31]	Azapagasi et al. [36]
Population	≤22 years with NDD (n = 178)	2-17 years with CP (n = 25)	5–18 years with disabilities (final study group n = 11)	PICU patients 3–78 months (n = 20, of whom 19/20 had a NDD)
Product	atropine 0.5% ophthalmic drop; atropine 1% ophthalmic drop; atropine 0.5% oral solution	atropine 0.5% ophthalmic drop	atropine 1% ophthalmic drop	atropine sulfate ampoule
Directions	Varied/retrospective observation, initial dosing	Give 1 drop SL TID at 6h intervals for patients 10–19 kg Give 2 drops SL TID at 6h intervals for patients ≥20 kg	After 3 weeks of no treatment, Give 1 drop QDay for 4 weeks followed by 1 drop BID for 4 weeks	0.02 mg/kg/dose 4-6 times daily for 7 days Minimum dose was 0.25 mg, Maximum dose was 0.03 mg/kg (per author)
Drops/dose	1–3 drops	10–19 kg: 1 drop ≥20 kg: 2 drop	1 drop	N/A
Frequency	QDay-6 times daily	TID	QDay-BID	4–6 times daily
mg/day	0.25–6 mg/day Average: 1.5 mg/day	10–19 kg: 0.75 mg/day * ≥20 kg: 1.5 mg/day *	0.5–1 mg/day †	1 mg/day ‡-range unknown
mg/kg/day	0.01–0.49 mg/kg/day Average: 0.091 mg/kg/day	10–19 kg: 0.04–0.075 mg/kg/day * ≥20 kg: ≤0.075 mg/kg/day *	NA	0.08–0.18 mg/kg/day §

* Calculations were made by extrapolating on the reported data to allow comparison in discussion with the primary author. † Calculation was made by extrapolating on the reported data to allow comparison. ‡ Dose based on reported 0.25 mg minimum dose given 4 times daily. § Dose based on giving 0.02 mg/kg/dose 4 times daily to 0.03 mg/kg/dose 6 times daily to determine minimum and maximum dosing strategies. Abbreviations: NDD, Neurodevelopmental Disability; CP, Cerebral Palsy; PICU, Pediatric Intensive Care Unit; SL, sublingual; TID, three times daily; h, hour; kg, kilogram, QDay, once daily; BID, twice daily.

When compared to other anticholinergic therapies used for sialorrhea, SLA was prescribed as a first or second line agent for the majority of patients in this study [Figure 1].

Eighty patients (44.9%) were on SLA in addition to at least one other anti-cholinergic therapy (atropine with glycopyrrolate, scopolamine, benztropine, and/or trihexyphenidyl) at some point during their course of treatment with atropine. Anticholinergic therapies trialed prior to atropine are summarized in Figure 2. Glycopyrrolate was used prior to SLA in 85 (47.8%) patients and scopolamine was used prior to atropine in 20 (11.2%).

Sixteen patients underwent more invasive therapies prior to the initiation of SLA. All patients who had medication data available in the chart (n = 13) trialed glycopyrrolate, while two patients trialed scopolamine in addition to glycopyrrolate prior to moving towards more invasive therapy options and, subsequently, onto SLA. Invasive treatments included: salivary gland ablation (n = 7 patients, 3.9%), submandibular salivary gland surgery (n = 4, 2.2%), botulinum toxin injection into the salivary glands (n = 3, 1.7%), salivary gland botulinum toxin followed by ablation (n = 1, 0.6%), and salivary gland surgery followed by ablation (n = 1, 0.6%).

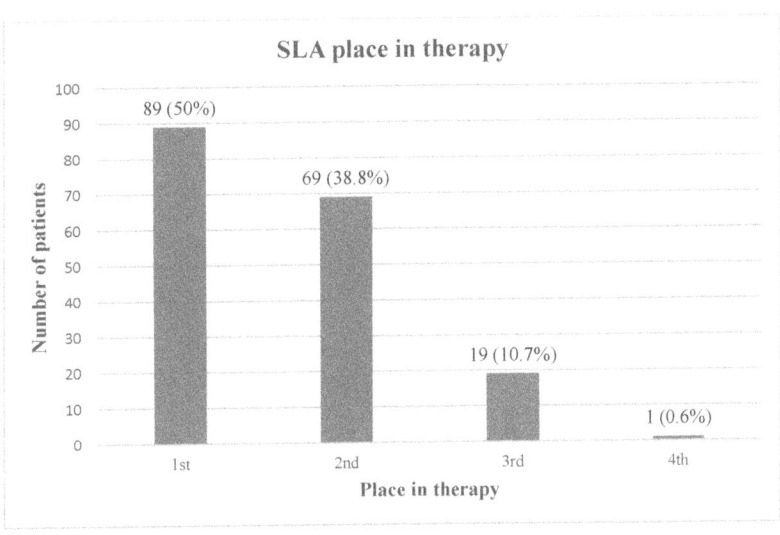

Figure 1. SLA place in therapy. SLA's place in therapy relative to alternative anticholinergic medications, including glycopyrrolate, scopolamine, benztropine, and trihexyphenidyl. Percentages do not total 100 due to rounding.

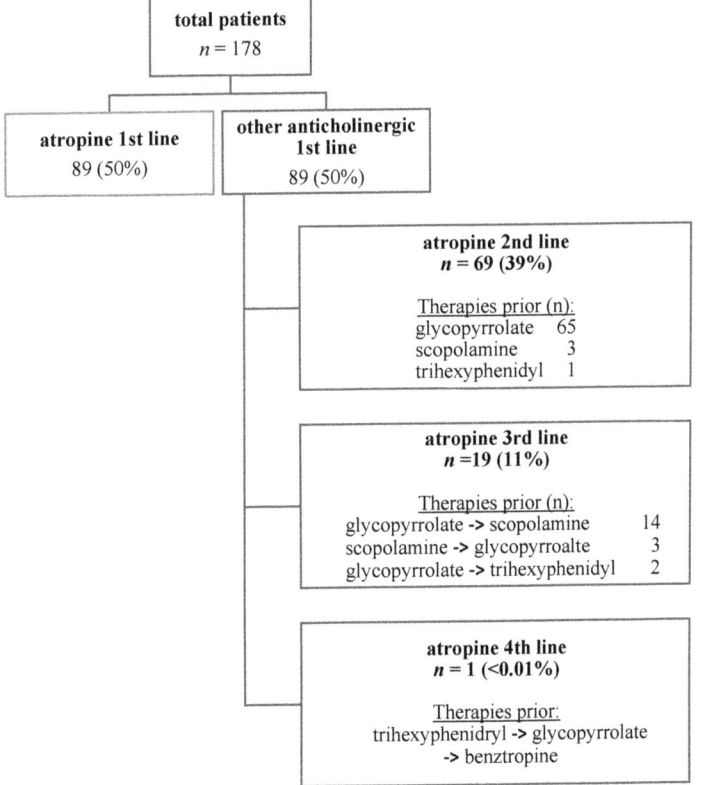

Figure 2. Pharmacologic sialorrhea treatment regimens in relation to SLA.

4. Discussion

This study presents a single institution's real-world practice in relation to already available literature in order to advance the breadth and depth of literature available regarding the use of SLA in the treatment of sialorrhea in children and young adults with NDD. Two previous prospective small cohort studies and one retrospective study suggest the potential efficacy of SLA for this purpose. Our study evaluated the current prescribing practice of SLA in children and young adults with NDD to understand the scope of need to establish prescribing guidance and safety profiles. We did not evaluate efficacy in drooling reduction, nor did we evaluate adverse events, as that information was not available through chart review in a standardized manner.

We found significant variability in actual practice among prescribers, and there was no institutional standardized dosing guidance. Initial doses ranged from one to three drops and frequencies ranged from as needed to six times daily. Although six times daily dosing was infrequent ($n = 14$, 7.9%), this same pattern was seen in the Azapagasi study [31]. The dosing range, in mg/day, documented in our study far exceeded that studied in the three previously mentioned cohorts [28,29,31]. However, our calculations assumed that all doses written for "as needed" were given at scheduled dosing intervals. Although this possibly falsely elevated upper limits of actual practice, the prescriptions were, importantly, written to allow for this possibility. Despite the wider range of dosing prescribed, most regimens were in keeping with the Dias and Norderyd studies [28,29]. More than 90% of regimens were written for 1–2 drops per dose of the atropine 1% solution (0.5 mg/drop), and >80% were written for up to TID dosing frequency. Overall, weight-based doses remained fairly stable from initial to final prescriptions, potentially reflecting the expected weight gain of growing children during the study period.

While it was not possible to assess for side effects in our study, those observed in other studies were reversible and of minimal impact [22,28,29]. Anticholinergic side effects, including urinary hesitancy or retention, constipation, flushing, and the desired effect of decreased saliva production, are the most commonly reported side effects from SLA in this setting. Some of the more serious potential side effects include arrhythmias, ataxia, and respiratory failure [20] and were not reported to date in this body of literature. The limited available data suggest that the dosing regimens explored thus far may be useful in defining a safe range for assessing efficacy and safety. Future studies will require monitoring for the full constellation of potential adverse effects.

Despite a lack of established safety or dosing guidance, SLA is a tool frequently used in the treatment of sialorrhea in children with NDD. At our institution, atropine was used as a first-line anti-cholinergic agent in patients 50% of the time, and second to other anticholinergic treatments 50% of the time, generally after glycopyrrolate, which is the only agent that carries an FDA approval for chronic drooling in children ages 3 to 16 years. Atropine in the dosage form described in this study is dispensed in a dropper bottle and is typically administered into the eyes. When prescribed for administration via the sublingual route, there is risk of misuse, accidental overdose, or toxicity. Prescribers, nursing staff, and consumers/patients should receive thorough education regarding SLA indication, use, administration, and side effects. It should also be recommended to store the dropper bottle in a child-proof container and keep out of reach of small children.

This descriptive medication use evaluation is a first step in examining actual SLA use in children and young adults with NDD. There are several limitations to this study. Our work reflects local prescribing habits at a single institution. However, SLA is used widely for this application without guidelines, and it is possible to surmise that similar variability in practice might exist more broadly. Based on the data available for this study, it was not possible to evaluate efficacy, side effects, adherence to therapy, or rationale for therapy cessation. Outside records were not reviewed to obtain previous exposure to anticholinergic agents, botulinum toxin, surgery, and/or ablation outside of our institution. Additionally, to capture the maximum potential dosing made by prescribers, our dosing may be overestimated as we rounded up on dosing intervals and assumed scheduled doses when prescriptions were written on an "as needed" basis.

5. Conclusions

Our study summarizes the data for SLA use within a single institution. It documents that SLA is commonly used to treat drooling in children and young adults with NDD and that the prescribing practices are highly variable. We identify a lack of consistency regarding dosing, schedule, and place in therapy for SLA use in this population. Importantly, it draws attention to the wide practice variation that often evolves in the absence of guidelines. Efficacy, dosing regimens and adverse events of SLA require additional exploration. Further rigorous prospective study is necessary to establish the safety and efficacy of SLA for the treatment of sialorrhea in children and young adults with NDD. We hope that this preliminary study will form the basis for a randomized control trial of SLA in comparison to a more established therapy, such as enteral glycopyrrolate.

Author Contributions: Conceptualization, L.G. and K.D.P.; methodology, K.D.P. and L.G.; validation, K.D.P., L.G. and G.N.; formal analysis, K.D.P., L.G. and G.N.; investigation, K.D.P.; resources, K.D.P. and L.G.; data curation, K.D.P.; writing—original draft preparation, K.D.P.; writing—review and editing, K.D.P., L.G. and G.N.; visualization, K.D.P. and L.G.; supervision, K.D.P. and L.G.; project administration, K.D.P. and L.G.; funding acquisition, L.G. All authors have read and agreed to the published version of the manuscript.

Funding: This research received no external funding.

Institutional Review Board Statement: The study was conducted according to the guidelines of the Declaration of Helsinki, and approved by the Institutional Review Board of Nationwide Children's (protocol code STUDY00002028, 8 November 2021) and a waiver of consent was granted.

Informed Consent Statement: Patient consent was waived.

Data Availability Statement: The data presented in this study are not publicly available due to privacy restrictions. Questions relating to the data may be addressed by contacting the corresponding author.

Conflicts of Interest: The authors declare no conflict or financial interest in any product or service mentioned in the manuscript, including grants, equipment, medications, employment, gifts, and honoraria. The authors had full access to all the data in the study and take responsibility for the integrity of the data and the accuracy of the data analysis.

Abbreviations

NDD, Neurodevelopmental Disability; CP, Cerebral Palsy; SLA, sublingual atropine; IM, intramuscular; IV, intravenous; SubQ, subcutaneous; Rx, prescription; PRN, as needed; QDay, once daily; BID, twice daily; TID, three times daily.

References

1. Speyer, R.; Cordier, R.; Kim, J.H.; Cocks, N.; Michou, E.; Wilkes-Gillan, S. Prevalence of drooling, swallowing, and feeding problems in cerebral palsy across the lifespan: A systematic review and meta-analyses. *Dev. Med. Child Neurol.* **2019**, *61*, 1249–1258. [CrossRef]
2. Rosenbaum, P.; Paneth, N.; Leviton, A.; Goldstein, M.; Bax, M.; Damiano, D.; Dan, B.; Jacobsson, B. A report: The definition and classification of cerebral palsy April 2006. *Dev. Med. Child Neurol Suppl.* **2007**, *109*, 8–14.
3. McGuire, D.O.; Tian, L.H.; Yeargin-Allsopp, M.; Dowling, N.F.; Christensen, D.L. Prevalence of cerebral palsy, intellectual disability, hearing loss, and blindness, National Health Interview Survey, 2009–2016. *Disabil. Health J.* **2019**, *12*, 443–451. [CrossRef]
4. Jongerius, P.H.; van Hulst, K.; van den Hoogen, F.J.; Rotteveel, J.J. The Treatment of Posterior Drooling by Botulinum Toxin in a Child with Cerebral Palsy. *J. Pediatr. Gastroenterol. Nutr.* **2005**, *41*, 351–353. [CrossRef]
5. Chiang, J.; Amin, R. Respiratory Care Considerations for Children with Medical Complexity. *Children* **2017**, *4*, 41. [CrossRef]
6. Russell, C.J.; Simon, T.D. Care of children with medical complexity in the hospital setting. *Pediatr. Ann.* **2014**, *43*, e157–e162. [CrossRef]

7. Marpole, R.; Blackmore, A.M.; Gibson, N.; Cooper, M.S.; Langdon, K.; Wilson, A.C. Evaluation and Management of Respiratory Illness in Children With Cerebral Palsy. *Front. Pediatr.* **2020**, *8*, 333. [CrossRef] [PubMed]
8. Blair, E.; Watson, L.; Badawi, N.; Stanley, F.J. Life expectancy among people with cerebral palsy in Western Australia. *Dev. Med. Child Neurol.* **2001**, *43*, 508–515. [CrossRef] [PubMed]
9. Blair, E.; Langdon, K.; McIntyre, S.; Lawrence, D.; Watson, L. Survival and mortality in cerebral palsy: Observations to the sixth decade from a data linkage study of a total population register and National Death Index. *BMC Neurol.* **2019**, *19*, 111. [CrossRef] [PubMed]
10. Walshe, M.; Smith, M.; Pennington, L. Interventions for drooling in children with cerebral palsy. *Cochrane Database Syst. Rev.* **2012**, *2*, CD008624.
11. Begley, K.A.; Braswell, L.E.; Noritz, G.H.; Murakami, J.W. Salivary gland ablation: Introducing an interventional radiology treatment alternative in the management of sialorrhea. *Pediatr. Radiol.* **2020**, *50*, 869–876. [CrossRef]
12. Alrefai, A.H.; Aburahma, S.K.; Khader, Y.S. Treatment of sialorrhea in children with cerebral palsy: A double-blind placebo controlled trial. *Clin. Neurol Neurosurg.* **2009**, *111*, 79–82. [CrossRef] [PubMed]
13. Schild, S.D.; Timashpolsky, A.; Ballard, D.P.; Horne, S.; Rosenfeld, R.M.; Plum, A.W. Surgical Management of Sialorrhea: A Systematic Review and Meta-analysis. *Otolaryngol. Head Neck Surg.* **2021**, *165*, 507–518. [CrossRef] [PubMed]
14. Rodwell, K.; Edwards, P.; Ware, R.S.; Boyd, R. Salivary gland botulinum toxin injections for drooling in children with cerebral palsy and neurodevelopmental disability: A systematic review. *Dev. Med. Child Neurol.* **2012**, *54*, 977–987. [CrossRef]
15. McInerney, M.S.; Reddihough, D.S.; Carding, P.N.; Swanton, R.; Walton, C.M.; Imms, C. Behavioural interventions to treat drooling in children with neurodisability: A systematic review. *Dev. Med. Child Neurol.* **2019**, *61*, 39–48. [CrossRef] [PubMed]
16. Reid, S.M.; Westbury, C.; Guzys, A.T.; Reddihough, D.S. Anticholinergic medications for reducing drooling in children with developmental disability. *Dev. Med. Child Neurol.* **2020**, *62*, 346–353. [CrossRef]
17. Parr, J.R.; Todhunter, E.; Pennington, L.; Stocken, D.; Cadwgan, J.; O'Hare, A.E.; Tuffrey, C.; Williams, J.; Cole, M.; Colver, A.F. Drooling Reduction Intervention randomised trial (DRI): Comparing the efficacy and acceptability of hyoscine patches and glycopyrronium liquid on drooling in children with neurodisability. *Arch. Dis. Child.* **2018**, *103*, 371–376. [CrossRef]
18. Camp-Bruno, J.A.; Winsberg, B.G.; Green-Parsons, A.R.; Abrams, J.P. Efficacy of benztropine therapy for drooling. *Dev. Med. Child Neurol.* **1989**, *31*, 309–319. [CrossRef]
19. Zeller, R.S.; Lee, H.M.; Cavanaugh, P.F.; Davidson, J. Randomized Phase III evaluation of the efficacy and safety of a novel glycopyrrolate oral solution for the management of chronic severe drooling in children with cerebral palsy or other neurologic conditions. *Ther. Clin. Risk Manag.* **2012**, *8*, 15–23. [CrossRef]
20. Mato, A.; Limeres, J.; Tomás, I.; Muñoz, M.; Abuín, C.; Feijoo, J.F.; Diz, P. Management of drooling in disabled patients with scopolamine patches. *Br. J. Clin. Pharmacol.* **2010**, *69*, 684–688. [CrossRef]
21. Mier, R.J.; Bachrach, S.J.; Lakin, R.C.; Barker, T.; Childs, J.; Moran, M. Treatment of sialorrhea with glycopyrrolate: A double-blind, dose-ranging study. *Arch. Pediatr. Adolesc. Med.* **2000**, *154*, 1214–1218. [CrossRef]
22. You, P.; Strychowsky, J.; Gandhi, K.; Chen, B.A. Anticholinergic treatment for sialorrhea in children: A systematic review. *Pediatr. Child. Health* **2021**, *27*, 82–87. [CrossRef]
23. McLendon, K.; Preuss, C.V. Atropine. In *StatPearls*; StatPearls Publishing: Treasure Island, FL, USA, 2023. Available online: https://www.ncbi.nlm.nih.gov/books/NBK470551/ (accessed on 8 July 2023).
24. Brown, J.; Brandl, K.; Wess, J. Muscarinic Receptor Agonists and Antagonists. In *Goodman & Gilman's: The Pharmacological Basis of Therapeutics*; Brunton, L.L., Knollmann, B.C., Eds.; McGraw Hill: New York, NY, USA, 2017; p. 13e. Available online: https://accesspharmacy.mhmedical.com/content.aspx?bookid=2189&sectionid=167889643 (accessed on 8 July 2023).
25. Atropine. In *Pediatric and Neonatal Lexi-Drugs*; Lexicomp: Hudson, OH, USA, 2023. Available online: http://online.lexi.com/ (accessed on 19 July 2023).
26. Volz-Zang, C.; Waldhäuser, T.; Schulte, B.; Palm, D. Comparison of the effects of atropine in vivo and ex vivo (radioreceptor assay) after oral and intramuscular administration to man. *Eur. J. Clin. Pharmacol.* **1995**, *49*, 45–49. [CrossRef]
27. Schwartz, M.D.; Raulli, R.; Laney, J.W.; Coley, W.; Walker, R.; O'Rourke, A.W.; Raine, K.; Horwith, G.; Gao, Y.; Eisnor, D.L.; et al. Systemic Bioavailability of Sublingual Atropine Ophthalmic Solution: A Phase I Study in Healthy Volunteers with Implications for Use as a Contingency Medical Countermeasure. *J. Med. Toxicol.* **2022**, *18*, 187–197. [CrossRef]
28. Sharma, A.; Ramaswamy, S.; Dahl, E.; Dewan, V. Intraoral application of atropine sulfate ophthalmic solution for clozapine-induced sialorrhea. *Ann. Pharmacother.* **2004**, *38*, 1538. [CrossRef]
29. De Simone, G.G.; Eisenchlas, J.H.; Junin, M.; Pereyra, F.; Brizuela, R. Atropine drops for drooling: A randomized controlled trial. *Palliat. Med.* **2006**, *20*, 665–671. [CrossRef] [PubMed]
30. Dias, B.L.S.; Fernandes, A.R.; de S Maia Filho, H. Treatment of drooling with sublingual atropine sulfate in children and adolescents with cerebral palsy. *Arq. Neuropsiquiatr.* **2017**, *75*, 282–287. [CrossRef] [PubMed]
31. Norderyd, J.; Graf, J.; Marcusson, A.; Nilsson, K.; Sjöstrand, E.; Steinwall, G.; Ärleskog, E.; Bågesund, M. Sublingual administration of atropine eyedrops in children with excessive drooling—A pilot study. *Int. J. Paediatr. Dent.* **2017**, *27*, 22–29. [CrossRef]
32. Protus, B.M.; Grauer, P.A.; Kimbrel, J.M. Evaluation of atropine 1% ophthalmic solution administered sublingually for the management of terminal respiratory secretions. *Am. J. Hosp. Palliat. Care.* **2013**, *30*, 388–392. [CrossRef]
33. Rapoport, A. Sublingual atropine drops for the treatment of pediatric sialorrhea. *J. Pain. Symptom Manag.* **2010**, *40*, 783–788. [CrossRef] [PubMed]

34. Van der Poorten, T.; De Hert, M. The sublingual use of atropine in the treatment of clozapine-induced sialorrhea: A systematic review. *Clin. Case Rep.* **2019**, *7*, 2108–2113. [CrossRef]
35. Reid, S.M.; Johnson, H.M.; Reddihough, D.S. The Drooling Impact Scale: A measure of the impact of drooling in children with developmental disabilities. *Dev. Med. Child Neurol.* **2010**, *52*, e23–e38. [CrossRef]
36. Azapağası, E.; Kendirli, T.; Perk, O.; Kutluk, G.; Öz Tunçer, G.; Teber, S.; Çobanoğlu, N. Sublingual Atropine Sulfate Use for Sialorrhea in Pediatric Patients. *J. Pediatr. Intensive Care* **2020**, *9*, 196–200. [CrossRef]
37. Pharmacy Auditing and Dispensing Job Aid: Billing Other Dosage Forms. Available online: https://www.cms.gov/Medicare-Medicaid-Coordination/Fraud-Prevention/Medicaid-Integrity-Education/Downloads/pharmacy-selfaudit-jobaid-billing-other.pdf (accessed on 1 March 2023).

Disclaimer/Publisher's Note: The statements, opinions and data contained in all publications are solely those of the individual author(s) and contributor(s) and not of MDPI and/or the editor(s). MDPI and/or the editor(s) disclaim responsibility for any injury to people or property resulting from any ideas, methods, instructions or products referred to in the content.

MDPI
St. Alban-Anlage 66
4052 Basel
Switzerland
www.mdpi.com

Journal of Clinical Medicine Editorial Office
E-mail: jcm@mdpi.com
www.mdpi.com/journal/jcm

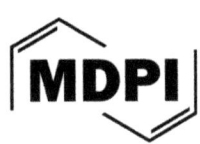

Disclaimer/Publisher's Note: The statements, opinions and data contained in all publications are solely those of the individual author(s) and contributor(s) and not of MDPI and/or the editor(s). MDPI and/or the editor(s) disclaim responsibility for any injury to people or property resulting from any ideas, methods, instructions or products referred to in the content.

www.ingramcontent.com/pod-product-compliance
Lightning Source LLC
LaVergne TN
LVHW070151100526
838202LV00015B/1933